METHODS IN MOLECULAR BIOLOGY™

Series Editor
John M. Walker
School of Life Sciences
University of Hertfordshire
Hatfield, Hertfordshire, AL10 9AB, UK

For further volumes:
http://www.springer.com/series/7651

The Complement System

Methods and Protocols

Edited by

Mihaela Gadjeva

Division of Infectious Diseases, Brigham and Women's Hospital, Harvard Medical School, Harvard University, Boston, MA, USA

Humana Press

Editor
Mihaela Gadjeva
Division of Infectious Diseases
Brigham and Women's Hospital
Harvard Medical School
Harvard University
Boston, MA, USA

ISSN 1064-3745 ISSN 1940-6029 (electronic)
ISBN 978-1-4939-6306-5 ISBN 978-1-62703-724-2 (eBook)
DOI 10.1007/978-1-62703-724-2
Springer New York Heidelberg Dordrecht London

Softcover reprint of the hardcover 1st edition 2014

Printed on acid-free paper

Humana Press is a brand of Springer
Springer is part of Springer Science+Business Media (www.springer.com)

Dedication

To Prof. Kenneth Reid in recognition of his outstanding and fundamental work in Complement Biology.

To Prof. Gerald Pier in gratitude for his continuous advice and generous support.

To my family who are my inspiration.

Preface

The complement system is a key system for immune surveillance and homeostasis. Discoveries during the past 20 years of complement research yielded detailed knowledge of the molecular structure of complement components, the mechanisms of activation, and regulation of the system in health and disease. The objective of the current book is to describe methods to study the soluble components and receptors involved in the complement system, including new methodological aspects to assay complement function and activation in humans and in model animals. This collection of more than 30 individual chapters describes variety of protocols to purify and analyze the activity of the individual complement components. Of particular interest to clinical workers are the sections focused on the detection of complement SNPs, the clinical methods to evaluate complement system activation, and data interpretation. The introduction portions of each of the chapters highlights the current concepts and scientific principles based on which the individual assays are build, whereas the references include key papers that are selected to broaden reader's knowledge of the specific topics.

I hope that this collection of well-established "classical" assays and recently developed "new" assays to analyze the complement system activation will be useful to a wide audience of scientists, interested in complement research including complementologists, new entrants to the field as well as clinician–scientists, biochemists, molecular biologists, and immunologists.

I would like to thank John Walker, Series Editor, and Humana Press, for the opportunity to assemble this outstanding collection of articles dedicated to analysis of the complement system. In addition, I would like to thank the contributing authors for taking time from their busy schedules to create easy-to-follow and well-presented chapters.

Boston, MA, USA *Mihaela Gadjeva*

Contents

Contributors

SCOTT ALDERUCCI • *Department of Biomolecular Research and Technologies, Shire Human Genetic Therapies, Cambridge, MA, USA*
GREGERS ROM ANDERSEN • *Department of Molecular Biology and Genetics, University of Aarhus, Aarhus C, Denmark*
GERARD J. ARLAUD • *CEA, DSV, Institut de Biologie Structurale (IBS), CNRS, UMR 5075, Université Joseph Fourier, Grenoble, France*
JAMES N. ARNOLD • *Department of Biochemistry, University of Oxford, Oxford, UK*
ISABELLE BALLY • *CEA, DSV, Institut de Biologie Structurale (IBS), CNRS, UMR 5075, Université Joseph Fourier, Grenoble, France*
NIRMAL K. BANDA • *Pediatrics, Massachusetts General Hospital, Boston, MA, USA*
CHARLES BEDARD • *Department of Cell Culture Process Development, Shire Human Genetic Therapies, Cambridge, MA, USA*
CAROLINE BLANC • *Cordeliers Research Center, INSERM UMRS 872, Université Pierre et Marie Curie, Université Paris Descartes, Paris, France*
ANNA M. BLOM • *Department of Laboratory Medicine, Section of Medical Protein Chemistry, The Wallenberg Laboratory, Lund University, Skåne University Hospital, Malmö, Sweden*
PAULINE BORDEREAU • *Service d'Immunologie Biologique, Hôpital Européen Georges Pompidou, Assistance Publique-Hôpitaux de Paris, Paris, France*
MICHAEL F. CONCINO • *Department of Biomolecular Research and Technologies, Shire Human Genetic Therapies, Cambridge, MA, USA*
LYNETTE C. COOK • *Department of Biomolecular Research and Technologies, Shire Human Genetic Therapies, Cambridge, MA, USA*
MOHAMED R. DAHA • *Department of Nephrology, Leiden University Medical Centre, Leiden, The Netherlands*
JÓZSEF DOBÓ • *Institute of Enzymology, RCNS, Hungarian Academy of Sciences, Budapest, Hungary*
ESWARI DODAGATTA-MARRI • *Centre for Infection, Immunity and Disease Mechanisms, Biosciences, School of Health Sciences and Social Care, Brunel University, London, UK*
LUKE R. DONIUS • *Department of Pathology, Division of Microbiology and Immunology, University of Utah School of Medicine, Salt Lake City, UT, USA*
MARIE-AGNÈS DRAGON-DUREY • *Cordeliers Research Center, INSERM UMRS 872, Paris, France; Université Paris Descartes, Sorbonne Paris Cité, Paris, France; Assitance Publique-Hopitaux de Paris Hopit al Europeen Georges-Pompidou, Service d'Immunologie Biologique, Paris Cedex, France*
EUGENIE DU • *Department of Biochemistry, University of Oxford, Oxford, UK*
MARKRYAN DWYER • *Division of Infectious Diseases, Brigham and Women's Hospital, Harvard Medical School, Harvard University, Boston, MA, USA*

Yuichi Endo • *Radioisotope Research Center, Fukushima Medical University, Fukushima, Japan*
Marina Fedorova • *Department of Biochemistry, University of Oxford, Oxford, UK*
Susan M. Fish • *Department of Biomolecular Research and Technologies, Shire Human Genetic Therapies, Cambridge, MA, USA*
Zvi Fishelson • *Department of Cell and Developmental Biology, Sackler School of Medicine, Tel Aviv University, Tel Aviv, Israel*
Vèronique Frèmeaux-Bacchi • *Assitance Publique-Hopitaux de Paris Hopit al Europeen Georges-Pompidou, Service d'Immunologie Biologique, APHP, Paris, France*
Teizo Fujita • *Fukushima General Hygiene Institute, Fukushima, Japan*
Mihaela Gadjeva • *Division of Infectious Diseases, Brigham and Women's Hospital, Harvard Medical School, Harvard University, Boston, MA, USA*
Peter Garred • *Laboratory of Molecular Medicine, Department of Clinical Immunology, Rigshospitalet, University of Copenhagen, Copenhagen, Denmark*
Berhane Ghebrehiwet • *The Department of Medicine, Stony Brook University, Stony Brook, NY, USA*
John Gill • *Department of Cell Culture Process Development, Shire Human Genetic Therapies, Cambridge, MA, USA*
Meike Heurich • *Institute of Infection and Immunity, Cardiff University, School of Medicine, Cardiff, UK*
Mihály Józsi • *Junior Research Group Cellular Immunobiology, Leibniz Institute for Natural Product Research and Infection Biology, Jena, Germany; MTA-ELTE "Lendületc" Complement Research Group, Department of Immunology, Eötvös Loránd University, Budapest, Hungary*
Najmunisa Karbani • *Centre for Infection, Immunity and Disease Mechanisms, Biosciences, School of Health Sciences and Social Care, Brunel University, London, UK*
Christian M. Karsten • *Institute for Systemic Inflammation Research, University of Lübeck, Lübeck, Germany*
Claudia Kemper • *Division of Transplantation Immunology and Mucosal Biology, MRC Centre for Transplantation, King's College London, Guy's Hospital, London, UK*
David Kilpatrick • *Scottish National Blood Transfusion Service, Edinburgh, UK*
Uday Kishore • *Centre for Infection, Immunity and Disease Mechanisms, Biosciences, School of Health Sciences and Social Care, Brunel University, London, UK*
Troels R. Kjaer • *Department of Biomedicine, Aarhus University, Aarhus, Denmark*
Jörg Köhl • *Division of Cellular and Molecular Immunology, Cincinnati Children's Hospital Medical Center and University of Cincinnati College of Medicine, Cincinnati, OH, USA*
Mihaela Kojouharova • *Department of Biochemistry, Sofia University "St. Kliment Ohridski", Sofia, Bulgaria*
Martin Kolev • *Division of Transplantation Immunology and Mucosal Biology, MRC Centre for Transplantation, King's College London, Guy's Hospital, London, UK*
Maria C. Faber Krol • *Department of Nephrology, Leiden University Medical Centre, Leiden, The Netherlands*
Monique Lacroix • *CEA, DSV, Institut de Biologie Structurale (IBS), CNRS, UMR 5075, Université Joseph Fourier, Grenoble, France*
Yves Laumonnier • *Institute for Systemic Inflammation Research, University of Lübeck, Lübeck, Germany*
Man Chung Li • *Department of Biochemistry, University of Oxford, Oxford, UK*

Yu Liu • *Department of Cell and Developmental Biology, Wuhan University, College of Life Sciences, Wuhan, China*
Dianna M. Lundberg • *Department of Biomolecular Research and Technologies, Shire Human Genetic Therapies, Cambridge, MA, USA*
Taruna Madan • *Innate Immunity Group, National Institute of Reproductive Health, Mumbai, India*
Priyaa Madhukaran • *Innate Immunity Group, National Institute of Reproductive Health, Mumbai, India*
Hans Ole Madsen • *Laboratory of Molecular Medicine, Department of Clinical Immunology, Rigshospitalet, University of Copenhagen, Copenhagen, Denmark*
Paolo G.V. Martini • *Department of Discovery, Shire Human Genetic Therapies, Cambridge, MA, USA*
Misao Matsushita • *Department of Applied Biochemistry, Tokai University, Hiratsuka, Japan*
Seppo Meri • *Department of Bacteriology and Immunology, Haartman Institute, University of Helsinki, Helsinki, Finland*
Beryl E. Moffatt • *Department of Biochemistry, University of Oxford, Oxford, UK*
Frida C. Mohlin • *Department of Laboratory Medicine, Section of Medical Protein Chemistry, The Wallenberg Laboratory, Lund University, Skåne University Hospital, Malmö, Sweden*
Oren Moskovich • *Department of Cell and Developmental Biology, Sackler School of Medicine, Tel Aviv University, Tel Aviv, Israel*
Lea Munthe-Fog • *Laboratory of Molecular Medicine, Department of Clinical Immunology, Rigshospitalet, University of Copenhagen, Copenhagen, Denmark*
Stèphanie Ngo • *Service d'Immunologie Biologique, Hôpital Européen Georges Pompidou, Assistance Publique-Hôpitaux de Paris, Paris, France*
Gitte Krogh Nielsen • *Biophysical Immunology Laboratory, Department of Biomedicine, The Lundbeck Foundation Nanomedicine Center for Individual Management of Tissue Damage and Regeneration, Aarhus University, Aarhus, Denmark*
Sara C. Nilsson • *Department of Laboratory Medicine, Section of Medical Protein Chemistry, The Wallenberg Laboratory, Lund University, Skåne University Hospital, Malmö, Sweden*
Angela W. Norton • *Department of Biomolecular Research and Technologies, Shire Human Genetic Therapies, Cambridge, MA, USA*
Joseph O'Flynn • *Department of Nephrology, Leiden University Medical Centre, Leiden, The Netherlands*
Ellinor I.B. Peerschke • *The Department of Laboratory Medicine, Memorial Sloan-Kettering Cancer Center, New York, NY, USA*
Nelly Poulain • *Service d'Immunologie Biologique, Hôpital Européen Georges Pompidou, Assistance Publique-Hôpitaux de Paris, Paris, France*
Asif S. Qaseem • *Centre for Infection, Immunity and Disease Mechanisms, Biosciences, School of Health Sciences and Social Care, Brunel University, London, UK*
Anja Roos • *Wieslab B.V., Eurodiagnostica, Nijmegen, The Netherlands*
Roxane Roquigny • *Cordeliers Research Center, Université Pierre et Marie Curie, Université Paris Descartes, Paris, France*
Véronique Rossi • *CEA, DSV, Institut de Biologie Structurale (IBS), CNRS, UMR 5075, Université Joseph Fourier, Grenoble, France*

LUBKA T. ROUMENINA • *Cordeliers Research Center, INSERM UMRS 872, Université Pierre et Marie Curie, and Université Paris Descartes, Paris, France*
MARIETA M. RUSEVA • *Department of Medicine, Centre for Complement and Inflammation research, Imperial College, London, UK*
ALI RYAN • *Department of Pharmacology, University of Oxford, Oxford, UK*
HIROSHI SHIRAKI • *Yokohama College of Pharmacy, Yokohama, Japan*
ROBERT B. SIM • *Department of Biochemistry, University of Oxford, Oxford, UK*
LARS SOTTRUP-JENSEN • *Department of Molecular Biology and Genetics, University of Aarhus, Aarhus C, Denmark*
ASTRID SWINKELS • *Department of Biochemistry, University of Oxford, Oxford, UK*
KAZUE TAKAHASHI • *Pediatrics, Massachusetts General Hospital, Boston, MA, USA*
KOICHIRO TATEISHI • *Department of Applied Biochemistry, Tokai University, Hiratsuka, Japan*
STEFFEN THIEL • *Department of Biomedicine, Aarhus University, Aarhus, Denmark*
NICOLE M. THIELENS • *CEA, DSV, Institut de Biologie Structurale (IBS), CNRS, UMR 5075, Université Joseph Fourier, Grenoble, France*
ANTHONY G. TSOLAKI • *Centre for Infection, Immunity and Disease Mechanisms, Biosciences, School of Health Sciences and Social Care, Brunel University, London, UK*
MITSUSHI TSUJIMURA • *Fukuoka Red Cross Blood Center, Chikushino, Japan*
ARTHUR O. TZIANABOS • *Department of Research, Shire Human Genetic Therapies, Cambridge, MA, USA*
CEES VAN KOOTEN • *Department of Nephrology, Leiden University Medical Centre, Leiden, The Netherlands*
LILIAN VARGA • *3rd Department of Internal Medicine, Semmelweis University, Budapest, Hungary*
CLAIRE G.S. VILLIERS • *Department of Biochemistry, University of Oxford, Oxford, UK*
THOMAS VORUP-JENSEN • *Biophysical Immunology Laboratory, Department of Biomedicine, The Lundbeck Foundation Nanomedicine Center for Individualized Management of Tissue Damage and Regeneration, and Interdisciplinary Nanoscience Center, Aarhus University, Aarhus, Denmark*
PATRICK WATERS • *Neuroimmunlogy Group, John Radcliffe Hospital, Oxford, UK*
JOHN H. WEIS • *Division of Microbiology and Immunology, Department of Pathology, University of Utah School of Medicine, Salt Lake City, UT, USA*
JÖRGEN WIESLANDER • *Eurodiagnostica, Malmö, Sweden*
BING-BIN YU • *Department of Biochemistry, University of Oxford, Oxford, UK*

Chapter 1

Overview

Mihaela Gadjeva

Key words Complement, Innate immunity

Studies in Complement swiftly progressed over the years to yield knowledge that paved the way to the current boom in the interest in Innate Immunity. Complement research generated novel therapeutics that successfully underwent clinical trials, demonstrating that this filed is among the most advanced in biomedical research. Today, we have a novel appreciation of the Complement System that comprises more than 50 fluid and membrane-associated proteins and functions to secure antimicrobial immunity, efficient removal of soluble immune complexes, and tissue regeneration to ensure homeostasis.

Complement activation is initiated via three distinct routes: the Classical, the Alternative, and the Lectin pathways which unite to trigger covalent deposition of Complement proteins onto the target surface with the ultimate goal to destroy the target either by lysis or phagocytosis [1] (Fig. 1). Although the Classical pathway is the first pathway discovered scientifically, evolutionary it is the most recently developed pathway. It requires immunoglobulins IgM and IgG for its activation. When antigen–antibody complexes containing IgG or IgM are formed they can be recognized by the first component of the Complement System, C1q (Chapter 3) [2–4]. C1q circulates with blood stream in complex with C1r and C1s (Chapter 4) [5]. C1q binding to immune complexes triggers autoactivation of the proteolytic activity of C1r, which then cleaves C1s. The next Complement component to be activated in the Classical pathway is C4 (*The Complement components were numbered before the pathway sequence was established and, therefore, their numbers do not correspond to the sequence of events*). C1s cleaves C4, releasing a small fragment, C4a, and a larger residual fragment,

Mihaela Gadjeva (ed.), *The Complement System: Methods and Protocols*, Methods in Molecular Biology, vol. 1100, DOI 10.1007/978-1-62703-724-2_1, © Springer Science+Business Media New York 2014

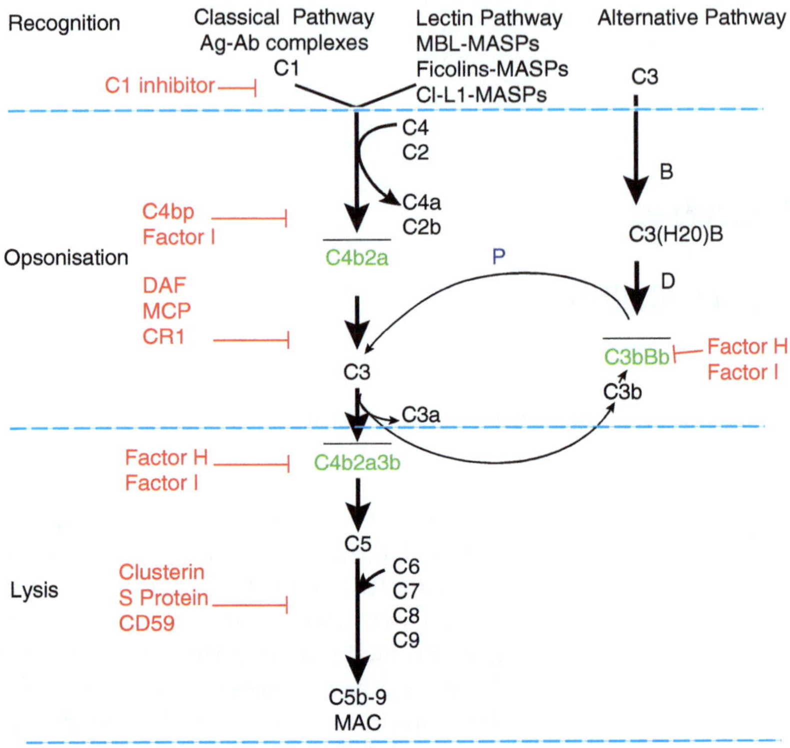

Fig. 1 Schematic diagram of the Complement System. The converatses of the Classical and Alternative pathways are shown in *green*; the Complement regulators are in *red*; the individual complement proteins are in *black*

C4b. The C4b molecule covalently attaches to the surface of the target (aka opsonisation of the target). In the presence of Mg^{2+}, C2 (Chapter 5) can form complexes with C4b, becoming a new substrate for C1s. C1s cleaves C2, releasing the C2b fragment from the complex. The remaining product—C4bC2a—is a vital complex known as C3 convertase. The C3 convertase cleaves C3, the most abundant Complement protein in serum (1–2 mg/ml) (Chapter 6). Binding of an immune complex to a single C1 complex can bring about proteolysis of 1,000-fold more C3 molecules, thus propagating greatly the activation signal [6]. Because the proteolytically cleaved form of C3–C3b is a highly reactive molecule with an exposed thioester, it covalently deposits onto the adjacent substrate, hence opsonizing the target [7, 8].

The Classical pathway C3 convertase (C4b2a) has the same substrate specificity as the Alternative pathway C3 convertase. The Alternative pathway provides a rapid, antibody-independent route for complement activation. Factor B, a single chain plasma protein, binds to C3b which renders Factor B susceptible to cleavage by Factor D, a serine protease circulating in serum in active form. The remaining complex C3bBb is the C3 convertase of the alternative pathway. The half-life of the C3 convertase can be extended via binding to Properdin [9] (Chapter 13), a positive regulator of the alternative pathway [10].

The Lectin pathway provides another antibody-independent way to activate the Complement System. This pathway is initiated either by binding of Mannan Binding Lectin (MBL) (Chapter 9) to mannose or *N*-acetylglucoseamine or by binding of Ficolins (Chapter 12) to acetylated carbohydrates on the surface of pathogens. MBL and Ficolins are found in circulation in complexes with mannan binding lectin-associated serine proteases (MASPs): MASP-1, MASP-2, MASP-3, and their truncated forms sMAP and MAp44 [11]. Similar to the C1 complexes, the MBL-MASP complexes cleave C4 and C2 resulting in C4 deposition (Chapter 11). MASP-1 and MASP-2 have enzymatic activity with defined substrates, whereas MASP-3, MAp19, and MAp44 function as regulators [12, 13]. The substrate for MASP-3 has been enigmatic for long time, but recent evidence suggests that it may mediate the activity of a novel collectin Cl-K1 [14].

C3 convertases of the classical or the alternative pathway generate a wealth of cleaved C3b molecules that bind to the convertases resulting in the formation of C4b2a3b or C3bBb3b complexes. These complexes cleave C5 (Chapter 7) and are termed C5 convertases. The subsequent binding events result in the formation of the membrane attack complex (MAC) containing the proteins C5b-8. Once formed, the soluble C5b-8 complex undergoes conformational change and transitions from a globular, hydrophilic form to an elongated, amphipathic form, which incorporates C9 [15]; the C5b-9 complex traverses the target membrane forming pores (Chapter 8).

Because the Complement System is a very effective killing machine, its activities are tightly regulated. The activation of the complement system is controlled by soluble molecules: C1 inhibitor (Chapter 16), Factor H (Chapter 17), Factor H-related proteins (Chapter 18), Factor I (Chapter 15), C4 binding protein (Chapter 14), S protein, clusterin or by membrane proteins: membrane cofactor protein (MCP, CD46) (Chapter 27), decay accelerating factor (DAF), CD35, CD59 (Chapters 28 and 29). These proteins either inhibit the activity of the serine proteases, promote the decay and destruction of the convertases, or control the assembly of MAC [16].

The versatile functions of Complement are mediated by an array of receptors of Complement proteins. Complement-opsonized targets that carry covalently attached C3b or C4b are recognized by complement receptor 1(CR1, CD35). Because CR1 has a Factor I cofactor activity, it promotes breaking down of C3b to iC3b, C3d, and C3dg. These fragments can be efficiently bound to complement receptor 2 (CR2), 3 (CR3), and 4 (CR4). Receptors exist for C1q, MBL, ficolins, lung collectins SP-D, and SP-A (which have structure and binding activity similar to MBL). They recognize either the collagenous portion of the molecules (e.g., calreticulin) or globular fragments (e.g., globular C1q receptor (gC1qR)). Complement split products C3a, C4a, and C5a act as anaphylatoxins via binding to C3aR and C5aR. This Book includes information on methods for detection and functional analysis of complement receptors. Chapters 24, 27, and 28 describe protocols for detection of CR1, CR2, CD46, and CD59 using standard flow cytometry approaches. These protocols can be easily adapted for detection of the rest of the complement receptors as reagents are available. We have also included protocols for well-established assays for complement receptor functionality in Chapters 23, 25, 26, and 29. It must be acknowledged that this list of protocols is by no means complete, mostly due to the great diversity in complement receptor activities.

One exciting example of Complement activities is the ability of Complement to act as an adjuvant, elegantly documented by series of studies [17]. This can be achieved by several distinct pathways: (1) Binding of Complement ligands to CR3, CR4, and C1qR facilitates antigen presentation and transport to the lymph nodes. (2) Binding of C3b, C3d, C3dg to CR2 lowers the threshold for B cell activation stimulating B cell proliferation, antibody somatic hypermutation, and class switching [18]. (3) Antigen capture on the surface of follicular dendritic cells (FDC) by CR1- and CR2-mediated recognition of Complement-opsonized particles promotes germinal center reaction and B cell memory. With the availability of X-ray structure of the C3d-CR2 co-crystal, the molecular interaction is understood in great detail allowing for design of targeted vaccine [19].

In this Book we include detailed protocols to measure each of the Complement activation pathways: Classical, Alternative, or Lectin. Traditionally, Complement activation is analyzed using hemolysis assays. They provide information about the integrity of the whole Complement cascade. The tests are based on the original protocol described in the 1970s by Rapp and colleagues [20, 21] and consist of serial dilutions of the sample in the presence of antibody-sensitized sheep erythrocytes at a defined temperature. The results are expressed as reciprocal dilutions of the samples required to produce 50 or 100 % lysis (CH50 or CH100) and provide information about the status of the classical pathway activation (Chapters 3 and 6). In contrast, the tests evaluating the integrity of the Alternative pathway (AH50) utilize rabbit, guinea pig, or chicken erythrocytes which stimulate assembly of the Alternative pathway C3 convertase and Complement deposition. In those assays the activation of the Classical pathway is blocked by depleting Ca^{2+} via adding EGTA (an efficient chelator for Ca^{2+}) and supplying Mg^{2+} [22]. However, the AH50 is frequently normal or only slightly reduced in the case of rare properdin deficiencies, which limits its use. Another major limitation of the hemolysis assays is that they do not allow for analysis of the lectin pathway activity.

Today, the classical hemolysis assays are substituted with ELISA-based assays, relying on the use of neoepitope-specific antibodies that recognize terminal C5b-9 complexes (Chapter 2) [23]. This ELISA-based approach allows for robust analysis of the functionality of all the three pathways. A similar assay can be carried out to quantify Complement activation in animals. We provide a chapter that describes protocols for detection of Complement activation in mice (Chapter 31). The assays make use of Complement-triggered C4 deposition, which is detected by neoepitope-specific antibodies to deposited C4. Because the assay relies on exogenously supplied C4, it is more sensitive than the hemolysis-based assays, which rely on the highly labile endogenous murine C4, thus circumventing the issue with low-level Classical pathway activation in mice.

When Complement deficiency is suspected in a patient (e.g., patient with recurrent infections), the initial screen should characterize the status of the three pathways (as described in Chapter 2) followed by quantification and functional analysis of the individual Complement components. A simple assay to detect functional deficiencies of a specific Complement protein is to analyze the ability of the sample to reconstitute Complement activity in a serum with known Complement deficiency [24]. Based on this principle is the assay frequently used to characterize MBL pathway deficiencies (Chapter 11) [25].

Analysis of the individual Complement components is especially advisable in patients with age-related macular degeneration (AMD) [26], membrano-proliferative glomerulonephritis (MPGN), atypical hemolytic uremic syndrome (aHUS) [27], which often present with functional deficiency of factor H and subsequent overactivation of Complement. We supply protocols for testing Factor H functionality based on analysis of the ability of Factor H to protect erythrocytes from lysis (Chapters 17 and 19).

Access to recombinant or plasma-derived Complement proteins facilitates generation of component-specific reagents that are used to precisely quantify the individual Complement components in healthy Caucasians (Table 1). Based on studies of patients with suspected immunodeficiency, a wealth of information is gathered to define Complement deficiencies. Deficiencies in the Classical Complement activation pathway often sensitize to development of Systemic Lupus Erythematosus (SLE) [28–30]. More than 90 % of individuals with homozygous C1q deficiency develop lupus-like disease. Similarly, deficiencies in C4 or C2 also associate with SLE [31]. These strong disease susceptibility associations are thought to depend on impaired immune complex clearance that occurs in the absence of Classical Complement proteins. An alternative

Table 1
Ranges of Complement proteins in circulation in healthy Caucasians

Pathway	Ranges in normal individuals
Classical pathway	
C1q	12–22 mg/dl
C2	1.1–3.0 mg/dl
C3	Males: 88–252 mg/dl
	Females: 88–206 mg/dl
C4	Males: 12–72 mg/dl
	Females: 13–75 mg/dl
Lectin pathway	
MBL	0.01–12.20 μg/ml
H-ficolin	8.9–54.9 μg/m [40]
L-ficolin	900–7,000 ng/ml [41]
MASP-1	6.27 ± 1.85 μg/ml [42]
MASP-2	321–747 μg/ml [43]
MASP-3	1.8–10.6 μg/ml [44]
MAp19	26–675 ng/ml [45]
Map44	0.8–3.2 μg/ml [44]
Alternative pathway	
Factor B	74–286 μg/ml [46]
Factor D	25–105 μg/ml [47]
Properdin	15–41 μg/ml [48]
Terminal pathway	
C5	10.6–26.3 mg/dl
C6	32–57 U/ml
C7	35.3–96.5 μg/ml
C8	33–58 U/ml
C9	37–61 U/ml
Fluid phase regulators	
Factor I	39–100 μg/ml [48]
Factor H	63.5–847 μg/ml [49]
	150–750 μg/ml [50]
C4bp	199–532 μg/ml [48]

explanation is that proteins of the Classical pathway are needed to capture self-antigens to promote B cell tolerance by enhancing the elimination of self-reactive lymphocytes [32].

Unlike Classical Complement deficiencies, MBL deficiency is surprisingly frequent. About 5 % of European Caucasions carry SNPs that result in low MBL protein levels in circulation (below 100 ng/ml) (Chapter 10) [33–35]. Low levels of MBL are associated with increased risk of infections [36], which may be exemplified in cases when cancer patients undergo chemotherapy, or organ-transplant patients are treated with immunosuppressive drugs [37]. Deficiencies in Alternative Complement components or MAC components are very rare in European populations and are typically associated with recurrent invasive infections caused by *N. meningitides* and *N. gonorrhoeae*.

These studies prompted ideas that reconstitutive therapies with recombinant complement proteins are viable strategic approaches [38]. An exciting example is the reconstitutive therapy with C1 inhibitor (Chapter 16). The C1 inhibitor deficiency causes an autosomal-dominant disorder termed hereditary angioedema (HAE), characterized by frequent episodes of angioedema [20]. This is one of the most common immune deficiencies (after the immunoglobulin deficiency) with frequency of occurrence 1:50,000. Interestingly, the angioedema is thought to be due to the absence of control over the kallikrein system, not a consequence of a failure to control the Classical or Lectin pathways. The treatment strategy for HAE is supplying the patients with recombinant C1 Inhibitor and is becoming available as the product successfully past clinical trials type II.

The discovery of strategies to modulate complement activation is of great interest to the Complement community and significant breakthroughs have been made in the recent years. One exciting example is Eculizumab (trade name Solaris), a humanized C5-blocking antibody, that is approved by FDA for use in patients with paroxysmal nocturnal hemoglobinurea (PNH). These patients experience high level of Complement activation due to deficiency in membrane bound Complement regulatory proteins CD59 and the monoclonal antibody prevents the cleavage of C5 to C5a and C5b, thus overriding the need for CD59 [39].

Without a doubt the tendency to discover and employ novel Complement regulators will govern the next decade of Complement research. We hope that this book will facilitate the process by providing well-established sets of protocols that define the molecular characteristics and functionality of individual Complement proteins and pathways.

References

1. Carroll MV, Sim RB (2011) Complement in health and disease. Adv Drug Deliv Rev 63:965–975
2. Reid KB, Day AJ (1990) Ig-binding domains of C1q. Immunol Today 11:387–388
3. Reid KB (1989) Chemistry and molecular genetics of C1q. Behring Inst Mitt 84:8–19
4. Reid KB, Lowe DM, Porter RR (1972) Isolation and characterization of C1q, a subcomponent of the first component of complement, from human and rabbit sera. Biochem J 130:749–763
5. Gaboriaud C, Thielens NM, Gregory LA, Rossi V, Fontecilla-Camps JC, Arlaud GJ (2004) Structure and activation of the C1 complex of complement: unraveling the puzzle. Trends Immunol 25:368–373
6. Cooper NR (1985) The classical complement pathway: activation and regulation of the first complement component. Adv Immunol 37:151–216
7. Gadjeva M, Dodds AW, Taniguchi-Sidle A, Willis AC, Isenman DE, Law SK (1998) The covalent binding reaction of complement component C3. J Immunol 161:985–990
8. Law SK, Dodds AW (1996) Catalysed hydrolysis: the complement quickstep. Immunol Today 17:105
9. Gotze O, Muller-Eberhard HJ (1974) The role of properdin in the alternate pathway of complement activation. J Exp Med 139:44–57
10. Goundis D, Reid KB (1988) Properdin, the terminal complement components, thrombospondin and the circumsporozoite protein of malaria parasites contain similar sequence motifs. Nature 335:82–85
11. Thiel S, Vorup-Jensen T, Stover CM, Schwaeble W, Laursen SB, Poulsen K, Willis AC, Eggleton P, Hansen S, Holmskov U, Reid KB, Jensenius JC (1997) A second serine protease associated with mannan-binding lectin that activates complement. Nature 386:506–510
12. Thiel S, Jensen L, Degn SE, Nielsen HJ, Gal P, Dobo J, Jensenius JC (2012) Mannan-binding lectin (MBL)-associated serine protease-1 (MASP-1), a serine protease associated with humoral pattern-recognition molecules: normal and acute-phase levels in serum and stoichiometry of lectin pathway components. Clin Exp Immunol 169:38–48
13. Sekine H, Takahashi M, Iwaki D, Fujita T (2013) The role of MASP-1/3 in complement activation. Adv Exp Med Biol 734:41–53
14. Selman L, Hansen S (2012) Structure and function of collectin liver 1 (CL-L1) and collectin 11 (CL-11, CL-K1). Immunobiology 217:851–863
15. Kolb WP, Muller-Eberhard HJ (1974) Mode of action of human C9: adsorption of multiple C9 molecules to cell-bound C8. J Immunol 113:479–488
16. Whaley K, Ruddy S (1976) Modulation of C3b hemolytic activity by a plasma protein distinct from C3b inactivator. Science 193:1011–1013
17. Dempsey PW, Allison ME, Akkaraju S, Goodnow CC, Fearon DT (1996) C3d of complement as a molecular adjuvant: bridging innate and acquired immunity. Science 271:348–350
18. Carroll MC, Isenman DE (2012) Regulation of humoral immunity by complement. Immunity 37:199–207
19. van den Elsen JM, Isenman DE (2011) A crystal structure of the complex between human complement receptor 2 and its ligand C3d. Science 332:608–611
20. Khan DA (2011) Hereditary angioedema: historical aspects, classification, pathophysiology, clinical presentation, and laboratory diagnosis. Allergy Asthma Proc 32:1–10
21. Nilsson UR, Nilsson B (1984) Simplified assays of hemolytic activity of the classical and alternative complement pathways. J Immunol Methods 72:49–59
22. Joiner KA, Hawiger A, Gelfand JA (1983) A study of optimal reaction conditions for an assay of the human alternative complement pathway. Am J Clin Pathol 79:65–72
23. Seelen MA, Roos A, Wieslander J, Mollnes TE, Sjoholm AG, Wurzner R, Loos M, Tedesco F, Sim RB, Garred P, Alexopoulos E, Turner MW, Daha MR (2005) Functional analysis of the classical, alternative, and MBL pathways of the complement system: standardization and validation of a simple ELISA. J Immunol Methods 296:187–198
24. Sjoholm AG, Selander B, Ostenson S, Holmstrom E, Soderstrom C (1991) Normal human serum depleted of C1q, factor D and properdin: its use in studies of complement activation. APMIS 99:1120–1128
25. Petersen SV, Thiel S, Jensenius JC (2001) The mannan-binding lectin pathway of complement activation: biology and disease association. Mol Immunol 38:133–149
26. Majewski J, Schultz DW, Weleber RG, Schain MB, Edwards AO, Matise TC, Acott TS, Ott J, Klein ML (2003) Age-related macular degeneration: a genome scan in extended families. Am J Hum Genet 73:540–550
27. Warwicker P, Goodship TH, Donne RL, Pirson Y, Nicholls A, Ward RM, Turnpenny P, Goodship JA (1998) Genetic studies into inherited and sporadic hemolytic uremic syndrome. Kidney Int 53:836–844

28. Truedsson L, Bengtsson AA, Sturfelt G (2007) Complement deficiencies and systemic lupus erythematosus. Autoimmunity 40:560–566
29. Trendelenburg M (2005) Antibodies against C1q in patients with systemic lupus erythematosus. Springer Semin Immunopathol 27:276–285
30. Manderson AP, Botto M, Walport MJ (2004) The role of complement in the development of systemic lupus erythematosus. Annu Rev Immunol 22:431–456
31. Yang Y, Chung EK, Zhou B, Lhotta K, Hebert LA, Birmingham DJ, Rovin BH, Yu CY (2004) The intricate role of complement component C4 in human systemic lupus erythematosus. Curr Dir Autoimmun 7:98–132
32. Carroll MC (2004) The complement system in B cell regulation. Mol Immunol 41:141–146
33. Garred P, Larsen F, Seyfarth J, Fujita R, Madsen HO (2006) Mannose-binding lectin and its genetic variants. Genes Immun 7:85–94
34. Heitzeneder S, Seidel M, Forster-Waldl E, Heitger A (2012) Mannan-binding lectin deficiency: good news, bad news, doesn't matter? Clin Immunol 143:22–38
35. Thiel S, Gadjeva M (2009) Humoral pattern recognition molecules: mannan-binding lectin and ficolins. Adv Exp Med Biol 653:58–73
36. Super M, Thiel S, Lu J, Levinsky RJ, Turner MW (1989) Association of low levels of mannan-binding protein with a common defect of opsonisation. Lancet 2:1236–1239
37. Thiel S, Frederiksen PD, Jensenius JC (2006) Clinical manifestations of mannan-binding lectin deficiency. Mol Immunol 43:86–96
38. Garred P, Pressler T, Lanng S, Madsen HO, Moser C, Laursen I, Balstrup F, Koch C, Koch C (2002) Mannose-binding lectin (MBL) therapy in an MBL-deficient patient with severe cystic fibrosis lung disease. Pediatr Pulmonol 33:201–207
39. Hillmen P, Hall C, Marsh JC, Elebute M, Bombara MP, Petro BE, Cullen MJ, Richards SJ, Rollins SA, Mojcik CF, Rother RP (2004) Effect of eculizumab on hemolysis and transfusion requirements in patients with paroxysmal nocturnal hemoglobinuria. N Engl J Med 350:552–559
40. Michalski M, Szala A, St Swierzko A, Lukasiewicz J, Maciejewska A, Kilpatrick DC, Matsushita M, Domzalska-Popadiuk I, Borkowska-Klos M, Sokolowska A, Szczapa J, Lugowski C, Cedzynski M (2012) H-ficolin (ficolin-3) concentrations and FCN3 gene polymorphism in neonates. Immunobiology 217:730–737
41. Cedzynski M, Atkinson AP, St Swierzko A, MacDonald SL, Szala A, Zeman K, Buczylko K, Bak-Romaniszyn L, Wiszniewska M, Matsushita M, Szemraj J, Banasik M, Turner ML, Kilpatrick DC (2009) L-ficolin (ficolin-2) insufficiency is associated with combined allergic and infectious respiratory disease in children. Mol Immunol 47:415–419
42. Terai I, Kobayashi K, Matsushita M, Fujita T (1997) Human serum mannose-binding lectin (MBL)-associated serine protease-1 (MASP-1): determination of levels in body fluids and identification of two forms in serum. Clin Exp Immunol 110:317–323
43. Moller-Kristensen M, Jensenius JC, Jensen L, Thielens N, Rossi V, Arlaud G, Thiel S (2003) Levels of mannan-binding lectin-associated serine protease-2 in healthy individuals. J Immunol Methods 282:159–167
44. Degn SE, Jensen L, Gal P, Dobo J, Holmvad SH, Jensenius JC, Thiel S (2010) Biological variations of MASP-3 and MAp44, two splice products of the MASP1 gene involved in regulation of the complement system. J Immunol Methods 361:37–50
45. Degn SE, Thiel S, Nielsen O, Hansen AG, Steffensen R, Jensenius JC (2011) MAp19, the alternative splice product of the MASP2 gene. J Immunol Methods 373:89–101
46. Oglesby TJ, Ueda A, Volanakis JE (1988) Radioassays for quantitation of intact complement proteins C2 and B in human serum. J Immunol Methods 110:55–62
47. Hiemstra PS, Langeler E, Compier B, Keepers Y, Leijh PC, van den Barselaar MT, Overbosch D, Daha MR (1989) Complete and partial deficiencies of complement factor D in a Dutch family. J Clin Invest 84:1957–1961
48. de Paula PF, Barbosa JE, Junior PR, Ferriani VP, Latorre MR, Nudelman V, Isaac L (2003) Ontogeny of complement regulatory proteins - concentrations of factor h, factor I, c4b-binding protein, properdin and vitronectin in healthy children of different ages and in adults. Scand J Immunol 58:572–577
49. Sofat R, Mangione PP, Gallimore JR, Hakobyan S, Hughes TR, Shah T, Goodship T, D'Aiuto F, Langenberg C, Wareham N, Morgan BP, Pepys MB, Hingorani AD (2013) Distribution and determinants of circulating complement factor H concentration determined by a high-throughput immunonephelometric assay. J Immunol Methods 390:63–73
50. Tan LA, Yu B, Sim FC, Kishore U, Sim RB (2010) Complement activation by phospholipids: the interplay of factor H and C1q. Protein Cell 1:1033–1049

Chapter 2

Evaluation of Complement Function by ELISA

Anja Roos and Jörgen Wieslander

Abstract

Evaluation of total complement function in human serum is an essential component of laboratory diagnostics of the human complement system. During recent years, established hemolytic assays for classical pathway and alternative pathway function, CH50 and AP50 assays, respectively, have been replaced in many diagnostic laboratories by ELISA assays. Next to an improved standardization, this assay platform also allows for functional analysis of the lectin pathway of complement. The present chapter describes the methodology of ELISA assays for assessment of the classical pathway, the alternative pathway, the MBL-dependent lectin pathway, and the Ficolin-3-dependent lectin pathway of complement in clinical laboratory diagnostics.

Key words Complement, CH50, AP50, MBL, Ficolin, Alternative pathway, Classical pathway, Lectin pathway, ELISA

1 Introduction

Genetic deficiencies for the large majority of complement factors have been described in patients [1, 2]. For molecules that function within the complement cascade, this would imply a block in the cascade. The spectrum of diseases that is associated with complement dysfunction is broad and still growing. Patients with genetic complement deficiency often present with apparent immune deficiency, suffering from recurrent infections with Neisseria species (alternative pathway and terminal pathway deficiencies), and/or encapsulated bacteria (classical pathway deficiencies) [1]. Therefore, screening for complement deficiency should be part of a regular protocol for immune deficiency screening. Patients with classical pathway deficiencies typically present also with systemic SLE (systemic lupus erythematosus)-like autoimmune disease, especially the deficiencies early in the cascade. Patients with a deficiency in the central component C3 usually suffer from severe infections, frequently in combination with immune complex disorders and glomerulonephritis. Patients with factor I deficiency may have a similar presentation due to a regulation defect, whereas patients

Mihaela Gadjeva (ed.), *The Complement System: Methods and Protocols*, Methods in Molecular Biology, vol. 1100,
DOI 10.1007/978-1-62703-724-2_2, © Springer Science+Business Media New York 2014

with factor H deficiency may show membranoproliferative glomerulonephritis type II or atypical hemolytic uremic syndrome, next to the infectious complications. These conditions warrant clinical analysis of complement function, which can be of key relevance in disease diagnosis.

Next to genetic complement disorders, also a number of acquired conditions may result in detectable deviations in the complement cascade. Autoantibodies to complement regulatory molecules (C1 inhibitor, factor H) or to complement convertases (C3 nephritic factor) may induce similar aberrations and clinical pictures as a genetic complement deficiency [3]. Patients with circulating immune complexes, with systemic autoimmune diseases, or with cryoglobulins may show clearly impaired complement activity due to in vivo consumption of complement factors. Analysis of complement function in these patients may be helpful in disease diagnosis and follow-up.

Functional assays have been developed that measure the complete pathway in order to detect abnormalities in the complement cascade in human serum. Traditionally, hemolytic assays have been used for that purpose; these have a well-established role in the assessment of the complete complement cascade for the classical pathway (CH50 assay) and the alternative pathway of complement (AP50 assay). However, for the lectin pathway of complement, a reliable and specific hemolytic assay for the complete cascade that is well-suitable for routine use has not been described.

In order to facilitate functional measurement of all complement activation pathways in a similar setting, assays have been developed using other platforms, i.e., based on ELISA format. These assays are designed in such a way that specificity is guaranteed both at the level of the plastic-coated activating ligand, as well as at the level of the buffer used for sample incubation. Functional and pathway-specific ELISA-based assays for complement activation have been described in several publications and can detect the complement activation cascade up to several levels, from the early step of conversion of C4 up to the final step of formation of C5b-9 [4–9].

The classical pathway can be activated via binding of C1q to its ligands, leading to activation of C1r and C1s, the complement-activating enzymes of the classical pathway. Likewise, the lectin pathway of complement can be activated via binding of mannose-binding lectin (MBL), ficolin-1, ficolin-2, or ficolin-3 to their ligands, respectively, leading to activation of the complement-activating enzyme MASP-2 (MBL-associated serine protease-2). Specific assays to assess complement activation via ficolin-1 and ficolin-2, suitable for routine use, have not yet been described. The alternative pathway of complement can be activated via interplay of complement factor C3 with factor D, factor B, properdin, and a suitable stabilizing ligand.

The present chapter describes a method for functional assessment of complement activation for four different pathways, i.e., the classical pathway, the alternative pathway, the MBL-mediated lectin pathway, and the ficolin-3-dependent lectin pathway, up to the level of C5b-9 [7]. This test is useful in a routine diagnostic setting in clinical laboratories without the need for detailed technical expertise in complementology. The current chapter provides support for basic data interpretation, and the tests described here can be used as a first diagnostic step in most clinical situations. However, complement-related disorders can be highly complex and thorough expertise is required in final interpretation of the current test results and smart selection of additional and follow-up-testing in individual clinical situations. Next to their use in a diagnostic setting, these assays can also be used in clinical trials, depending on the requirements of the study.

2 Materials

2.1 Materials for Sample Collection

1. Regular equipment for collection of patient blood by venipuncture.
2. Blood collection tubes, either serum tube without additives, or, preferably, serum tube with separator gel.
3. Box with crushed ice.
4. Centrifuge that is able to cool up to +5 °C.
5. Aliquotting tubes for serum that can be frozen at −70 °C.
6. Adequate freezer-resistant labels.

2.2 Required Equipment

1. Set of calibrated precision pipettes (minimum volume 5 μl, maximum volume 500 μl).
2. Disposable tips.
3. Multichannel pipette suitable for 300 μl.
4. Laboratory shaker.
5. Graduated cylinder 500 ml.
6. Paper towels.
7. Laboratory ice machine.
8. Water bath (37 °C).
9. Incubator (37 °C).
10. Timer.
11. Absorbance plate reader suitable to measure at 405 nm.
12. Freezer (preferably < −70 °C).
13. Refrigerator.

2.3 Assay Materials

1. Wieslab® Complement system Classical pathway (COMPL CP 310) (Eurodiagnostica, Malmö, Sweden). The kit contains pre-coated wells (coated with human IgM) as well as all necessary buffers and reagents.
2. Wieslab® Complement system Alternative pathway (COMPL AP 330) (Eurodiagnostica, Malmö, Sweden). The kit contains pre-coated wells (coated with LPS) as well as all necessary buffers and reagents. The buffer contains EGTA to allow activation of the alternative pathway but not the classical pathway or lectin pathway.
3. Wieslab® Complement system MBL pathway (COMPL MP 320) (Eurodiagnostica, Malmö, Sweden). The kit contains pre-coated wells (coated with mannan) as well as all necessary reagents. The buffer contains a blocking antibody against C1q to allow activation of the lectin pathway but not the classical pathway.
4. Wieslab® Complement system Ficolin 3 (COMPLF3) (Eurodiagnostica, Malmö, Sweden). The kit contains pre-coated wells (coated with acetylated BSA) as well as all necessary reagents. The buffer contains a blocking antibody against C1q to allow activation of the lectin pathway but not the classical pathway.
5. Distilled water.
6. Wash solution. A 30× concentrated wash solution is supplied in the kit. Dilute 1/30 with distilled water and store at 2–8 °C until kit expiration.

All kits should be stored at 2–8° C except for the positive control. The positive control should be stored below –18° C.

3 Methods

3.1 Specimen Collection, Pre-analysis

1. Prepare the patient or donor and draw venous blood in accordance to established protocols. Please note that only serum can be used for complement function ELISA's described below, NOT plasma.
2. Mix the tube thoroughly by turning it around at least five times. Place the tube on crushed ice (*see* **Notes 1** and **2**).
3. Take care of the donor following regular procedures.
4. Allow the tube to clot for 1–2 h on ice. Centrifuge the tube in a cooled centrifuge. Collect the serum and divide in at least six tubes with at least 250 μl per tube, when possible. Keep cool while handling.
5. Freeze the aliquots as soon as possible, preferably at –70 °C or less. Freezing at –20 °C is acceptable for a period of around 4 weeks.

6. When the test starts, thaw the samples, preferably in a shaking water bath (37 °C) until a small piece of ice is left, and place on ice during the complete procedure. Do not use samples that have been thawed more than once. Mix on laboratory shaker before use.

3.2 Assay Startup

1. Decide which assay(s) will be performed (*see* **Notes 3** and **4**). A full interpretation of results as described in Subheading 3.8.2 is only possible if all four tests described here have been performed on (a comparable aliquot of) the same sample. A selection of tests, however, can give a relevant answer to a specific question.
2. Calculate the number of wells required for the analysis and remove the number of strips required from the aluminum package. Reseal the package properly and store at 4 °C.
3. Equilibrate all required wells and kit reagents to room temperature (*see* **Note 5**).
4. Thaw suitable samples.
5. Reconstitute positive control present in the kit. Make sure all lyophilized material is on the bottom of the tube by gently tapping the tube. Remove the cap and add 200 μl of distilled water. Replace cap, incubate for 5 min on ice and mix on the shaker until completely dissolved. Keep on ice until use. Please note that the assay reproducibility is to a considerable extent dependent on the quality of this positive control (*see* **Note 6**).

3.3 Sample Incubation for Assessment of the Classical Pathway of Complement

1. Dilute the sample 1/101 by adding 5 μl of sample to 500 μl of Diluent CP (*see* **Note 5**). Mix well on the vortex. Keep diluted samples preferably on ice until further processing for 60 min at maximum.
2. Treat the reconstituted positive control as a sample: dilute 1/101. The negative control is ready to use.
3. Add adequate samples for internal quality control, according to requirements of the quality system of the laboratory (*see* **Note** 7).
4. Start to fill the microtiter plate when all samples and controls are ready. Always add all controls on every plate (*see* **Note 8**). Pipet samples in the plate column-wise and pipet all samples and controls in duplicate: start at A1 and B1, next C1 and D1, etc. Start with diluent CP as a blank, then diluted positive control, then negative control (which is ready to use) and then diluted samples. Add 100 μl per well for each sample or control. Do not interrupt the process until all samples are in the plate and incubation has been started.
5. Incubate the plate with lid for 60–70 min at 37 °C. Continue at Subheading 3.7, **step 1**.

3.4 Sample Incubation for Assessment of the Alternative Pathway of Complement

1. Dilute the sample 1/18 by adding 20 µl of sample to 340 µl of Diluent AP (*see* **Note 5**). Mix well on the vortex. Keep diluted samples preferably on ice until further processing for 60 min at maximum.
2. Treat the reconstituted positive control as a sample: dilute 1/18. The negative control is ready to use.
3. Add adequate samples for internal quality control, according to requirements of the quality system of the laboratory (*see* **Note 7**).
4. Start to fill the microtiter plate when all samples and controls are ready (*see* **Note 8**). Pipet samples in the plate column-wise and pipet all samples and controls in duplicate: start at A1 and B1, next C1 and D1, etc. Start, e.g., with diluent AP as a blank, then diluted positive control, then negative control (which is ready to use) and then diluted samples. Add 100 µl per well for each sample or control. Do not interrupt the process until all samples are in the plate and incubation has been started.
5. Incubate the plate with lid for 60–70 min at 37 °C. Continue at Subheading 3.7, **step 1**.

3.5 Sample Incubation for Assessment of the MBL Pathway of Complement

1. Dilute the sample 1/101 by adding 5 µl of sample to 500 µl of Diluent MP (*see* **Note 5**). Mix well on the vortex.
2. Treat the reconstituted positive control as a sample: dilute 1/101. The negative control is ready to use.
3. Incubate diluted samples and controls, preferably on ice, during 15–60 min before further processing to allow proper classical pathway inhibition.
4. Add adequate samples for internal quality control, according to requirements of the quality system of the laboratory (*see* **Note 7**).
5. Start to fill the microtiter plate when all samples and controls are ready (*see* **Note 8**). Pipet samples in the plate column-wise and pipet all samples and controls in duplicate: start at A1 and B1, next C1 and D1, etc. Start with diluent MP as a blank, then diluted positive control, then negative control (which is ready to use) and then diluted samples. Add 100 µl per well for each sample or control. Do not interrupt the process until all samples are in the plate and incubation has been started.
6. Incubate the plate with lid for 60–70 min at 37 °C. Continue at Subheading 3.7, **step 1**.

3.6 Sample Incubation for Assessment of the Ficolin-3-Pathway of Complement

1. Dilute the sample 1/50 by adding 10 µl of sample to 490 µl of Diluent F3 (*see* **Note 5**). Mix well on the vortex.
2. Treat the reconstituted positive control as a sample: dilute 1/50. The negative control is ready to use.

3. Incubate diluted samples and controls, preferably on ice, during 15–60 min before further processing to allow proper classical pathway inhibition.
4. Add adequate samples for internal quality control, according to requirements of the quality system of the laboratory (*see* **Note 7**).
5. Start to fill the microtiter plate when all samples and controls are ready (*see* **Note 8**). Pipet samples in the plate column-wise and pipet all samples and controls in duplicate: start at A1 and B1, next C1 and D1, etc. Start with diluent F3 as a blank, then diluted positive control, then negative control (which is ready to use) and then diluted samples. Add 100 μl per well for each sample or control. Do not interrupt the process until all samples are in the plate and incubation has been started.
6. Incubate the plate with lid for 60–70 min at 37 °C. Continue at Subheading 3.7, **step 1**.

3.7 Assay Development

1. Wash the plate: empty the wells by flicking the plate over a sink and patting it on paper towels (*see* **Note 9**). Add 300 μl of washing solution, empty the wells. Repeat this procedure twice. After the last step, remove the remaining drops by patting the plate on a pile of paper towels. Avoid cross-contamination. Proceed to **step 2** and avoid further drying of the plate.
2. Add 100 μl of ready-to-use conjugate to each well, preferably using a multichannel pipette. The conjugate is an alkaline phosphatase-labeled antibody directed against a neoantigen exposed at the membrane attack complex. Cover the plate.
3. Incubate for 30 min at room temperature (20–25 °C).
4. Wash the plate: empty the wells by flicking the plate over a sink and patting it on paper towels. Add 300 μl of washing solution, empty the wells. Repeat this procedure twice. After the last step, remove the remaining drops by patting the plate on a pile of paper towels. Proceed to **step 5** and avoid further drying of the plate.
5. Add 100 μl of ready-to-use substrate solution to each well, preferably using a multichannel pipette. Cover the plate.
6. Incubate for 30 min at room temperature (20–25 °C).
7. Remove the lid. Read the absorbance (optical density) of the wells at 405 nm in an absorbance plate reader (*see* **Note 10**). Use shaker function of the reader before measurement, if available.

3.8 Data Calculation and Interpretation

3.8.1 Data Calculation

For each pathway the calculations are based on optical density (OD) values (absorbances) of samples, positive controls, negative controls, and blanks *from the same pathway and from the same plate*.

Subtract the OD of the blank (diluent) from the OD of the negative control, positive control, and samples. The net OD of the positive control (PC) and the negative control (NC) should be >1 and <0.2, respectively (*see* **Note 11**).

The negative and positive controls can be used in a semiquantitative way to calculate complement activity, expressed as a percentage of the value of the positive control. Calculate the mean OD values of duplicate measurements for the samples, PC and NC. Subsequently, calculate the % complement activity of the samples:

$$100 \times \left((Sample - NC) / (PC - NC) \right).$$

3.8.2 Data Interpretation

Data are interpreted on basis of the result in relation to the reference range (*see* **Note 12**). For the classical pathway, alternative pathway, and MBL pathway, reference values have been determined in an international study, based on measurements in 120 sera of healthy controls, 60 male and 60 female, distributed between 20 and 70 years old [7]. For the classical pathway, the cutoff was set at 74 %, and for the alternative pathway, the cutoff was set at 39 %. Values in patient samples below this value are considered to be decreased.

Due to the large genetic variation in the human *mbl2* gene, the observed variation in MBL pathway activity is also large. An arbitrary cutoff was defined at 10 % [7].

For Ficolin-3-pathway activity, a cutoff at 25 % was defined, based on measurements in 120 sera of healthy controls (see kit insert for data).

Results that are below the cutoff can be divided into at least two groups: acquired complement deficiencies and genetic complement deficiencies. Furthermore, pre-analytical errors are a frequent cause of complement function results below the cutoff and should always be excluded. In most patient sera the alternative pathway is most sensitive to pre-analytical errors.

Genetic deficiencies are usually characterized by very low values, usually below 3 % of activity, often below 1 %, although exceptions are possible. Acquired deficiencies usually show up in more than one pathway and are usually associated with low levels of complement molecules such as C3, C4, and/or C1q, which can be measured by common immunochemical methods. A suspected genetic deficiency should always be confirmed using a new sample of the same patient, collected at a later moment with special care for required pre-analysis conditions (*see* Subheading 3.1). When the results are comparable between both measurements and an acquired defect can be ruled out with a high degree of probability, further analysis is warranted.

Based on the pattern of the deficiency, i.e., the pathways that do work and the pathways that do not work, the complement factor(s) most likely involved can be figured out (Table 1). Since the assays as described above measure the complete cascade, any deficiency in the shared terminal pathway of complement (C3, C5,

Table 1
Interpretation of complement function results in case of suspected genetic deficiency of complement

CP result	AP result	MBL-P[a] result	Fic-3-P result	Possible deficiencies[b]
Deficient	Normal	*Normal*[a]	Normal	C1q, C1r, C1s
Normal	**Deficient**	*Normal*[a]	Normal	Properdin, factor D, *factor B*[c]
Normal	Normal	**Deficient**	Normal	MBL
Normal	Normal	*Normal*[a]	**Deficient**	Ficolin-3
Normal	Normal	**Deficient**	**Deficient**	(MASP-2) or (Ficolin-3 and MBL[a])
Deficient	Normal	**Deficient**	**Deficient**	C4, C2, C1 inhibitor
Deficient	**Deficient**	**Deficient**	**Deficient**	C3, C5, C6, C7, C8, C9, factor H, factor I

[a]MBL deficiency is common and can be combined with any other deficiency
[b]Possible complement deficiencies in patients with the described pattern of complement function. For example, a patient with deficient function of the classical pathway only may be genetically deficient for C1q *or* C1r *or* C1s. Acquired deficiencies of complement function should be excluded
[c]Factor B deficiency has not yet been described

C6, C7, C8, C9) will affect all pathways to a similar extent. Specific classical pathway deficiency can be due to a defect at C1q, C1r, and C1s. Specific alternative pathway deficiency can be due to a defect at properdin, factor D or factor B. Specific MBL pathway deficiency will be due to MBL deficiency, which is a common trait in the human population. Specific ficolin-3-pathway deficiency will be due to a genetic deficiency of ficolin-3. A deficiency in both MBL-dependent and ficolin-3-dependent lectin pathway activation can be due to a MASP-2 defect. When the alternative pathway alone does work normally and all others do not, the defect most likely resides at the level of C4 or C2. Since MBL deficiency is common, this defect can occur in combination with every other defect, thus further complicating the interpretation. Furthermore, also genetic deficiencies of regulatory molecules can result in a complete dysfunction of the complement cascade, such as for Factor H and factor I (activity in all pathways almost unmeasurable due to consumption of C3) and for C1 inhibitor (impaired classical pathway and lectin pathway activation due to consumption of C4 and C2).

For follow-up analysis, assays for single components that are suspected to be deficient, in accordance with Table 1, should be performed to identify the defect. These assays should in principle be performed on a functional basis. For example, reconstitution experiments can be performed using defined complement-deficient sera. Usually as a next step, genetic analysis can be performed to identify the defect at a genetic basis. Such extended analysis steps can be limited or extended, based on the clinical needs.

Results could be used for clinical management of the patient, for example by offering additional antimicrobial protection (vaccination, antibiotic prophylaxis), as well as for family analysis and genetic counseling, if desired.

If the pattern of complement function deviations is more consistent with an acquired defect, it is helpful to define the pathway(s) of complement consumption. Supporting analysis can include concentration measurements of individual components, such as C1q, C4, and C3, and measurements of complement activation products of different pathways. Further interpretation of the results should be made on basis of the combination of clinical picture, complement profile, and other (laboratory) analysis and could require more specialized knowledge and testing.

4 Notes

1. Storage of blood samples on ice is preferable to prevent ongoing in vitro complement activation, resulting in consumption of complement factors and reduced complement function. Each laboratory may perform validation studies in order to develop feasible pre-analysis protocols that sufficiently prevent artifacts by in vitro complement activation. In a number of situations, immediate cooling of samples could be not essential and serum samples that have been taken by regular procedures might also suffice. However, reference values should be determined in samples of healthy controls that have been treated in a similar way. Furthermore, it is important to realize that clinical samples may differ fundamentally from samples from healthy controls in their capacity to trigger and maintain in vitro complement activation, related for example to the presence of immune complexes, defects in complement regulation, autoantibodies to complement molecules, and cryoglobulins (*see* **Note 2**). Therefore, protocols described above are based on treating the samples as cold as possible, in order to prevent artifacts in individual patient sera.
2. Cryoglobulins may induce complement activation in vivo and in vitro. In vitro complement activation and consumption may be extensive, even during the execution of the test. When a cryoglobulin is suspected to be present, the sample can be centrifuged in a cooled Eppendorf centrifuge immediately following thawing of the sample and before warming up. The supernatant can be transferred to another tube and used for the complement testing as described above. This treatment will deliver results that are closer to the in vivo situation.
3. The current chapter describes the methodology for functional complement assessment based on ELISA kits produced by

Eurodiagnostica, Malmö, Sweden, and manual performance of the test. Next to performance by hand, also automation of complement function ELISA's is possible on instruments for ELISA automation. For example Eurodiagnostica kits are harmonized for usage on Dynex instruments. Validation of automated tests should include the pre-analytical effects of automation on sample quality, using samples that are comparable to the samples of the population to be tested.

4. For the sake of clarity, all four complement activation tests (classical pathway (CP), alternative pathway (AP), MBL pathway (MBL-P), and Ficolin-3-pathway (Fic-3-P) will be described here separately. For experienced technicians, it is however possible to perform the four different complement tests on a number of samples in parallel. This could be of relevance since every thawed sample can in principle be used only once. If a sample is used that has been thawed for a second time, the sample will generally show a decreased complement activity as compared to a fresh sample. This decrease of complement function can be dependent on the condition of the patient. If the sample protocol as described in Subheading 3.1 is followed, there will be six samples available for each patient or donor, i.e., one for every test, one in case something needs to be repeated and one for follow-up-testing.
5. Do not mix the constituents of the different kits unless the lot numbers on the vials are identical. *Make sure that the sample diluent in each kit is only used for the specific pathway of the kit*, since the sample diluent contains specific inhibitors to ensure pathway specificity. Plates and diluents are color coded to help in identification.
6. The reproducibility of the assay is dependent on a number of factors, including pipetting, incubation times and temperatures, and, to a large extent, the quality of the positive control. In order to increase analytical reproducibility, it is recommended to standardize the reconstitution of the positive control as precise as possible. Furthermore, take a fresh vial of the control for each separate experiment and do not store these controls after reconstitution. Extra vials with positive control can be ordered from Eurodiagnostica, Malmö, Sweden, when required. It is also possible to produce a home-made positive control by collecting a large volume of serum, e.g., pooled from several healthy donors, collected in a well-controlled way as described in Subheading 3.1. Make sure that complement activity, especially for the lectin pathway, is high enough to serve as positive control (i.e., exclude MBL-deficient donors). Freeze the material in a high number of identical aliquots at less than −70 °C and determine a calculation factor by calibration against the positive control of the kit. Take a fresh vial for

every test and use as positive control as a basis for calculations. Such a procedure may increase reproducibility. However, final calibration may differ from the units based on the positive controls supplied in the kits, with consequences for the lab-to-lab comparability. If used, this calibration method should be well validated, including self-established reference ranges. Overall, these ELISA assays are semiquantitative and an inter-assay coefficient of variation of around 15 % is acceptable.

7. For internal QC, home-made samples, e.g., from pooled serum, can be used that are prepared and stored as described in **Note 6**. Optimally, such controls have complement activity that is around the assay cutoffs. This can be reached by, e.g., sample dilution, by preparing a sample mixture, by sample maltreatment in the pre-analytical phase, or by using pooled samples from patients. However, the last two options may result in samples that do not have a stable complement function upon long-term storage and use. Preparation of a suitable internal control can be a matter of trial and error. Depending on the requirements of the quality system of the laboratory, e.g., Westgard rules (http://www.westgard.com/westgard-rules-and-multirules.htm) can be used for internal monitoring and control of test performance.

8. If more than one plate is required for the number of samples to test, always put all controls (blank, positive control, negative control, internal QC) on every single plate.

9. Plate washing can also be performed by a plate washer, which is available on the market from simple to fully automated formats. Plate washers generally use more washing buffers and therefore additional buffer can be ordered from the producer. Plate washers may increase assay reproducibility. In general, the quality of washing, including the efficient removal of fluid from the well in between washing steps, may positively influence both the background and the positive signal of the test.

10. Make sure to remove any air bubbles in the wells before measurement of optical density. A simple hairdryer can be used to remove air bubbles. Make sure the bottom of the plate is clean and clear. Do not write on the bottom of plates or in close proximity of the wells.

11. A failure of the test can take place when the protocol is not followed properly. When the negative control is too high, the washing procedure might be suboptimal or cross-contamination may have taken place. When the positive control is too low, the kit constituents might be expired or not well stored. When performing more than one assay in parallel, a mix-up of diluents may occur and will result in erroneous results in all pathways. Further information for troubleshooting is available in the kit inserts.

12. Determination of reference values should optimally be performed in each laboratory, using sera from healthy controls that resemble the patient population of the hospital. Please note that reference values described above do only refer to adult patients. Children may have different reference values depending on their age. For complement function, the upper value of the reference range is of limited importance. Complement function can be increased, e.g., as a result of acute phase response. In most clinical situations, only low complement values are of importance and therefore only a single cutoff value is used. This value is usually determined on basis of the mean minus 2 SD of the results of a healthy population. This method is only useful for normally distributed results. With respect to MBL pathway function, the distribution is not normal, and the results cannot easily be divided into normal and abnormal, in view of the high frequency of MBL deficiency and the biological advantages that are associated with MBL deficiency in many clinical situations. Although the cutoff has been chosen at 10 %, a sample with a complete MBL deficiency, such as related to homozygous or compound heterozygous expression of MBL variant alleles, presents with MBL function below 3 % and in principle below 1 %. Samples with results between 3 and 10 % could be from patients with heterozygous expression of MBL variant alleles or from patients with low expression of MBL protein due to genetic variants in the MBL promoter. Such deficiencies are in most cases clinically not relevant.

References

1. Skattum L, van Deuren M, van der Poll T et al (2011) Complement deficiency states and associated infections. Mol Immunol 48: 1643–1655
2. Degn SE, Jensenius JC, Thiel S (2011) Disease-causing mutations in genes of the complement system. Am J Hum Genet 88:689–705
3. Daha NA, Banda NK, Roos A et al (2011) Complement activation by (auto-)antibodies. Mol Immunol 48:1656–1665
4. Fredrikson GN, Truedsson L, Sjöholm AG (1993) New procedure for the detection of complement deficiency by ELISA. Analysis of activation pathways and circumvention of rheumatoid factor influence. J Immunol Methods 166:263–270
5. Petersen SV, Thiel S, Jensen L et al (2001) An assay for the mannan-binding lectin pathway of complement activation. J Immunol Methods 257:107–116
6. Roos A, Bouwman LH, Munoz J et al (2003) Functional characterization of the lectin pathway of complement in human serum. Mol Immunol 39:655–668
7. Seelen MA, Roos A, Wieslander J et al (2005) Functional analysis of the classical, alternative, and MBL pathways of the complement system: standardization and validation of a simple ELISA. J Immunol Methods 296:187–198
8. Munthe-Fog L, Hummelshoj T, Honore C et al (2009) Immunodeficiency associated with FCN3 mutation and ficolin-3 deficiency. N Engl J Med 360:2637–2644
9. Hein E, Honore C, Skjoedt MO et al (2010) Functional analysis of Ficolin-3 mediated complement activation. PLoS One 5:e15443

Chapter 3

Classical Complement Pathway Component C1q: Purification of Human C1q, Isolation of C1q Collagen-Like and Globular Head Fragments and Production of Recombinant C1q—Derivatives. Functional Characterization

Mihaela Kojouharova

Abstract

The classical complement pathway (CCP) activation is a multimolecular complex, composed of three subcomponents namely C1q, C1r, and C1s. C1q is the recognition subunit of this complex and its binding to the specific targets leads to the formation of active C1, which in turn activates the CCP in an immunoglobulin-dependent or -independent manner. C1q is a hexameric glycoprotein composed of 18 polypeptide chains of three different types (A, B, and C), organized in two fragments—collagen-like (CLR) and globular head (gC1q) possessing different functional activity. The contemporary knowledge of the C1q structure allows the isolation and purification of a C1q molecule from serum by combination of different chromatography procedures including ion-exchange, size-exclusion, and affinity chromatography, as well as the isolation of CLR and gC1q by limited enzymatic hydrolysis of the native C1q molecule. In this chapter, we described methods for purification of human C1q and its CLR and gC1q fragments, as well as methods for their biochemical and functional characterization. The production and purification of recombinant C1q derivatives ghA, ghB, and ghC (globular fragments of the individual C1q chains) are also presented.

Key words Complement component C1q, Purification, Pepsin and collagenase digestion, Expression of recombinant globular heads of A, B, and C chains of C1q

1 Introduction

The classical complement pathway (CCP) activation involves a sequentially acting multistep cascade initiated by the first component C1, which is a multimolecular complex, composed of three subcomponents namely C1q, C1r, and C1s that associate together in a calcium-dependent macromolecular protease ($C1q + C1r_2 + C1s_2$). The binding of C1q to its targets leads to activation of C1, which in turn activates the CCP in an immunoglobulin-dependent (via binding IgG1 or IgM) or immunoglobulin-independent manner.

Mihaela Gadjeva (ed.), *The Complement System: Methods and Protocols*, Methods in Molecular Biology, vol. 1100, DOI 10.1007/978-1-62703-724-2_3, © Springer Science+Business Media New York 2014

C1q, the recognition subunit, is a hexameric 460-kDa glycoprotein with the overall shape of a bouquet of tulips. It is composed of 18 polypeptide chains of three different types A, B, and C (6A, 6B, and 6C), consisting of 223, 236, and 217 residues, respectively. Each chain has a short N-terminal region flanked by a collagen-like region (CLR) and a C-terminal heterotrimeric ligand-binding globular domain (gC1q). The structure of the C1q molecule allows the isolation of these fragments by limited enzymatic hydrolysis (pepsin or collagenase digestion of C1q) leading to the CLR and gC1q, respectively. Inter-chain disulfide bonding yields 6(A–B) and 6(C–C) dimer subunits. These dimers and the collagen-like sequences in the C1q chains form a triple-helical collagen-like structural unit of the arrangement ABC–CBA, which is held together by both covalent and non-covalent bonds [1].

C1q is of interest to many laboratories investigating structural–functional relationships since it is a remarkable multifunctional molecule, which possesses the ability to recognize and bind an amazing variety of structurally different self- and non-self-target molecules and thus participates in immunological processes with great importance [2]. Such studies ultimately require biochemically pure and functionally active C1q. Furthermore, laboratories involved in clinical research (e.g., immune complex detection, detection of anti-C1q autoantibodies) also rely on the isolation of highly purified C1q and/or its purified fragments (gC1q and CLR).

The aim of this chapter is to describe methods for isolation and purification of human C1q and assays to test its functional activity. In general, three main types of procedures have been developed for C1q purification [3]. They include (a) conventional purification involving euglobulin precipitation, ion-exchange chromatography, and size-exclusion chromatography; (b) affinity chromatography on IgG-Sepharose 4B, followed by additional purification step (e.g., FPLC ion-exchange chromatography, affinity chromatography on Protein-A Sepharose); and (c) precipitation procedures with different agents (DNA, 1,3 diaminopropan, polyethylene glycol or low ionic strength buffers containing chelating agents EDTA, EGTA) to precipitate out C1q. Here we present two widely used, rapid, simple, and reproducible methods. Each of them could be chosen depending on the laboratory needs. The isolation of the fragments (CLR and gC1q), derived from serum C1q, based on limited enzymatic hydrolysis of C1q is also described [4, 5].

C1q is a very complicated molecule and so far the whole recombinant C1q molecule or even its individual recombinant A, B, and C chains are still not available. The investigation of the recognition properties mainly attributed to the gC1q fragment of Clq lead to the development of recombinant forms of its globular head fragments (ghA, ghB, and ghC). Here their production from culture supernatants, based on affinity chromatography is also presented [6].

2 Material

2.1 Preparation of Human Serum

1. Human citrated plasma.
2. 1 M $CaCl_2$ (stock solution).
3. NPGB (*p*-nitrophenyl-*p′*-guanidinobenzoate) and/or PMSF (phenyl methyl–sulfonyl fluoride).
4. Muslin.

2.2 Purification of C1q by Chromatography on BioRex70 and Biogel A5m

1. 200 mM EDTA (stock solution).
2. Starting buffer: 50 mM sodium phosphate buffer, pH 7.3, 2 mM EDTA, 82 mM NaCl.
3. 50 mM sodium phosphate buffer, pH 7.3, 2 mM EDTA, 300 mM NaCl.
4. 50 mM Tris–HCl, pH 7.3, 1 mM EDTA, 500 mM NaCl (buffer for size exclusion chromatography).
5. Ammonium sulfate (for protein precipitation) (*see* **Note 1**).
6. Column matrixes: BioRex 70 column and Biogel A5m column.
7. Protease inhibitors (*see* **Note 2**).

2.3 Purification of C1q by Chromatography on IgG-Sepharose 4B and FPLC on Mono S

1. 200 mM EDTA (stock solution).
2. 5 mM phosphate-buffered saline (PBS), pH 7.4.
3. PBSE (PBS containing 10 mM EDTA).
4. PBSE, pH 7.4, 1 M NaCl, 30 % (w/w) ethylene glycol (elution buffer).
5. 20 mM HEPES, pH 7.8, 60 mM NaCl, 10 mM EDTA, 10 mM 1, 3 diaminopropane (buffer I for FPLC).
6. 20 mM HEPES, pH 7.8, 300 mM NaCl, 10 mM EDTA, 10 mM 1, 3 diaminopropane (buffer II for FPLC).
7. Protease inhibitors (*see* **Note 2**).
8. Column matrixes: IgG-Sepharose 4B and Mono S column for FPLC. A human IgG-Sepharose column ((50 mL) G/mL Sepharose) has to be made incubating human IgG with CNBr-activated sepharose (Pharmacia) according to the manufacturer's instructions (*see* **Note 3**).

2.4 Isolation of the Collagen-Like Region (CLR) of C1q by Pepsin Digestion

1. Purified C1q.
2. 100 mM sodium acetate buffer, pH 4.45.
3. 1 M Tris.
4. 150 mM Tris–HCl, pH 7.6 (TB), 5.0 mM $CaCl_2$.
5. Column matrixes Sepharose 4B or Superose 12.
6. Pepsin (Sigma-Aldrich).

2.5 Isolation of the Globular Head Fragment (gC1q) of C1q by Collagenase Digestion

1. Purified C1q.
2. Collagenase Sigma-Aldrich.
3. 200 mM EDTA (stock solution).
4. 20 mM Tris–HCl, pH 7.4, 200 mM NaCl, 10 mM $CaCl_2$.
5. 20 mM Tris–HCl, pH 7.4, 360 mM NaCI, 10 mM $CaCI_2$ (buffer for size exclusion chromatography).
6. Column matrixes Sephacryl S-200 or Superdex 200 10/300 GL.

2.6 Preparation of Competent Cells of E. coli BL21 and Transformation with the Recombinant Plasmids pKBM-a, pKBM-b, and pKBM-c

1. *E. coli BL21(DE3)* cells.
2. 2xTY medium: 16 g bacto tryptone, 10 g yeast extract, 5 g NaCl/L, pH 7.4.
3. 2xTY medium, 1.5 % (w/v) bactoagar, 100 μg/mL ampicillin.
4. 1 M $CaCl_2$ (stock solution).
5. Plasmid DNA (recombinant plasmids pKBM-a, pKBM-b, and pKBM-c) (*see* **Note 4**).

2.7 Expression and Purification of Recombinant Globular Fragments of A, B, and C Chains of C1q

1. *E. coli* BL21 cells containing the recombinant plasmid pKBM-a, pKBM-b, or pKBM-c.
2. Luria-Bertini broth (1 L) containing ampicillin (100 μg/mL).
3. 0.4 mM isopropyl β-D-thiogalactoside (IPTG).
4. Lysis buffer: 20 mM Tris–HCl, pH 8.0, 500 mM NaCl, 0.2 % v/v Tween 20, 1 mM EGTA, 1 mM EDTA, 5 % v/v glycerol, 100 μg/mL lysozyme, 0.1 mM PMSF.
5. Buffer I: 20 mM Tris–HCl, pH 8.0, 100 mM NaCl, 0.2 % v/v Tween 20, 1 mM EDTA, 5 % v/v glycerol.
6. Buffer II: 20 mM Tris–HCl, pH 8.0, 100 mM NaCl, 1 mM EDTA, 5 % v/v glycerol.
7. 10 mM maltose.
8. 20 mM Tris–HCl, pH 8.0, 100 mM NaCl.
9. 20 mM Tris–HCl, pH 8.0, 1 M NaCl.
10. 20 mM Tris–HCl, pH 7.4, 100 mM NaCl, 1 mM EDTA (equilibrium buffer for size exclusion chromatography).
11. 20 mM Tris–HCl, pH 8.0, 100 mM NaCl, 2 mM $CaCl_2$, 5 % v/v glycerol (factor Xa buffer).
12. Chromatography matrixes: Amylose resin column, Q-Sepharose ion-exchange column and Superose 12 size exclusion chromatography column.
13. Human aggregated IgG (HAIgG) (*see* **Note 5**).

2.8 Western Blot Analysis

Western blot analysis is used for identification of purified C1q chains, fragments, and recombinant derivatives.

1. Protein to be tested (suitable concentration as determined by SDS-PAGE).
2. All the reagents for SDS-PAGE (*Laemmli*) 12 or 15 % (w/v) gel under reducing conditions.
3. 2 % BSA (bovine serum albumin).
4. Polyvinyl difluoride transfer membrane.
5. Protein-specific antibody (IgG) (rabbit Ab specific toward the human C1q, C1q individual chains, or C1q-fragments).
6. Goat anti-rabbit IgG-alkaline phosphatase conjugate.
7. Substrates—*p*-nitroblue tetrazolium chloride and 5-bromo-4-chloro-3-indolyl phosphate.

2.9 C1q Hemolytic Assay

1. C1q depleted serum (C1qD)—the effluent of the IgG-Sepharose column, used for C1q purification.
2. Normal human serum (standard).
3. Erythrocytes (EA)—sheep red blood cells (SRBC) sensitized with hemolysin (purified anti-sheep red blood cells IgG or IgM).
4. Dextrose gelatin Veronal-buffered saline ($DGVB^{++}$)—0.5× VBS, 167 mM glucose 0.1 % gelatin, 0.15 mM $CaCl_2$, 0.5 mM $MgCl_2$. VBS is supplied in tablet form by Oxoid Ltd.

2.10 Inhibition of C1q-Dependent Hemolysis

1. C1q-deficient human serum (C1qD).
2. C1q.
3. $DGVB^{++}$.
4. EA_{IgG} (10^7 cells) in $DGVB^{++}$.
5. Purified recombinant C1q-fragments (MBP-ghA, or MBP-ghB, or MBP-ghC).

2.11 ELISA for the Detection of the Interaction of C1q (or C1q Fragments) with Human Aggregated IgG

1. HAIgG (20 mg/mL) in PBS.
2. Purified C1q.
3. Recombinant fusion C1q-proteins (MBP-ghA, MBP-ghB, or MBP-ghC).
4. MBP (maltose-binding protein).
5. Sodium carbonate buffer, pH 9.6.
6. 2 % (w/v) BSA.
7. TBS-NTC buffer: 50 mM Tris–HCl, 150 mM NaCl, 0.05 % (w/v) NaN_3, 0.05 % (v/v) Tween 20, 5 mM $CaCl_2$.

8. Goat antihuman IgG antibody conjugated to peroxidase.
9. 3,3′,5,5′-tetramethylbenzidine (TMB) in aqueous dimethylformamide.
10. Hydrogen peroxide.
11. 1 M H_2SO_4.

3 Methods

Here we present two widely used methods for purification of human C1q. The usual starting material for C1q purification is outdated human plasma, although the fresh citrated plasma is better in order to avoid some degree of proteolysis. To prevent the C1q degradation plasma should be stored at −70 °C and all purification steps have to be carried out at 4 °C unless mentioned otherwise. Even when a rapid method such as fast protein liquid chromatography (FPLC) is used, it is advisable to run the procedure in a 4 °C cold room. Protease inhibitors should be also included during the process of purification, especially in the early steps of purification when plasma proteases are still present in the crude C1q preparations (*see* **Note 2**). More rarely the purification procedure aims to purify all the components of C1 (C1q, C1r, and C1s) from a single pool of plasma (*see* **Note 6**). In such cases the starting material for C1 purification is fresh citrated plasma, which has to be recalcified by addition of $CaCl_2$ since C1 is Ca^{2+}-dependent complex.

3.1 Preparation of Human Serum

1. Add $CaCl_2$ from 1 M stock solution (up to a final concentration 20 mM) and protease inhibitors NPGB and/or PMSF (up to a final concentration 0.1 mM) to human citrated plasma and allow plasma to clot for 4 h at room temperature, then overnight at 4 °C.
2. Fragment the fibrin clot into small pieces and remove it by centrifugation at 16,000 × *g* for 20 min at 4 °C followed by filtration through muslin.
3. Store the resulting serum at −70 °C until use.

3.2 Purification of C1q by Chromatography on BioRex70 and Biogel A5m

This method involves purification of C1q from human serum by two conventional chromatography steps: ion-exchange chromatography on week cation exchanger BioRex70 and size exclusion chromatography on Biogel A5m [7]. The concentration of the C1q preparations is calculated from the absorbance at 280 nm using extinction coefficient of = 6.82. The yield is usually at ~3–5 mg C1q per 100 mL serum. The obtained C1q (*see* **Note 7**) is homogeneous when tested by SDS-PAGE, although trace amounts of contaminations (less than 2 %) can be detected by ELISA. In such cases it is advisable to perform additional purification procedure (*see* **Note 8**).

1. Equilibrate BioRex 70 column (5.6 cm × 18 cm) with starting buffer.
2. Prepare human serum from fresh human plasma (as in Subheading 3.1), adjust to 5 mM EDTA (with 200 mM EDTA stock solution) and load onto a BioRex 70 column.
3. Then wash the column with the same buffer until OD_{280} is reduced to the background levels.
4. Elute the bound material, containing C1q with few contaminating proteins (Factor D and some lipoproteins) with ionic strange linear gradient made from equal amounts of starting buffer and 50 mM sodium phosphate buffer, pH 7.3, containing 2 mM EDTA and 300 mM NaCl.
5. Pool the C1q-containing fractions (shown in a typical run profile in Fig. 1a), detected by A_{280} measuring and by hemolytic assay (*see* Subheading 3.9.1). Concentrate by ammonium sulfate precipitation at 33 % saturation. Redissolve the precipitate in 50 mM Tris buffer, pH 7.2, containing 1 mM EDTA and 500 mM NaCl.
6. Equilibrate Biogel A5m (2 cm × 140 cm) column for size exclusion chromatography with the same buffer and apply the C1q containing material.
7. Elute fractions, pool those containing C1q (Fig. 1b) and concentrate as above. After precipitation redissolve the pellet in 5–10 mL 50 mM Tris buffer, pH 7.2 containing 500 mM NaCl and dialyze against the same buffer.
8. Store purified C1q at −70 °C (*see* **Note 9**).

3.3 Purification of C1q by Chromatography on IgG-Sepharose 4B and FPLC on Mono S

This method has been developed to rely on the affinity of C1q for human aggregated IgG and involves affinity chromatography on IgG-Sepharose 4B followed by FPLC on strong cation exchanger Mono S [8] (Fig. 2). The obtained C1q is biochemically pure, hemolytically active and free of any immunoglobulins. For better results add protease inhibitors during all the procedures (*see* **Note 2**). The C1q concentration is calculated as in (Subheading 3.2) and the yield is usually at ~3–5 mg (max. 10 mg) C1q per 100 mL serum.

1. Equilibrate IgG-Sepharose 4B column (50 mL affinity matrix, 30 mg IgG per mL Sepharose 4B) with PBSE (*see* **Note 10**).
2. Saturate the column with rabbit IgG by repeated passage of rabbit antihuman IgG antiserum containing 10 mM EDTA (~50 mL) over the column.
3. Wash the column with PBS containing 1 M NaCl to remove unbound protein and equilibrate with PBSE.

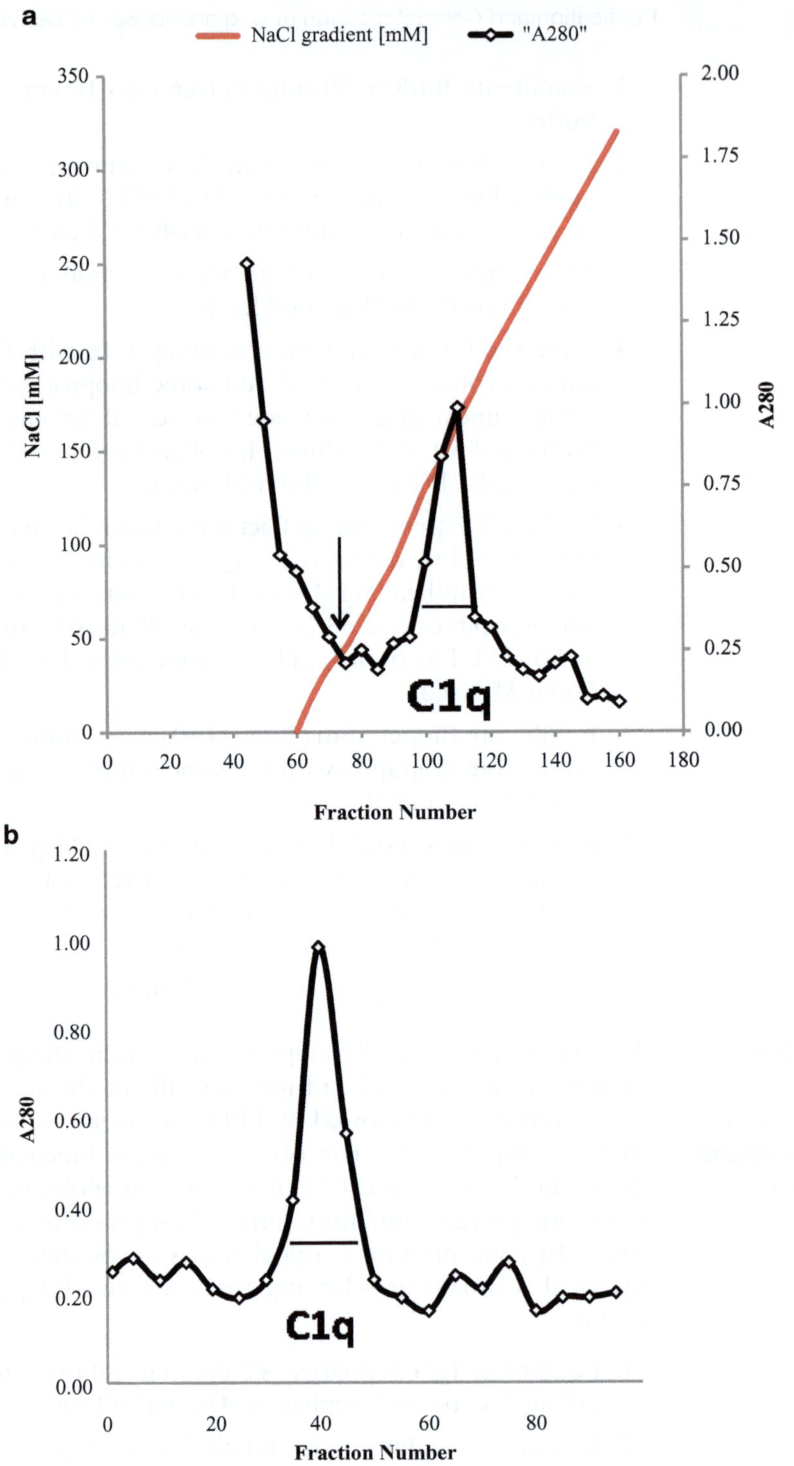

Fig. 1 Purification of human C1q by ion-exchange and size exclusion chromatography. (**a**) Chromatography of EDTA human serum on BioRex 70. Human serum (850 mL) was applied to a BioRex 70 column (5 cm × 18 cm). The proteins were eluted using a linear salt gradient (600 mL of starting buffer and 600 mL of 50 mM sodium phosphate buffer, pH 7.3, containing 2 mM EDTA and 300 mM NaCl). C1q containing fractions were pooled and concentrated; (**b**) Size exclusion chromatography on a Biogel A5m. The partially purified C1q preparation was additionally purified by Biogel A5m chromatography (column 2 cm × 140 cm). The C1q containing fractions were pooled and concentrated

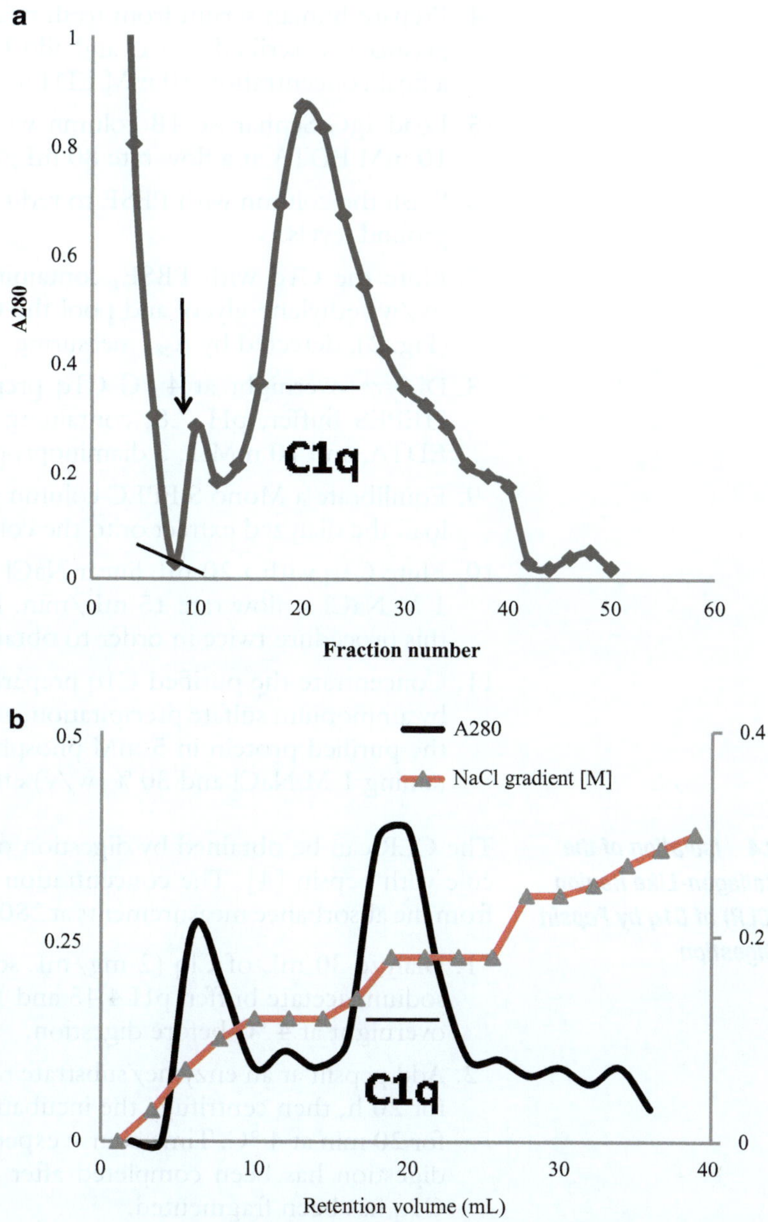

Fig. 2 Purification of C1q by affinity chromatography and FPLC ion-exchange chromatography. (**a**) IgG-Sepharose 4B affinity chromatography. NHS (100 mL) containing 10 mM EDTA was applied to an IgG-Sepharose column (50 mL), and 5-mL fractions were collected. The column was eluted with PBSE, pH 7.4, 1 M NaCl, 30 % (w/w) ethylene glycol. The starting point for the elution was indicated by *arrow*. The C1q containing fractions, assayed for protein concentration (A_{280}) and hemolytic activity were pooled and concentrated. (**b**) FPLC chromatography on Mono S. C1q purified by affinity chromatography was dialyzed against buffer I for FPLC and loaded onto the column. C1q was eluted with a 20-mL linear NaCl gradient form from buffer I and buffer II for FPLC (60 mM to 1 M NaCl salt gradient) at flow rate 15 mL/min

4. Prepare human serum from fresh or outdated citrated human plasma as described above, and add EDTA (stock solution) to a final concentration 10 mM EDTA.
5. Load IgG-Sepharose 4B column with the serum, containing 10 mM EDTA at a flow rate 80 mL/h.
6. Wash the column with PBSE to reduce the OD_{280} at the background levels.
7. Elute the C1q with PBSE, containing 1 M NaCl and 30 % (w/w) ethylene glycol and pool the C1q-containing fractions (Fig. 2), detected by A_{280} measuring and by hemolytic assay.
8. Dialyze overnight at 4 °C C1q preparation against 20 mM HEPES buffer, pH 7.8, containing 60 mM NaCl, 10 mM EDTA, and 10 mM 1, 3 diaminopropane.
9. Equilibrate a Mono S FPLC column with the same buffer and load the dialyzed extract onto the column.
10. Elute C1q with a 20-mL linear NaCl gradient from 60 mM to 1 M NaCl at flow rate 15 mL/min. It is advisable to perform this procedure twice in order to obtain higher yield.
11. Concentrate the purified C1q preparation by ultrafiltration or by ammonium sulfate precipitation, and store small portions of the purified protein in 5 mM phosphate buffer, pH 7.4, containing 1 M NaCl and 30 % (w/v) ethylene glycol at −70 °C.

3.4 Isolation of the Collagen-Like Region (CLR) of C1q by Pepsin Digestion

The CLR can be obtained by digestion of the purified C1q molecule with pepsin [4]. The concentration of CLR was determined from the absorbance measurements at 280 nm using E1cm1 % = 2.1.

1. Dialyze 30 mL of Clq (2 mg/mL solution) against 100 mM sodium acetate buffer, pH 4.45 and 150 mM sodium chloride overnight at 4 °C before digestion.
2. Add pepsin at an enzyme/substrate ratio 1:30 (w/w) at 37 °C for 20 h, then centrifuge the incubation mixture at 30,000 × *g* for 20 min at 4 °C. Time course experiments indicated that the digestion has been completed after this period and 95 % of C1q has been fragmented.
3. Wash the precipitate with approximately 2.0 mL digestion buffer twice and pool the resulted supernatants.
4. Stop the enzyme reaction by adjusting the supernatant at room temperature to pH 8.0 with 1 M Tris solution and concentrate by ultrafiltration YM10 membrane.
5. Apply the concentrated material to size exclusion chromatography column (Sepharose 4B or Superose 12) (2 cm × 100 cm) equilibrated with 0.15 M Tris–HCl buffer, pH 7.6 (TB), containing 5.0 mM $CaCl_2$. Run the chromatography procedure at 4 °C.

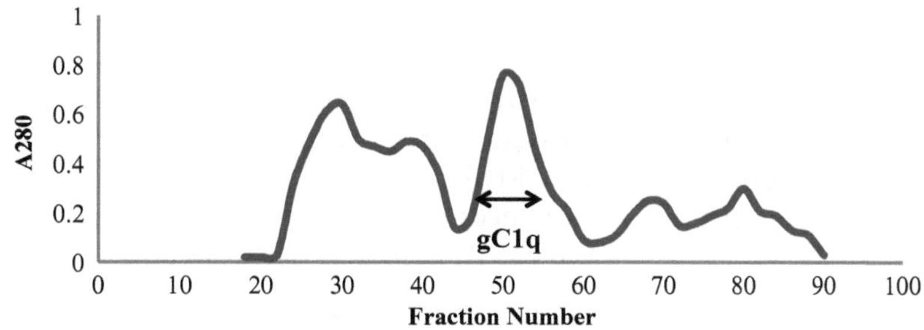

Fig. 3 Size exclusion chromatography on Sephacryl S200 of pepsin digested C1q

6. Elute the protein fraction by the same buffer. CLR is obtain as the protein eluting in the void volume of the column. Store in aliquots at −70 °C. Depending of the purposes of the micro-variant of purification procedure can be used instead of this described above (*see* **Note 11**).

3.5 Isolation of the gC1q Fragment

The gC1q fragment can be obtained by collagenase digestion of the collagen-like fragment of purified C1q [5]. The collagenase and undigested C1q is removed from the incubation mixture by size-exclusion chromatography.

1. Dialyze (10 mg C1q in 2 mL) against 20 mM Tris buffer, pH 7.4, containing 200 mM NaCl and 10 mM $CaCl_2$ at 4 °C.
2. Add collagenase in weight ratio C1q/enzyme 15:1 to the C1q and incubate the mixture by shaking for 16 h at 37 °C.
3. Stop the reaction by adding cold 200 M EDTA (stock solution) to a final concentration 10 mM.
4. Separate the precipitate from the mixture by centrifugation at 10,000 × *g* for 15 min.
5. Equilibrate the Sephacryl S-200 (1 cm × 90 cm) column with 20 mM Tris–HCl buffer, pH 7.4, containing 360 mM NaCI and 10 mM $CaCI_2$.
6. Apply the supernatant on the Sephacryl S-200 and elute the fractions with the same buffer (Fig. 3). For better purification repeat this step. Any residual undigested C1q (observed on SDS-PAGE) can be removed by chromatography on IgG-Sepharose 4B as described above (*see* Subheading 3.2).
7. Concentrate the purified gC1q by ultrafiltration and store at −70 °C.
8. Depending of the purposes of the micro-variant of purification procedure can be used instead of this described above (*see* **Note 11**).

3.6 Preparations of Competent Cells of E. coli BL21 and Transformation with Plasmids pKBM-A, pKBM-B, and pKBM-C

The expression vectors pKBM-A, pKBM-B, and pKBM-C, containing the ghA, ghB, and ghC sequences of C1q chains linked to MBP are used for the transformation of competent *E. coli* BL21 cells and for the expression of the recombinant fusion proteins, ghA-MBP, ghB-MBP, and ghC-MBP. The expressed polypeptide sequences correspond to residues 88–223 of ghA, 90–226 of ghB, and 87–217 of ghC, respectively.

1. Inoculate *E. coli BL21* cells (1: 100 dilution), precultured and shaken overnight at 37 °C in 100 ml of 2xTY medium.
2. Incubate and shake at 37 °C by till A_{600} ~0.9.
3. Then chill the culture on ice, pellet and suspend the cells in half volume of 0.1 M $CaCl_2$, cool on ice for 30 min, and re-pellet and resuspend in 5 mL 0.1 M $CaCl_2$.
4. Store the competent cells at 4 °C or as 100 μL aliquots in 10 % glycerol at −70°C.
5. For transformation mix ~5–10 ng of plasmid DNA with 100 μL of competent cells, incubate for 30 min on ice, spread onto selective agar plates, pre-warmed to 37 °C, and incubate overnight at 37 °C.
6. Store the obtained transformed cells at −70 °C.

3.7 Expression and Purification of Recombinant Globular Fragments of A, B, and C Chains of C1q

1. Grow transformed *E. coli* BL21 cells in 1L Luria-Bertani medium containing ampicillin (100 μg/ml) to A_{600}=0.5 at 37 °C.
2. Induce the cells with 0.4 mM isopropyl β-D-thiogalactoside for 3 h, and centrifuge (3,000×*g*) at 4 °C for 5 min.
3. Suspend the pellet (~2.5 mg) in 50 mL of lysis buffer and incubate over ice for 30 min.
4. Sonicate the cell lysate at 60 Hz for 30 s with an interval of 1 min (15 cycles) to disrupt the cells and shear the bacterial chromosomal DNA.
5. Centrifuge the lysate after sonication (16,000×*g* for 30 min), collect the supernatant and dilute fivefold using buffer I .
6. Apply the diluted supernatant on an amylose resin column (50 mL). Wash the column first with buffer I (150 mL), followed by buffer II.
7. Elute each fusion protein with 100 mL of buffer II containing 10 mM maltose. At this stage of isolation the recombinant fusion proteins ghA-MBP, ghB-MBP, and ghC-MBP contain minor contaminating proteins and DNA.
8. To further remove the contaminants, apply the fusion proteins to a Q-Sepharose ion exchange column. Wash extensively the column with buffer containing 20 mM Tris–HCl, pH 8.0, 100 mM NaCl to remove MBP-bound maltose.
9. Elute the fusion protein using a 0.1–1 M NaCl gradient in 20 mM Tris–HCl, pH 8.0.

10. To examine their oligomeric forms, load each fusion protein individually over a Superose 12 size exclusion chromatography column equilibrated with buffer containing 20 mM Tris–HCl, 100 mM NaCl, and 1 mM EDTA, pH 7.4.
11. In order to obtain ghA, ghB, and ghC from their fusion counterparts ghA-MBP, ghB-MBP, ghC-MBP protein dialyze at 4 °C fusion proteins individually against factor Xa buffer 1 U per 50 μg of the fusion protein. This step allows cleaving MBP form recombinant fusion proteins and isolation of ghA, ghB, and ghC alone.

3.8 Biochemical Analysis

The purity of all preparations (serum derived and recombinant C1q proteins) is checked by electrophoretic analysis, using sodium dodecyl sulfate polyacrylamide gel electrophoresis (SDS-PAGE) performed according to the standard procedure of Laemmli. SDS-PAGE (12 or 15% gel) after silver staining of the purified C1q preparations demonstrates two protein bands, corresponding to A–B and C–C dimers (under nonreducing conditions), and three protein bands, corresponding to the individual A, B, and C chains (under reducing conditions) with MW of 29, 27, and 22 kDa, respectively [6, 9, 10].

The electrophoretic analysis, Western blot (*see* **Note 11**) and/or ELISA are also used for identification of the isolated proteins using antibodies, specific toward C1q, C1q chains, C1q fragments (gC1q and CLR) or the purified recombinant fusion proteins ghA-MBP, ghB-MBP, and ghC-MBP.

3.9 Functional Assays

The functional activity of the whole C1q molecule is usually assessed by a hemolytic assay, which is the most sensitive monitor of its biological activity. This assay demonstrates the ability of purified C1q to play both, the immunoglobulin binding activity and the activation role to form a C1 complex, able to activate the CCP. Under the experimental conditions used, the functional activity is demonstrated by the amount of released hemoglobin detected at OD_{414}. The method presented here is based on a procedure described in ref. 11 with slight modifications. The functional activity of the recombinant globular fragments of the individual C1q chains is detected by analysis of their ability to inhibit C1q-dependent hemolysis. The ligand-binding activity of C1q, attributed mostly to the gC1q fragment, is more often tested by ELISA. Here the ligand-binding activity of C1q fragments or recombinant derivatives is estimated by using human aggregated IgG as a typical C1q ligand.

3.9.1 C1q Hemolytic Assay

1. Incubate EA, diluted in $DVBS^{++}$ (50 μL 2 %) in wells of a microtiter plate with 50 μL C1qD (C1q depleted serum), diluted 1/10 in the same buffer and 50 μL of the test fractions, containing purified C1q or its derivatives (properly diluted in $DVBS^{++}$) for 30 min at 37 °C.

2. Spin, and read the absorbance of the supernatant at 414 nm.
3. Run in parallel the sample with normal human serum (standard serum) as a positive control, a sample containing EA incubated with buffer only as a negative control and a sample containing EA incubated with water only. Total hemolysis is assessed as the amount of hemoglobin released upon cell lysis with water. The C1q-dependent hemolytic activity is expressed as a percentage of total hemolysis.

3.9.2 Inhibition of Hemolysis

1. To detect of the inhibitory potential of C1q, dilute C1qD (*see* Subheading 3.7, **step 1**) 1:40 in $DGVB^{++}$ and add various concentrations of purified C1q to a final volume of 100 μL.
2. Incubate the mixture at 37 °C for 1 h.
3. Add 100 μL of EA_{IgG} (10^7 cells) in $DGVB^{++}$ and incubate for another hour.
4. Stop the reaction by transferring the tubes to an ice-bath and add 0.6 ml of ice cold $DGVB^{++}$.
5. Pellet the unlysed cells by centrifugation and measure the A_{414} values of 100 μL aliquots of the supernatant to monitor hemoglobin release.
6. For the detection of the inhibitory potential of the recombinant C1q-fragments, incubate 100 μL of the appropriate dilutions of recombinant proteins (MBP-ghA, or MBP-ghB, or MBP-ghC, respectively) with 100 μL EA_{IgG} (10^7 cells) in $DGVB^{++}$ for 1 h.
7. Pellet the pretreated cells gently by centrifugation at 3,000 × *g* for 2 min, wash and resuspend in 100 μL of $DGVB^{++}$.
8. Add each aliquot of EA_{IgG} to a mixture, composed of 1 μg of C1q in 10, 2.5 μL of C1qD (*see* Subheading 2.9, **step 1**) and 87.5 μL of $DGVB^{++}$ and incubate another hour at 37 °C.
9. Pellet the unlysed cells and estimate the amount of released hemoglobin spectrophotometrically from the A_{414} of the supernatant. Total hemolysis is assessed as the amount of hemoglobin released upon cell lysis with water. Express the C1q-dependent hemolytic activity as a percentage of total hemolysis.

3.9.3 ELISA for the Detection of the Interaction of C1q (or C1q Fragments) with Human Aggregated IgG

1. Incubate human IgG (20 mg/mL) at 63 °C for 30 min for obtaining heat-aggregated IgG.
2. Coat different concentrations of C1q (0–1 μg/mL), recombinant fusion C1q-proteins (MBP-ghA, MBP-ghB, or MBP-ghC) (0–3 μg/mL) and MBP alone in sodium carbonate buffer, pH 9.6, on to wells of polysorb ELISA plates and leave overnight at 4 °C.

3. Block the wells with 2 % (w/v) BSA for 2 h and wash.
4. Add 10 μg/mL of HAIgG in TBS-NTC buffer to the plates and incubate at 21 °C for 2 h.
5. Wash the wells and add goat antihuman IgG conjugated to peroxidase.
6. Incubate for 1 h at 37 °C, and wash the microtiter wells three times.
7. Add 100 μL of 3,3′,5,5′-tetramethylbenzidine (TMB) in aqueous dimethylformamide mixed with one-tenth volume of hydrogen peroxide added to each well.
8. Incubate the plates for 20 min at room temperature.
9. Stop the reaction by adding 150 μL of 1 M H_2SO_4 to each well and read the absorbance at 450 nm.

4 Notes

1. The purified preparations of C1q can be concentrated by ammonium sulfate precipitation at 33 % saturation. This method avoids the loss of material that occurs upon concentration of C1q by ultrafiltration.
2. During the purification procedure, particularly at the first step of purification when plasma enzymes are present as well as during the storage of plasma/serum, protease inhibitors should be included. The widely used protease inhibitors are NPGB (*p*-nitro phenyl *p*′-guanidinobenzoate) dissolved as a 100× concentrated stock solution (100 mM) in dimethyl formamide (DMF) and phenyl methyl sulfonyl fluoride (PMSF), dissolved as a 100× stock solution (100 mM) in isopropanol. The two inhibitors are used at a final concentration of 0.1 mM. The protease inhibitors are toxic to varying degrees and should be handled with caution. EDTA in buffers also serves as an inhibitor of the activation of Ca^{2+}- and Mg^{2+}-dependent metalloproteases in the serum/plasma. It has to be kept in mind that the addition of EDTA will induce the dissociation of Ca^{2+}- and Mg^{2+}-dependent multimolecular complex C1 and also inhibits Ca^{2+}-dependent collagenase, used for limited hydrolysis of C1q.
3. When C1q is purified by affinity chromatography on IgG-Sepharose 4B, better results are obtained by preparing the column matrix containing 30 (or even more) mg IgG/mL Sepharose. Solve human IgG in 0.1 M $NaHCO_3$ and 0.5 M NaCl to a final concentration 30 or 40 mg/mL and dialyze against the same buffer overnight at 4 °C. Then incubate IgG with CNBr-activated Sepharose 4B according to the manufacturer's instructions.

4. The cDNA encoding the globular fragments of the individual A, B, and C chains of C1q may be purchased from the IMAGE libraries and recloned into pMAL-c2expression vector, which contains maltose-binding protein (MBP) under the Ptac promoter.

   The following primers are used to PCR-amplify the DNA sequences corresponding to ghA, ghB, and ghC:

   ghA forward primer (FP) 5-GCCCGAGGCCTAAGGACCAGCCGAGGC-3 and

   ghA reverse primer (RP) 5-GCCCGGCTGCAGCTAGGCAGATGGGAAGATG-3;

   ghB FP 5-GCCCGGAGGCCTAAGGCCACCCAGAAAT C-3 and

   ghB RP 5-GCCCGGCTGCAGCTAGGCCTCCATATCTGG-3;

   ghC FP 5-GCCCGGAGGCCTAAGCAGAAATTCCAGTC-3 and

   ghC RP 5-GCCCGGCTGCAGCTAGTCGGGGAAGAGCAG-3.

   This includes also the last Gly-Xaa-Yaa triplet of the C1q collagen-like region.

5. Human aggregated IgG (HAIgG) is often used for the detection of the IgG-binding property of C1q and its derivatives (serum derived and recombinant). HAIgG can be prepared by incubation of human IgG (20 mg/mL) solution in PBS at 63 °C for 30 min and then the soluble fractions are used.

6. In cases when the purification procedure of C1q aims to purify all the components of C1 (C1q, C1r, and C1s) from a single batch, the starting material is a recalcified human plasma. The C1 complex can be isolated by affinity chromatography on IgG-Sepharose 4B, then C1 components can be separated from one another by FPLC on Mono Q by using the elution with linear (0–1 M) NaCl gradient. C1r elutes before C1s. C1q which remains bound to the column matrix is eluted with high ionic strength (1 M NaCl). For detailed information, concerning the purification of C1r and C1s see Chapter 2.

7. When obtaining of biochemically pure C1q is required and is more important than the yield, it is best to pool fractions tightly, discarding fractions on the edges of the protein peak which may contain contaminants.

8. The trace amounts of contaminants (more often IgG) in the purified C1q preparation can be additionally removed by specific clean-up steps by affinity chromatography (e.g., chromatography on protein-A or protein-G columns, or IgG-Sepharose 4B).

9. The repeated freezing and thawing of C1q preparations (especially at neutral pH) leads to the irreversible denaturation of the

protein. For better storing of the purified C1q it is advisable to keep C1q in acidic buffers containing 0.25 M NaCl, pH 5.3 at −70 °C, or in buffers which do not freeze under the storage conditions (e.g., PBS, pH 7.2 in 30 % ethylene glycol at −20 to −70 °C or C1q in 50 mM NaCl, containing 40 % glycerol).

10. If the micro-variant [12] for the isolation of CLR is more suitable for the laboratory purposes use 200 μg of C1q, instead of 2 mg/mL and dialyze it against sodium acetate buffer, pH 4.45, add 14 μg pepsin and incubate for 20 h at 37 °C. Then centrifuge the digest for 20 min at 35,000 × *g* and apply the supernatant on a size exclusion column (Superdex 200 10/300 GL). Use FPLC for the separation of CLR.

    If the micro-variant for isolation of gC1q is preferable, incubate 200 μg of C1q with 800 μg collagenase (Sigma-Aldrich) for 16 h at 37 °C and centrifuge at 14,000 × *g* for 10 min at 4 °C. Then apply the incubation mixture on Superdex 200 10/300 GL and separate by FPLC the C1q from the collagenase and the undigested C1q. The assessment of the concentration of the obtained CLR and gC1q can be performed by NanoDrop 1000 spectrophotometer at OD_{280}nm and the degree of purity of both protein preparations can be confirmed by SDS-PAGE (12 % gel) followed by silver staining.

11. In addition to the electrophoretic analysis Western blot of the C1q or C1q derivatives can be successfully used for the identification of purified proteins, isolated according to the methods described above. Briefly, the protein of interest (e.g., C1q, 1–2 μg) is fractionated by SDS-PAGE under reducing conditions (with DTT) on a 15 % (w/v) gel, then electrotransfered to polyvinyl difluoride transfer membrane, blocked with 2 % (w/v) BSA, and probed with rabbit IgG antibodies with appropriate specificity (antihuman C1q, antihuman C1q chains, anti-C1q-fragments, or recombinant derivatives). Then the membrane is incubated with a goat anti-rabbit IgG-alkaline phosphatase conjugate. The blot is developed using the substrates, *p*-nitroblue tetrazolium chloride and 5-bromo-4-chloro-3-indolyl phosphate. BSA and other non-related to C1q proteins are used negative control proteins.

References

1. Kojouharova M, Reid K, Gadjeva M (2010) New insights into the molecular mechanisms of classical complement activation. Mol Immunol 47:2154–2160
2. Nayak A, Pednekar L, Reid KB, Kishore U (2012) Complement and non-complement activating functions of C1q: a prototypical innate immune molecule. Innate Immun 18: 350–363
3. Reid KB (1982) C1q. Methods Enzymol 82(Pt A):319–324
4. Reid KB, Porter RR (1976) Subunit composition and structure of subcomponent C1q of the first component of human complement. Biochem J 155:19–23
5. Hughes-Jones NC, Gardner B (1979) Reaction between the isolated globular sub-units of the

complement component C1q and IgG-complexes. Mol Immunol 16:697–701
6. Kojouharova MS, Gadjeva MG, Tsacheva IG, Zlatarova A, Roumenina LT, Tchorbadjieva MI, Atanasov BP, Waters P, Urban BC, Sim RB, Reid KB, Kishore U (2004) Mutational analyses of the recombinant globular regions of human C1q A, B, and C chains suggest an essential role for arginine and histidine residues in the C1q-IgG interaction. J Immunol 172:4351–4358
7. Tenner AJ, Lesavre PH, Cooper NR (1981) Purification and radiolabeling of human C1q. J Immunol 127:648–653
8. Stemmer F, Loos M (1984) Purification and characterization of human, guinea pig and mouse C1q by fast protein liquid chromatography (FPLC). J Immunol Methods 74:9–16
9. Kishore U, Gupta SK, Perdikoulis MV, Kojouharova MS, Urban BC, Reid KB (2003) Modular organization of the carboxyl-terminal, globular head region of human C1q A, B, and C chains. J Immunol 171:812–820
10. Kojouharova MS, Panchev ID, Tchorbadjieva MI, Reid KB, Hoppe HJ (1998) Differential binding of IgG and of a HIV gp41 peptide by the B chain and A chain globular head sequences of C1q, respectively. J Immunol 161:4325–4331
11. Berg V (2009) Purification of complement components, regulators, and receptors by classical methods. Methods Mol Biol 150: 15–52
12. Schaller M, Bigler C, Danner D, Ditzel HJ, Trendelenburg M (2009) Autoantibodies against C1q in systemic lupus erythematosus are antigen-driven. J Immunol 183: 8225–8231

Chapter 4

Classical Complement Pathway Components C1r and C1s: Purification from Human Serum and in Recombinant Form and Functional Characterization

Véronique Rossi, Isabelle Bally, Monique Lacroix, Gérard J. Arlaud, and Nicole M. Thielens

Abstract

C1r and C1s are the proteases responsible for the activation and proteolytic activity of the C1 complex of the classical complement pathway, respectively. They are assembled into a Ca^{2+}-dependent C1s–C1r–C1r–C1s tetramer which in turn associates with the recognition protein C1q. The C1 complex circulates in serum as a zymogen and is activated upon binding of C1q to appropriate targets, such as antigen–antibody complexes. This property is used for the purification of C1r and C1s from human serum after binding of C1 to insoluble immune complexes. Disruption of the bound C1 complex by EDTA releases C1r and C1s which are further separated by ion-exchange chromatography; both proteins can be reassembled in the presence of calcium ions and the reconstituted tetramer isolated by gel filtration. In this chapter, we describe the purification of the activated and proenzyme forms of C1r and C1s and of the proenzyme C1s–C1r–C1r–C1s tetramer as well as methods for their biochemical and functional characterization. The production of recombinant C1s and of the proenzyme tetramer in a baculovirus–insect cell system, and their purification by affinity chromatography is also presented.

Key words Complement protease, C1r, C1s, Purification, Activation, Enzymatic activity, C1 reconstitution

1 Introduction

The first component of the classical complement pathway, C1, is a multimolecular protease assembled from two functional entities, the recognition protein C1q and the catalytic subunit C1s–C1r–C1r–C1s, a Ca^{2+}-dependent tetrameric complex of two homologous serine protease zymogens, C1r and C1s. Binding of C1q to suitable targets (pathogenic microorganisms, immune complexes) triggers self-activation of proenzyme C1r to its activated form which in turn activates C1s. Activated C1s then cleaves complement components C2 and C4, thereby initiating the complement proteolytic cascade. Activation of C1r and C1s occurs through

Mihaela Gadjeva (ed.), *The Complement System: Methods and Protocols*, Methods in Molecular Biology, vol. 1100, DOI 10.1007/978-1-62703-724-2_4, © Springer Science+Business Media New York 2014

cleavage of a single Arg-Ile bond, resulting in the conversion of both single-chain proenzymes into active proteases comprising two disulfide-linked chains [1, 2]. The C-terminal B-chain corresponds to the serine protease domain, whereas the N-terminal A chain comprises two CUB modules, initially identified in C1r/C1s, sea urchin epidermal growth factor (EGF), and bone morphogenetic protein; an EGF-like module; and two complement control protein (CCP) modules. The three N-terminal CUB–EGF–CUB modules constitute the interaction region responsible for Ca^{2+}-dependent interaction between C1r and C1s and association of the tetramer with C1q. The catalytic domains encompass the two adjacent CCP modules and the B-chain and, in the case of C1r, associate as stable non-covalent dimers that form the core of the C1s–C1r–C1r–C1s tetramer. Each of the interaction regions of C1r is engaged in a Ca^{2+}-dependent interaction with the corresponding region of a C1s molecule, the catalytic domains of C1s being located at both extremities of the tetramer. In the absence of C1r, isolated C1s forms a Ca^{2+}-dependent homodimer through association of its interaction regions.

This chapter describes the purification of the activated and proenzyme forms of both C1r and C1s from serum as well as the purification of the proenzyme C1s–C1r–C1r–C1s tetramer based on the affinity of the C1 complex for insoluble antigen–antibody complexes [3]. Both proteases are selectively released from bound C1 and further separated by anion-exchange chromatography or can be reassembled to purify the tetramer by size-exclusion chromatography. The production of recombinant C1r, C1s, and the tetramer stabilized in a proenzyme form using a baculovirus/insect cell system are also presented as well as their purification from the culture supernatants, based on affinity chromatography. We also describe assays to test the functionality of the purified proteins, based on their enzymatic activity or on activation of the reconstituted C1 complex [4].

2 Materials

2.1 Preparation of Insoluble IgG–Ovalbumin Complexes

1. Rabbit antiserum against ovalbumin from chicken egg white (Sigma).
2. Anhydrous Na_2SO_4.
3. Immune complex (IC) buffer: 20 mM Tris–HCl, 150 mM NaCl, pH 7.0.
4. 0.1 N NaOH.
5. 10 % (w/v) sodium azide (NaN_3) (*see* **Note 1**).
6. Centrifuge (Beckman Coulter); polycarbonate centrifuge bottles (50, 250, and 500 mL).

2.2 Purification from Human Serum of C1r, C1s, and the C1s–C1r–C1r–C1s Tetramer

1. Pooled human citrated plasma.
2. 1 M $CaCl_2$ standard solution (Fluka).
3. 0.4 M EDTA, pH 7.8 (*see* **Note 2**).
4. Protease inhibitor stock solutions: 25 mg/mL soybean trypsin inhibitor (SBTI) (Sigma) in H_2O; 0.5 M diisopropylfluorophosphate (DFP) (Sigma) in isopropyl alcohol (*see* **Note 3**); 0.1 M 4-nitrophenyl-4′-guanidinobenzoate (NPGB) (Sigma) in dimethylformamide (DMF) (*see* **Note 4**).
5. Pre-swollen diethylaminoethyl cellulose (DE52) resin (Whatman).
6. Econo-column Bio-Rad (2.5 × 20 cm).
7. CNBr-activated Sepharose 4B (GE Healthcare).
8. Rabbit antiserum against C1r.
9. Protein purification system for size-exclusion chromatography (Bio-Rad).
10. Superose 12 10/300 GL column (GE Healthcare).
11. IC washing buffer: 20 mM Tris–HCl, 120 mM NaCl, 5 mM $CaCl_2$, pH 7.0.
12. Extraction buffer for activated C1r and C1s: 50 mM Tris–HCl, 60 mM NaCl, 20 mM EDTA, pH 7.0.
13. Extraction buffer for proenzyme C1r and C1s: 40 mM Tris–HCl, 56 mM EDTA, pH 7.0.
14. C1q extraction buffer: 50 mM Tris–HCl, 700 mM NaCl, pH 10.0.
15. DE 52 equilibration buffer: 20 mM sodium phosphate, 5 mM EDTA, pH 7.4 (activated C1r and C1s) or pH 6.1 (proenzyme C1r and C1s).
16. DE 52 gradient buffer: 20 mM sodium phosphate, 250 mM NaCl, 5 mM EDTA, pH 7.4 (activated C1r and C1s) or pH 6.1 (proenzyme C1r and C1s).
17. C1r and C1s storage buffer: 50 mM triethanolamine-HCl, 145 mM NaCl, pH 7.4.
18. 1 M propionic acid.
19. Superose 12 equilibration buffer and tetramer storage buffer: 50 mM triethanolamine-HCl, 145 mM NaCl, 2.5 mM $CaCl_2$, pH 7.4.
20. Protein concentration: Amicon® Ultra-4 and -15 centrifugal filters (30 K) and Amicon® stirred ultrafiltration cells (10 and 50 mL) with YM 30 disc membranes (Millipore).

2.3 Recombinant Protein Expression in Baculovirus-Infected Insect Cells

1. C1r and C1s plasmid expression vectors (*see* **Note 5**).
2. Bac-to-Bac® baculovirus expression system (Life Technologies™) (*see* **Note 6**).
3. LB agar (Miller or Lennox) and LB medium broth.

4. Antibiotics (stock concentrations in sterile H_2O unless otherwise stated): 100 mg/mL ampicillin, 50 mg/mL kanamycin, 50 mg/mL gentamycin, 5 mg/mL tetracycline (in 50 % (v/v) ethanol), 200 mg/mL isopropyl-thio-β-galactopyranoside (IPTG), 100 mg/mL Bluo-gal (Life Technologies™) (in DMF).
5. pUC/M13 forward and pUC/M13 reverse primers, PCR master mix 2× (Promega).
6. HiSpeed Plasmid Midi Kit (Qiagen).
7. Insect cells (serum-free medium (SFM)-adapted Sf9 cells, High Five™ cells) (Life Technologies™).
8. Cell culture medium: Sf-900 II SFM, TC-100 insect medium, heat-inactivated fetal bovine serum (FBS), penicillin–streptomycin (Life Technologies™) (*see* **Note 7**).
9. C1s- and C1q-Sepharose equilibration buffer: 50 mM triethanolamine-HCl, 145 mM NaCl, 2 mM $CaCl_2$, pH 7.4.
10. C1s- and C1q-Sepharose elution buffer: 50 mM triethanolamine-HCl, 145 mM NaCl, 5 mM EDTA, pH 7.4.

2.4 Protein Analysis by Sodium Dodecyl Sulfate-Polyacrylamide Gel Electrophoresis and Western Blot

1. Unreduced sample preparation buffer: 8 M urea, 2 % (w/v) sodium dodecyl sulfate (SDS), 0.2 M Tris–HCl, pH 8.0 containing 20 mM iodoacetamide (Sigma).
2. Reduced sample preparation buffer: 8 M urea, 2 % (w/v) SDS, 0.2 M Tris–HCl, pH 8.0 containing 100 mM dithiothreitol (Sigma).
3. SDS-polyacrylamide separation gel: 10 or 12.5 % (w/v) acrylamide/bis-acrylamide (37.1:1 ratio), 0.375 M Tris–HCl, pH 8.8, 0.1 % (w/v) SDS, 0.025 % (w/v) ammonium persulfate, 0.2 % (v/v) *N,N,N′,N′*-tetramethyl-ethylenediamine (TEMED).
4. SDS-polyacrylamide stacking gel: 3 % (w/v) acrylamide/bis-acrylamide (37.1:1 ratio), 0.125 M Tris–HCl, pH 6.8, 0.1 % (w/v) SDS, 0.04 % (w/v) ammonium persulfate, 0.4 % (v/v) TEMED.
5. Running buffer: 25 mM Tris–HCl, 192 mM glycine, 0.1 % (w/v) SDS.
6. InstantBlue stain (Expedeon).
7. SDS-polyacrylamide gel electrophoresis (PAGE) molecular standards (pre-stained protein ladder, Euromedex).
8. LMW-SDS marker kit (GE Healthcare), for preparation of unreduced and reduced protein standards.
9. Transfer membranes (Protran® BA85 nitrocellulose membranes, Whatman).
10. Transfer buffer: 25 mM Tris–HCl, 192 mM glycine, 20 % (v/v) ethanol.

11. Tris-buffered saline (TBS): 10 mM Tris–HCl, 200 mM NaCl, pH 7.2.
12. Blocking solution: 5 % (w/v) skimmed milk in TBS.
13. TBS-T: TBS containing 0.05 % (w/v) Tween-20.
14. 1-Step™ NBT/BCIP (Thermoscientific).
15. Rabbit polyclonal anti-C1s antibody.
16. Goat anti-rabbit IgG, alkaline phosphatase conjugate (Sigma).

2.5 Esterolytic Assays

1. UV/visible thermostated spectrophotometer.
2. N-acetylglycine-L-lysine methyl ester (AGLMe) (Sigma).
3. 100 mM K_2PO_4, pH 7.5.
4. Alcohol oxidase (AO) from *Pichia pastoris* (Sigma).
5. Horseradish peroxidase (HRP) type VI (Sigma).
6. 2,2′-Azino-bis(3-ethylbenzothiazoline-6-sulfonic acid) (ABTS) (Sigma).
7. N_α-benzoyl-L-arginine ethyl ester hydrochloride (BAEe) (Sigma).
8. BAEe buffer: 25 mM Tris, 75 mM tetrasodium diphosphate, 300 mM semicarbazide dihydrochloride, 50 mM glycine, pH 8.5.
9. L-glutathione, reduced (Sigma).
10. β-nicotinamide adenine dinucleotide hydrate (NAD).
11. Alcohol dehydrogenase (ADH) from yeast, ≥300 U/mg protein (Sigma) solution: 30 mg/mL in 0.1 % (w/v) bovine serum albumin (BSA).

3 Methods

3.1 Preparation of Insoluble Immune Complexes

3.1.1 Immunoglobulin Purification

1. Centrifuge the immune serum (volume V) at 16,000 × *g* for 15 min at 25 °C.
2. Add 16 % (w/v) Na_2SO_4 and, after complete dissolution, incubate for 1 h at 37 °C.
3. Centrifuge at 5,000 × *g* for 10 min at 25 °C.
4. Discard the supernatant, and dissolve the pellet in preheated distilled water (final volume: V) (*see* **Note 8**).
5. Repeat **steps 2–4** twice, and dissolve the third pellet in the IC buffer (final volume: V).
6. Dialyze the solution extensively (three changes) against the IC buffer.
7. Measure the absorbance at 280 nm (A_{280}) of a 1/30 dilution of the immunoglobulin (IgG) solution (the A_{280} of a 1 mg/mL solution is 1.40). A concentration close to 10 mg/mL is expected.

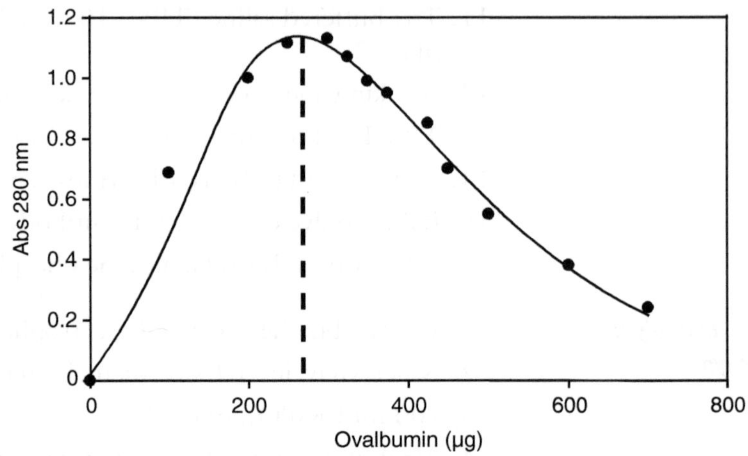

Fig. 1 Precipitation curve of anti-ovalbumin antibodies. Fixed amounts of Igs were incubated with increasing amounts of ovalbumin and the resulting insoluble immune complexes measured as indicated in Subheading 3.1.2. The plot of A_{280} versus the ovalbumin amount gives the equivalence point (amount of antigen yielding the maximal A_{280})

3.1.2 Titration of Anti-ovalbumin Antibodies

1. Mix fixed amounts of IgG (4 mg in 2 mL of IC buffer) with increasing amounts of ovalbumin (0.1–0.7 mg in 1 mL of IC buffer); incubate for 1 h at 37 °C and then overnight at 4 °C.
2. Centrifuge the ICs at 1,500 × *g* for 10 min at 4 °C to eliminate nonspecific IgGs.
3. Discard the supernatant, and suspend the ICs in 2 mL of the IC buffer.
4. Repeat **steps 2** and **3** three times, and dissolve the pellet in 2.5 mL of 0.1 N NaOH (*see* **Note 9**).
5. Measure the A_{280} values of the samples and plot them versus the ovalbumin quantity. A bell-shaped precipitation curve is obtained, allowing determination of the equivalence point (amount of antigen yielding the maximal A_{280} value) (Fig. 1).

3.1.3 Preparation of ICs at Equivalence

1. Add the appropriate amount of ovalbumin (from a 10 mg/mL stock solution in the IC buffer) to the IgG solution (volume V); incubate for 1 h at 37 °C and then overnight at 4 °C.
2. Centrifuge the ICs at 7,500 × *g* for 15 min at 4 °C, discard the supernatant, and suspend the ICs in the IC buffer (volume V).
3. Repeat **step 2** three times, and suspend the last pellet in the same volume of the IC buffer.
4. Calculate the concentration of the IC suspension by measuring the A_{280} of a 1/30 dilution in 0.1 N NaOH (a 1 mg/mL solution has an A_{280} of 1.30).
5. Adjust the IC concentration to 10 mg/mL and store at 4 °C in the presence of 0.1 % (w/v) NaN_3. The ICs are very stable and can be stored for a few years under these conditions.

3.2 Purification of Activated C1r and C1s from Human Serum

3.2.1 Blood Serum Preparation

1. Add 1 M $CaCl_2$ to human pooled citrated plasma to a final concentration of 20 mM.
2. Allow plasma to clot for 4 h at room temperature and then overnight at 4 °C.
3. Fragment the fibrin clot into small pieces and remove it by centrifugation at 16,000 × *g* for 20 min at 4 °C followed by filtration through muslin.
4. Store at –80 °C until use.

3.2.2 Binding of C1 to Immune Complexes and Extraction of Activated C1r and C1s

Unless otherwise stated, all steps are performed at 4 °C, and centrifugation conditions are 10,000 × *g* for 8 min.

1. Thaw 1 L (*see* **Note 10**) of serum and centrifuge at 12,500 × *g* for 15 min.
2. Add SBTI (50 μg/mL), and adjust the pH to 7.0.
3. Suspend 1 g of ICs (100 mL) in the serum and incubate for 45 min with occasional shaking.
4. Centrifuge and then re-suspend the ICs in 200 mL of washing buffer containing 40 μg/mL SBTI. Repeat this step twice, and suspend the ICs in 150 mL of washing buffer (*see* **Note 11**).
5. Incubate the suspension for 35 min at 30 °C to achieve full activation of the IC-bound C1 complex. Cool on ice, and centrifuge.
6. Suspend the pellet in 50 mL of the C1r/C1s extraction buffer, centrifuge, and collect the supernatant. Repeat this step twice.

3.2.3 Isolation of C1r and C1s

1. Centrifuge the extracts at 25,000 × *g* for 20 min and dialyze overnight against 2 L of the DE52 equilibration buffer.
2. Load the dialyzed extract at 45 mL/h onto a DE 52 column (50 mL) equilibrated in the same buffer (*see* **Note 12**). Wash with 150 mL of the equilibration buffer.
3. Elute the bound proteins with a linear NaCl gradient to 250 mM (2 × 350 mL).
4. Pool the C1r-containing fractions (shown in a typical elution profile in Fig. 2), dialyze against 2 × 1 L of storage buffer, and concentrate by ultrafiltration to about 0.5 mg/mL. Store purified C1r (6–8 mg) at 4 °C (*see* **Note 13**).
5. The C1s-containing fractions (Fig. 2) are contaminated by trace amounts of C1r (up to 5 %) that can be eliminated by chromatography on a column of anti-C1r IgG-Sepharose 4B (obtained by coupling 25 mg of anti-C1r IgGs (purified from rabbit immune serum as described in Subheading 3.1) to 15 mL of CNBr-activated Sepharose according to the supplier's instructions). Dialyze the C1s pool against 2 L of the C1s storage buffer, apply at 20 mL/h to the anti-C1r IgG-Sepharose

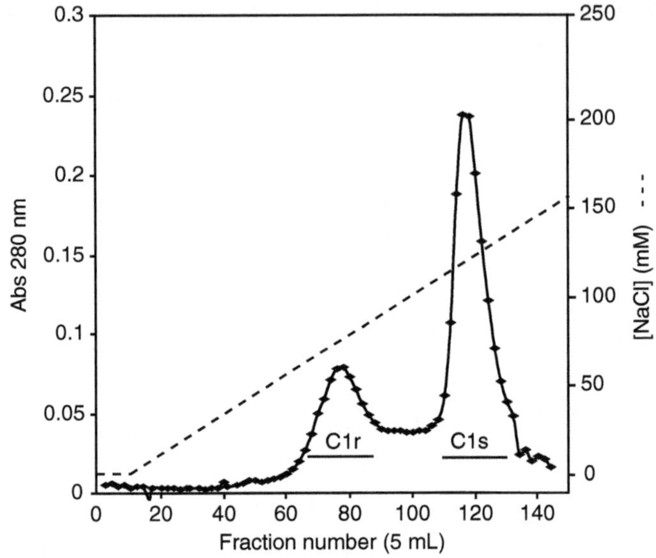

Fig. 2 Separation of activated C1r and C1s by anion-exchange chromatography. The dialyzed EDTA extract obtained from 2 L of serum was applied to the DE52 column, and C1r and C1s were eluted by a linear NaCl gradient (*see* Subheading 3.2.3). Fractions (5 mL) containing C1r and C1s were pooled as indicated

column equilibrated in the same buffer, and collect the flow-through fractions.

6. Concentrate the C1s pool to 1 mg/mL by ultrafiltration, and store purified C1s (6.5–8.5 mg) at −20 °C.

3.2.4 Recycling of the ICs

Extraction of C1r and C1s with EDTA leaves C1q bound to the ICs. The following steps (performed at 4 °C and using the centrifugation conditions described in Subheading 3.2.2) allow C1q to be removed.

1. Suspend the IC pellet (obtained in **step 5** of subheading 3.2.2) in 50 mL of the C1q extraction buffer, centrifuge, and collect the supernatant. Repeat this step twice. C1q can be further purified from the pooled supernatants by cation-exchange chromatography [3].
2. The pellet is washed once with 100 mL of the IC buffer, suspended in 100 mL of the same buffer, and incubated for 30 min at 30 °C in the presence of 5 mM DFP (*see* **Note 2**).
3. The ICs are washed twice in the IC buffer, and their concentration is adjusted to 10 mg/mL (by measuring the A_{280} of a 1/30 dilution in 0.1 N NaOH as described in **step 5** of Subheading 3.1.2). These ICs are stored at 4 °C in the presence of 0.1 % NaN_3 and can then be used for a new purification after reconstitution of the initial amount using fresh ICs.

3.3 Purification of Proenzyme C1r and C1s from Serum

Purification of the proenzyme forms of C1r and C1s is achieved as described for their activated forms (*see* Subheading 3.2), except that all steps are performed as close to 0 °C as possible and that the following modifications are introduced to prevent activation. The serine protease inhibitors DFP and NPGB should be added in the buffers extemporarily.

1. Fresh ICs (1 g) are incubated for 30 min at 30 °C in the presence of 2 mM DFP and washed once in the IC buffer prior to use.
2. The pH of the thawed serum is adjusted to 7.0 without adding SBTI.
3. The serum is preincubated in the presence of 1 mM DFP and 1 mM NPGB for 15 min at 0 °C before addition of the ICs, and the suspension is then incubated for 25 min only.
4. The three washes of the ICs before C1r/C1s extraction are performed in the presence of 1 mM DFP and 1 mM NPGB.
5. Four extraction steps (instead of two) using the proenzyme C1r/C1s extraction buffer containing 5 mM DFP and 1 mM NPGB are used to solubilize the proteases.
6. The EDTA extracts are dialyzed against the DE 52 equilibration buffer in the presence of 1 mM DFP and 0.1 mM NPGB. The ion-exchange chromatography step on DE 52 is performed in the presence of 1 mM DFP at pH 6.1, which helps prevent activation of the proteases [5].
7. The final affinity purification of proenzyme C1s on anti-C1r IgG-Sepharose is performed in the presence of 1 mM DFP.
8. After C1r/C1s extraction, the ICs are suspended in 200 mL of ICs buffer, incubated for 30 min at 30 °C, and centrifuged; this step is repeated two more times before extraction of C1q (*see* **Note 14**).
9. The ICs are washed and stored as described in Subheading 3.2.4. A yellow color may develop upon storage due to hydrolysis of residual NPGB. It will be removed upon pretreatment of the ICs with DFP before starting a new purification of proenzyme C1r and C1s.

3.4 Purification of the Proenzyme C1s–C1r–C1r–C1s Tetramer from Serum

1. Binding of the proenzyme C1 complex to the ICs, extraction of proenzyme C1r and C1s, and recycling of the ICs are performed essentially as described in Subheading 3.3. We usually start from 500 mL of serum instead of 1 L and adjust the amounts of ICs and the volumes of the washing and extraction buffers accordingly.
2. Dialyze the C1r/C1s extracts extensively against the Superose 12 equilibration buffer to reconstitute the tetramer by replacing EDTA by $CaCl_2$. Four dialysis batches are used, the first

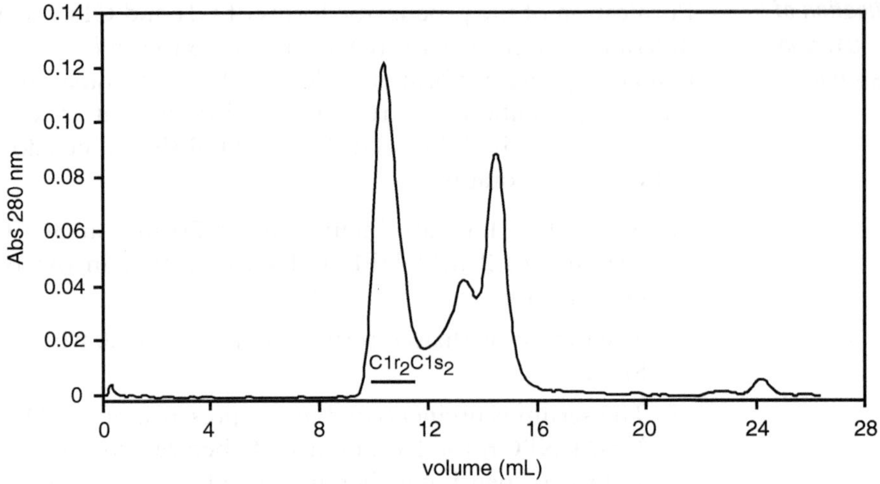

Fig. 3 Separation of the proenzyme C1s–C1r–C1r–C1s tetramer by size-exclusion chromatography. 0.5 mL of the dialyzed EDTA extract obtained from 0.5 L of serum was applied to the Superose 12 column (*see* Subheading 3.4), and fractions (1 mL) containing the tetramer were pooled as indicated

two containing 0.5 mM DFP and 0.1 mM NPGB and the last two containing 0.25 mM DFP and no NPGB.

3. Concentrate the dialyzed extracts to about 5 mL in the presence of 1 mM DFP.
4. Apply 0.5 mL fractions to the Sepharose 12 column equilibrated in the dialysis buffer at a flow rate of 30 mL/h.
5. Pool the fractions containing the tetramer (shown in a typical run profile in Fig. 3) from the different runs. Concentrate by ultrafiltration to about 1 mg/mL, and store the purified tetramer (2–4 mg) at 0 °C in the presence of 1 mM DFP.

3.5 Production and Purification of Recombinant C1s

Recombinant full-length C1r and C1s are expressed in baculovirus-infected insect cells [6–9]. We use the Bac-to-Bac™ system from Life Technologies to generate recombinant baculoviruses. This method is based on site-specific transposition of an expression cassette (contained in a donor plasmid) into a baculovirus shuttle vector (bacmid) propagated in *Escherichia coli* DH10Bac™. The isolated recombinant bacmid is then transfected into insect cells to generate recombinant baculovirus particles that are amplified and used to infect insect cells for protein expression (see user manual for more details).

We use Sf9 cells in Sf900-II serum-free medium for transfection and virus amplification and High Five™ cells cultivated in TC100 medium supplemented with 10 % FBS for recombinant protein production. Details are provided below in case of differences with the manufacturer's protocol.

3.5.1 Production of the Recombinant Baculovirus and Infection of Insect Cells

1. Clone the cDNA encoding full-length C1s into the multiple cloning site of the pFast-Bac™1 donor plasmid. The presence of the native signal peptide will result in secretion of the recombinant protein in the insect cell culture supernatant.
2. Transform DH10Bac™ cells with the pFast-Bac1-C1s plasmid, and select colonies containing the recombinant bacmid. You will need LB (Miller) agar plates containing 50 μg/mL kanamycin, 7 μg/mL gentamicin, 10 μg/mL tetracycline, 300 μg/mL Bluo-gal, and 40 μg/mL IPTG for selection of DH10Bac™ transformants. Positive clones have a white phenotype when re-streaked on the agar plates and should be sensitive to ampicillin. However, we usually analyze the recombinant bacmid DNA by PCR, which can be done directly on colonies (dispersed in H_2O using a sterile Eppendorf tip). The expected PCR fragment size using pUC/M13 forward and reverse primers is 2,300 bp + the size of the C1s insert (2,067 bp). The bacmid alone yields a PCR fragment of 300 bp.
3. Purify recombinant bacmid DNA from a 150-mL overnight culture containing the appropriate antibiotics using a plasmid Midiprep DNA kit, and recover the purified bacmid in 100 μl sterile water.
4. Transfect Sf9 cells (4×10^6 cells in a 25 cm^2 culture flask) using 20 μL of bacmid and 20 μL of Cellfectin®. Collect the supernatant (P1 viral stock) after 4 days at 27 °C.
5. Amplify the virus by incubating Sf9 cells (10^7 cells per 75 cm^2 culture flask) with 0.4 mL P1 (in 2 mL medium) for 1 h at room temperature (RT). Add 13 mL of Sf900-II SFM, and collect the supernatant (P2 viral stock) after 6 days at 27 °C.
6. Seed High Five cells (maintained in TC100 medium containing 10 % FBS) in 175 cm^2 culture flasks (1.75×10^7 cells per flask) and wash twice with Sf900-II SFM. Incubate for 2 h at RT with 3.5 mL of P2, and replace the virus by 35 mL of medium per flask. Collect the supernatant after 48 h at 27 °C for further purification or store at −80 °C.

3.5.2 Purification of Recombinant C1s from the Cell Culture Supernatant

1. Dialyze 100 mL of supernatant against 3×2 L of the C1s-Sepharose equilibration buffer.
2. Add 1 mM DFP and load onto a C1s-Sepharose column (prepared by coupling 40 mg of activated C1s (purified from serum) to 30 mL of CNBr-activated Sepharose 4B) equilibrated in the dialysis buffer at 8 mL/min, wash the column with the equilibration buffer, and elute with the same buffer containing 5 mM EDTA instead of $CaCl_2$. Regenerate the column by applying 100 mL of 1 M NaCl and 10 mM EDTA, wash with the equilibration buffer, and store at 4 °C in the presence of 0.1 % NaN_3.

3. Dialyze the EDTA eluate against the C1s storage buffer, concentrate to 0.5 mg/mL using centrifugal filters, and store at –20 °C. About 750 μg of recombinant C1s in the proenzyme form are recovered from 100 mL of cell culture supernatant.

3.6 Production of Recombinant Proenzyme C1r and Purification of the Recombinant C1s–C1r–C1r–C1s Tetramer

1. The baculovirus for expression of recombinant C1r is generated and amplified as described in Subheading 3.4. The PCR fragment size expected for C1r is 2,118 bp. High Five cells are infected for 55 h.
2. Attempts to purify recombinant C1r alone from the culture supernatant have proved unsuccessful, essentially due to low expression yield, considerable loss of protein during purification trials, and degradation of the protein.
3. Mutation of the active site serine 637 to alanine allows production of recombinant C1r stabilized in the proenzyme form by preventing self-activation. Using this C1r variant, it is possible to reconstitute a recombinant C1s–C1r–C1r–C1s tetramer that will not undergo activation upon incubation with C1q [8] and to purify it as follows:
   (a) Mix culture supernatants containing the C1r S637A variant (produced as described in **step 1** for its wild-type counterpart) and recombinant C1s to obtain equimolar amounts of both proteases, based on the estimation of their relative contents by SDS-PAGE gel analysis and Coomassie blue staining (*see* Subheading 3.7). Dialyze against the C1q-Sepharose equilibration buffer.
   (b) Load onto a C1q-Sepharose column (prepared by coupling 30 mg of C1q to 30 mL of CNBr-activated Sepharose 4B), wash the column, and elute the bound tetramer with the same buffer containing 5 mM EDTA instead of $CaCl_2$. Regenerate and store the column as described in Subheading 3.5.1 for the C1s-Sepharose column.
   (c) Dialyze the EDTA eluate extensively in the tetramer storage buffer, concentrate to 0.2–0.4 mg/mL, and store at 4 °C.

3.7 Biochemical Characterization of C1r, C1s, and the C1s–C1r–C1r–C1s Tetramer

1. SDS-PAGE analysis is used at different purification stages to identify the C1r- and/or C1s-containing fractions and to quantify the C1r and C1s protein contents of insect cell culture supernatants before reconstitution of the recombinant tetramer. Performing this analysis under reducing conditions allows discrimination between the single-chain proenzymes and the two-chain activated proteases. In addition, the activated forms migrate slightly slower than their proenzyme counterparts under nonreducing conditions.

   Samples are denatured by incubation for 1 h at 37 °C with an equivalent volume of the reduced or the unreduced sample preparation buffer, and the reduced samples are then alkylated

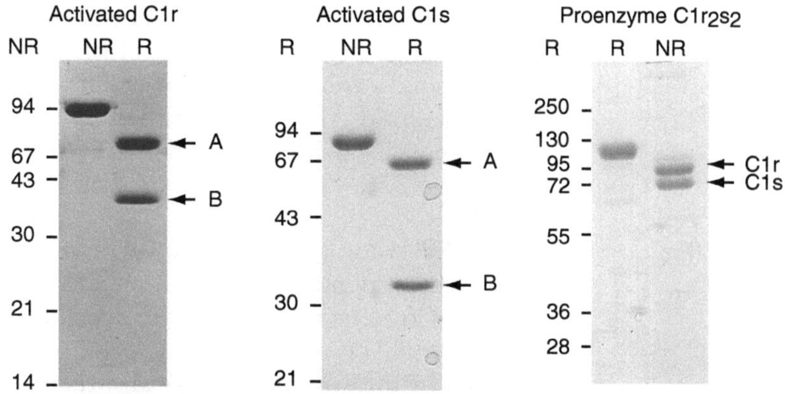

Fig. 4 SDS-PAGE analysis of purified activated C1r, activated C1s, and the proenzyme tetramer isolated from serum. The positions of reduced (R) and unreduced (NR) samples and standard proteins (in kDa) are indicated. The acrylamide % of the gels are 12.5 (isolated C1r and C1s) and 10 (tetramer)

by incubation with 140 mM iodoacetamide for 20 min at 37 °C.

Figure 4 illustrates analyses of activated Clr, activated Cls, and the proenzyme tetramer under both nonreducing and reducing conditions. Scanning of the bands allows calculation of the % of activation of the proteases, which is typically below 5 % for purified proenzyme Clr (not shown).

2. The concentrations of the purified proteins are determined using the following absorption coefficients (Abs 0.1 % (=1 mg/mL) at 280 nm) and molecular weights: serum-derived Cls monomer, 1.45 and 79,800; recombinant Cls monomer, 1.45 and 77,500; serum-derived Clr monomer, 1.24 and 86,300; serum-derived Cls–Clr–Clr–Cls tetramer, 1.35 and 332,200; recombinant Cls–Clr–Clr–Cls tetramer, 1.35 and 321,700.

3.8 Esterolytic Activities

3.8.1 AGLMe

The following assay uses the AGLMe substrate and is based on indirect measurement of methanol released upon cleavage of the methyl ester. Oxidation of methanol by AO produces H_2O_2, which is used by peroxidase (HRP) to convert the chromogenic substrate ABTS to its oxidized, blue-green-colored form. The conversion is followed by measurement of the increase in absorbance at 414 nm.

1. Prepare the reaction mixture containing 1 mM AGLMe, 1.6 U/mL AO (*see* **Note 15**), 1 U/mL HRP, and 0.5 mg/mL ABTS in 100 mM K_2HPO_4, pH 7.5. Filter the solution.
2. Incubate the mixture in two spectrophotometer cuvettes at 30 °C for 5 min.
3. Initiate the reaction by adding the protease sample in one cuvette and an equivalent volume of buffer in the reference cuvette. Monitor the increase of absorbance against the reference sample at 414 nm for 5–10 min.

4. Calculate the esterolytic activity by converting the absorbance change per minute in μmol of ABTS converted per minute, using a molar extinction coefficient of 36,000 M^{-1} cm^{-1} for oxidized ABTS. Under these conditions, the specific activity and sensitivity limits are 2–4 U/mg and 500 ng for pure C1r and 32 U/mg and 50 ng for pure C1s.

3.8.2 BAEe

The following assay uses the BAEe substrate and is based on indirect measurement of ethanol released upon cleavage of the ethyl ester. Conversion of ethanol to acetaldehyde by ADH in the presence of NAD^+ results in the generation of NADH, which is monitored by measurement of the absorbance increase at 340 nm. This assay is less sensitive than the AGLMe assay but is specific for C1s since BAEe is not cleaved by C1r.

1. In two spectrophotometer cuvettes, mix 2.3 mL of the BAEe buffer, 0.5 mL of 6 mM BAEe, 0.1 mL of 30 mM NAD, 0.01 mL of 1.3 mM reduced glutathione, and 0.02 mL of the ADH solution. Incubate the mixture at 30 °C for 5 min.
2. Initiate the reaction by adding the protease sample in one cuvette and an equivalent volume of buffer in the reference cuvette. Record the increase of absorbance against the reference sample at 340 nm for 5–10 min.
3. Calculate the esterolytic activity by converting the absorbance change per minute in μmol of NADH generated per minute, using a molar extinction coefficient of 6,220 M^{-1} cm^{-1}. Under these conditions, the specific activity is 2 U/mg for pure C1s and the sensitivity limit is 0.5 μg C1s.

3.9 Functional Characterization

1. The ability of purified proenzyme C1r to self-activate when incubated at 37 °C is monitored by SDS-PAGE analysis under reducing conditions as described in Subheading 3.7. Activation is complete after incubation for 1 h at 37 °C [10].
2. The ability of activated C1r to cleave proenzyme C1s is assayed by incubating C1s in the presence of 5 % (w/w) C1r for 1 h at 37 °C. C1s activation is followed by SDS-PAGE analysis as described above [11].
3. The proteolytic activity of activated C1s toward its physiological substrates C4 and C2 can be assayed by incubating the protein substrates with 2 % (w/w) protease at 37 °C [12, 13]. The conversion of the α chain of C4 to the α' chain of fragment C4b and the generation of the C2a and C2b fragments are monitored by SDS-PAGE analysis under reducing conditions as described above.
4. The biological activity of the serum-derived proenzyme C1s–C1r–C1r–C1s tetramer can be assayed by its ability to reconstitute the C1 complex in the presence of C1q and the subsequent

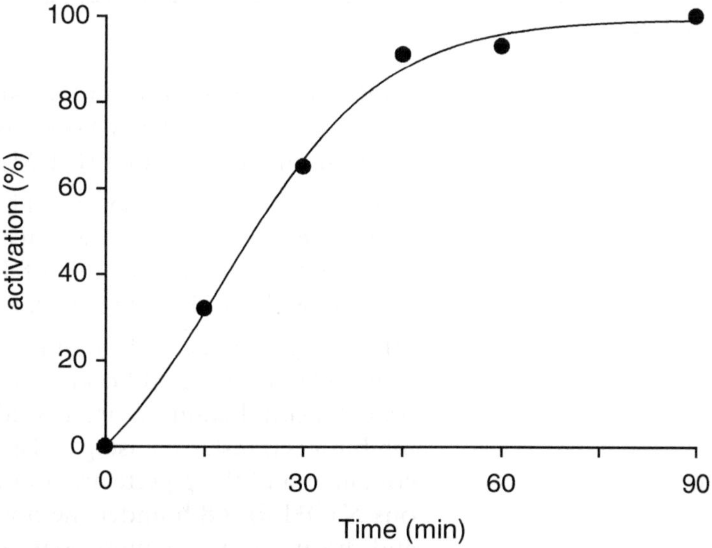

Fig. 5 Activation of C1s within the C1 complex. C1 (0.25 μM) was reconstituted from equimolar amounts of C1q and the proenzyme C1s–C1r–C1r–C1s tetramer and incubated at 37 °C. C1s activation was measured by SDS-PAGE and western blot analyses (*see* Subheading 3.9)

capacity of reconstituted C1 to undergo self-activation (C1 reconstitution assay):

(a) Incubate purified C1q and C1s–C1r–C1r–C1s in a 1:1 molar ratio (0.25 μM) in the tetramer storage buffer for 5 min at 4 °C to reconstitute the C1 complex (*see* **Note 16**).

(b) Incubate at 37 °C to allow spontaneous activation, which is complete within 90 min.

(c) Analyze the reaction mixture by SDS-PAGE under reducing conditions as described in Subheading 3.7.

(d) Since Coomassie blue staining is not sensitive enough to accurately measure activation of the proteases under these conditions, western blot analysis is performed after electrotransfer of the proteins to a nitrocellulose membrane.

(e) Saturate the membrane with the blocking buffer, and visualize C1s activation using a polyclonal anti-C1s antibody, followed by immunostaining (alkaline phosphatase).

(f) Scan the membrane to determine the % of activation (Fig. 5).

5. The interaction properties of the recombinant and serum-derived tetramers can be analyzed by surface plasmon resonance spectroscopy, using C1q as the immobilized ligand and the tetramer as the soluble analyte [8, 14].

4 Notes

1. NaN_3 is extremely toxic, and the stock solution should be prepared under a ventilated hood. Alternatively, a ready-to-use solution can be purchased (0.1 M, Fluka).
2. EDTA is difficult to dissolve in H_2O when the pH is below 7. To ensure fast dissolution, we mix 58.44 g of EDTA and 25 g of NaOH pellets in 500 mL of H_2O, which yields a 0.4 M solution with a pH of approximately 7.8.
3. DFP is highly toxic and should be handled with extreme caution under a ventilated hood. The DFP container and the isopropyl alcohol solution are placed in an ice bucket, and the inhibitor is transferred using a glass transfer pipette. The empty container and the pipette are immersed in a bath of 2 % aqueous NaOH for 48 h under the hood before rinsing with water and discarding in an appropriate disposal system. The 0.5 M DFP solution is stored at −20 °C.
4. The NPGB solution is stored at −20 °C; NPGB should be added extemporarily to aqueous solutions because of its tendency to hydrolyze, which will result in yellow coloring.
5. The cDNAs encoding C1s and C1r may be purchased from the Origene Trueclone human collection (C1s: SC119071; C1r: SC 126504).
6. The components of the system may be purchased individually (Max Efficiency® DH10Bac™ competent bacteria with S.O.C medium; pFast-Bac1 donor plasmid; cellfectin™).
7. FBS is inactivated by heating at 56 °C for 30 min. We do not freeze again heat-inactivated fetal calf serum, but keep it at 4 °C in sterile 50 mL Falcon tubes. Penicillin–streptomycin may be added in the media to prevent bacterial contamination of cell cultures.
8. Using preheated (37 °C) water will facilitate subsequent dissolution of Na_2SO_4.
9. NaOH is used to solubilize the antigen–antibody aggregates for A_{280} measurement.
10. The protocol described starts from 1 L of serum but can be adapted to 2 L of serum by doubling the ICs amount and buffer volumes and using a 70 mL DE52 column with a 2 × 500 mL NaCl gradient.
11. Vigorous shaking is required to maintain the IC suspension as homogeneous as possible (no aggregates should be visible). The initial serum + IC suspension (1.1 L) needs to be split into several bottles for the first centrifugation. During the first wash (200 mL of buffer), it is recommended to suspend each pellet

in a small volume of buffer and to collect them all in a single bottle after rinsing the other bottles, which facilitates the subsequent extraction steps.

12. The DE 52 slurry is prepared according to the manufacturer's instructions (10 g of dry resin yield about 55 mL of wet resin). The column should be washed in the equilibration buffer for at least 6 h at 4 °C.
13. Freezing of C1r should be avoided since this results in extensive precipitation of the protein. The protein is stable for a few months at 0 °C, even though slight precipitation occurs upon storage.
14. The supernatants should not be used for further purification of C1q due to the presence of large amounts of contaminating proteins.
15. One enzyme unit is defined as the amount that cleaves 1 μmol of substrate per minute.
16. It is important to dialyze the proenzyme tetramer prior to C1 reconstitution in order to eliminate DFP from the storage buffer. The presence of trace amounts of inhibitor can block activation of the reconstituted complex.

Acknowledgments

We thank Thomas Lunardi and Sarah Ancelet for help in preparing the figures. Part of the described work was supported by the Agence Nationale de la Recherche (grants ANR-05-MIIM-023-01 and ANR-09-PIRI-0021).

References

1. Gaboriaud C, Thielens NM, Gregory LA et al (2004) Structure and activation of the C1 complex of complement: unraveling the puzzle. Trends Immunol 25:368–373
2. Gal P, Dobo J, Zavodszky P et al (2009) Early complement proteases: C1r, C1s and MASPs. A structural insight into activation and functions. Mol Immunol 46:2745–2752
3. Arlaud GJ, Sim RB, Duplaa AM et al (1979) Differential elution of C1q, C1r and C1s from human C1 bound to immune aggregates. Use in the rapid purification of C1 subcomponents. Mol Immunol 16:445–450
4. Arlaud GJ, Thielens NM (1993) Human complement serine proteases C1r and C1s and their proenzymes. Methods Enzymol 223:61–82
5. Lane PD, Schumaker VN, Tseng Y et al (1991) Isolation of human complement subcomponents C1r and C1s in their unactivated, proenzyme forms. J Immunol Methods 141: 219–226
6. Gal P, Sarvari M, Szilagyi K et al (1989) Expression of hemolytically active human complement component C1r proenzyme in insect cells using a baculovirus vector. Complement Inflamm 6:433–441
7. Luo C, Thielens NM, Gagnon J et al (1992) Recombinant human complement subcomponent C1s lacking beta-hydroxyasparagine, sialic acid, and one of its two carbohydrate chains still reassembles with C1q and C1r to form a functional C1 complex. Biochemistry 31: 4254–4262
8. Bally I, Rosssi V, Lunardi T et al (2009) Identification of the C1q-binding sites of human C1r and C1s: a refined three-dimensional model of the C1 complex of complement. J Biol Chem 284:19340–19348

9. Rossi V, Teillet F, Thielens NM et al (2005) Functional characterization of complement proteases C1s/mannan-binding lectin-associated serine protease-2 (MASP-2) chimeras reveals the higher C4 recognition efficacy of the MASP-2 complement control protein modules. J Biol Chem 280:41811–41818
10. Arlaud GJ, Villiers CL, Chesne S et al (1980) Purified proenzyme C1r. Some characteristics of its activation and subsequent proteolytic cleavage. Biochim Biophys Acta 616:116–129
11. Arlaud GJ, Reboul A, Colomb MG (1977) Proenzymic C1s associated with catalytic amounts of C1r. Study of the activation process. Biochim Biophys Acta 485:227–235
12. Reboul A, Thielens N, Villiers MB et al (1979) Purification of human complement subcomponent C4. C4 cleavage by C1s. FEBS Lett 103:156–161
13. Thielens NM, Villiers MB, Reboul A et al (1982) Human complement subcomponent C2: purification and proteolytic cleavage in fluid phase by C1s, C1r2-C1s2 and C1. FEBS Lett 141:19–24
14. Phillips AE, Toth J, Dodds AW et al (2009) Analogous interactions in initiating complexes of the classical and lectin pathways of complement. J Immunol 182:7708–7717

Chapter 5

Expression and Purification Methods for the Production of Recombinant Human Complement Component C2

Angela W. Norton, Paolo G.V. Martini, Lynette C. Cook, Scott Alderucci, Dianna M. Lundberg, Susan M. Fish, Charles Bedard, John Gill, Arthur O. Tzianabos, and Michael F. Concino

Abstract

Human complement component C2 is a critical factor of the classical complement pathway. Here we provide a method for the production of recombinant human C2 (rhC2) protein for research purposes. The human complement component C2 (hC2) is cloned from a human cDNA library by polymerase chain reaction and inserted in a mammalian expression vector (Martini et al., BMC Immunol 11:43, 2010). Transient transfection is utilized to express hC2 in a mammalian cell line, and the expressed C2 is harvested from the conditioned media. rhC2 is purified from the conditioned media by sequential steps of cation exchange and affinity column chromatography. The purified hC2 is characterized for protein purity, stability, and enzymatic activity. The recombinant hC2 activity is tested in a complement activation ELISA assay that measures classical, alternative, and lectin complement pathway activity in C2-depleted serum.

Key words Recombinant human C2, Complement component C2, Expression of C2, Purification of C2

1 Introduction

Complement component 2 (C2) is a carbohydrate-containing protein containing an enzymatic domain that is critical to the early activation phase of the classical complement pathway [1–3]. The C2 protein is produced as an inactive zymogen which binds to C4b and is cleaved to form C2a and C2b [4–6]. C2a is the enzymatic domain of the protein which is used in the formation of the C3 and C5 convertases [5, 7, 8]. Recombinant full-length C2 is cloned by polymerase chain reaction (PCR) using a human liver-derived cDNA library. The human C2 cDNA is cloned into a mammalian expression plasmid and transiently transfected in human HEK293 cells in a serum-free environment [7, 9]. Harvest media is collected, and the protein is purified over two consecutive columns [3, 6, 10–12].

Mihaela Gadjeva (ed.), *The Complement System: Methods and Protocols*, Methods in Molecular Biology, vol. 1100,
DOI 10.1007/978-1-62703-724-2_5, © Springer Science+Business Media New York 2014

An SP Sepharose column serves as the capture step for the protein and effectively removes any C2a in the culture media from the desired full-length C2 protein product. Fractions from this column containing full-length recombinant human C2 (rhC2) are pooled and further purified over a heparin Sepharose column. The fractions are analyzed, and those containing purified recombinant hC2 are selected as the final product.

2 Materials

2.1 Protein Purification and C2 Storage Buffer

MilliQ water is defined as deionized water which has been further purified through a Millipore water system to attain a sensitivity of 18 MΩ and 5 ppm TOC at 25 °C.

1. SP equilibration buffer: 25 mM Sodium phosphate, pH 6.5, 2 mM EDTA in Milli Q water. Combine 2.4 g/L of sodium phosphate dibasic with 2.09 g/L sodium phosphate monobasic and 0.744 g/L EDTA and dissolve in MilliQ water. Check pH and bring to 6.5. If necessary, adjust the pH using 10 N sodium hydrozide or 6 N hydrochloric acid. Add MilliQ water to the final required volume and filter with a 0.2 μm filter before use.
2. SP elution buffer: 25 mM Sodium phosphate, pH 6.5, 2 mM EDTA, and 1 M sodium chloride in MilliQ water. Combine 2.4 g/L of sodium phosphate dibasic with 2.09 g/L sodium phosphate monobasic, 0.744 g/L EDTA, and 58.44 g/L sodium chloride and dissolve in MilliQ water. Check pH and bring to 6.5 if necessary. Add MilliQ water to the final required volume and filter with a 0.2 μm filter before use.
3. SP Sepharose storage buffer: 20 % ethanol in MilliQ water.
4. Heparin equilibration buffer: 25 mM Sodium phosphate, pH 6.5 in MilliQ water. Combine 2.4 g/L of sodium phosphate dibasic with 2.09 g/L sodium phosphate monobasic and dissolve in MilliQ water. Check pH and bring to 6.5 if necessary. Add MilliQ water to the final required volume and filter with a 0.2 μm filter before use.
5. Heparin elution buffer: 25 mM Sodium phosphate, pH 6.5 and 1 M sodium chloride in MilliQ water. Combine 2.4 g/L of sodium phosphate dibasic with 2.09 g/L sodium phosphate monobasic and 58.44 g/L sodium chloride and dissolve in MilliQ water. Check pH and bring to 6.5 if necessary. Add MilliQ water to the final required volume and filter with a 0.2 μm filter before use.
6. C2 storage buffer: 10 mM Sodium phosphate pH 7.0, 137 mM sodium chloride. 10× PBS (Gibco Cat. # 70013) diluted to 1X and adjusted to pH 7.

2.2 BCA Protein Assay

1. BCA protein assay kit.
2. Microtest tissue culture 96 wells.
3. Molecular Devices SPECTRAmax PLUS 384 Microplate Spectrophotometer.

2.3 SDS-PAGE and Western Blotting Buffer Components

1. Polyacrylamide 8–16 % Tris–glycine gels.
2. 6X Sample buffer: 1.0 mL 0.5 M Tris–HCl, pH 6.8, 0.8 mL glycerol, 1.6 mL 10 % SDS, and 0.2 mL 0.5 % bromophenol blue.
3. Protein molecular weight markers.
4. Gel running buffer: 24.8 mM Tris base, 0.125 % SDS, 191 mM glycine. Combine 3 g Tris base, 14.3 g of glycine, 1.25 g of SDS and bring to 1 L with MilliQ water.
5. Gel transfer buffer: 12.4 mM Tris base, 95.6 mM glycine, 10 % methanol, 0.01 % SDS. Combine 1.5 g Tris base, 7.18 g glycine, 100 mL methanol, and 0.1 g SDS and bring to 1 L with MilliQ water.
6. ECL wash buffer: 20 mM Tris, 0.15 M NaCl, 0.05 % Tween 20. Combine 2.42 g Tris base, 8.77 g sodium chloride, and 0.5 g Tween-20 and bring to 2 L with MilliQ water.
7. Western blot blocking buffer: 5 % Nonfat milk in ECL wash buffer. Combine 5 g of nonfat milk with 100 mL of ECl wash buffer.
8. ECL Western blotting detection reagents: Use according to the manufacturer's recommendations.
9. Coomassie-based staining solution: GelCode Blue Stain Reagent.

2.4 ELISA Buffer Components

1. ELISA coating buffer: 50 mM Sodium bicarbonate, pH 9.6. Add 4.2 g of sodium bicarbonate to a 1 L beaker. Add approximately 800 mL of MilliQ water. Check the pH and adjust to 9.6. Bring the total volume to 1 L with MilliQ water and filter with a 0.2 μm filter.
2. ELISA wash buffer: Add 10 mL of Tween 20 into a 1 L bottle of 10× Dulbecco's phosphate-buffered saline (DPBS). Add a stir bar and stir gently until Tween 20 is thoroughly mixed in. Add 4 L of MilliQ water to a 10 L carboy. Pour the 1 L Tween 20/DPBS mix into the carboy. Rinse the bottle which contained the Tween 20/DPBS mix with 1 L of MilliQ water, and add it to the carboy. Add an additional 4 L of MilliQ water to the carboy (total volume 10 L). Stir the solution for 30 min with a large stir bar. Store at room temperature.
3. ELISA blocking buffer: 1× PBS, 0.05 % Tween-20, 2 % BSA. Add 2 g of BSA to a 1 L beaker along with 0.5 g of Tween 20. Bring the total volume to 1 L with 1× PBS (Gibco 70013 diluted to 1×) and mix with a stir bar. Filter through a 0.2 μm filter.

4. TMB substrate reagent: TMB peroxidase EIA substrate kit. Use the substrate reagent according to the manufacturer's recommendations.
5. ELISA stop solution: 2 N Sulfuric acid. Add 800 mL of MilliQ water to a 1 L graduated cylinder. Fill to 1 L with 200 mL of 10 N sulfuric acid. Mix the graduated cylinder by inversion, and store the solution in a glass bottle.

2.5 HPLC Buffer Components

1. RP-HPLC mobile phase buffer A: 0.1 % Trifluoroacetic acid.
2. RP-HPLC mobile phase buffer B: 0.085 % TFA, 90 % acetonitrile.
3. SEC mobile phase buffer: 25 mM Sodium phosphate, 500 mM sodium chloride pH 6.5.

3 Methods

3.1 C2 Protein Production

1. C2 protein is produced via a transient expression system in 293-F cells. The complement component C2 can be cloned from a human liver cDNA library by PCR using primers synthesized based on the complement C2 published mRNA sequence (NM_000063) including restriction enzyme NheI on the forward primer and XhoI on the reverse primer, suitable for cloning into the recipient vector. Generate primers as follows: 5′ GCT AGC GAC ACC ATG GGC CCA ACT GAT GGT T; 3′ CTC GAG CTA GAG GGG TAA AAA ATT CAG GAC ATC C. Run the PCR reaction at 95 °C for 3 min, 27 cycles at 95 °C for 1 min, 65 °C for 30 s, 72 °C for 2.30 min, and 72 °C for 10 min, 4 °C. Insert the amplified cDNA by ligation after digestion with restriction enzymes NheI and XhoI into the pCEP4 vector containing a CMV promoter.
2. Expand the 293-F cells in Freestyle 293 culture medium in a series of batch cultures of increasing volume from shake-flask to WAVE. Maintain the vented shake-flask cultures at 37 °C under air with 8 % CO_2. During the culture, keep the WAVE cultures at 37 °C, and adjust the headspace pCO_2 daily (range 0.5–8 %) to maintain pH in the 6.8–7.2 range. Monitor the pO_2 in the WAVE cultures and keep it ≥60 mmHg by adjusting the rocking speed and angle. Once the viable cell density of the 12.5 L WAVE stage reached $> 1 \times 10^6$/mL, transfect the cells.
3. Use 1 μg of C2-pCEP4 per 10^6 cells to transfect using a polyethylenimine (PEI) mixture prepared in Optimem medium with a 1:3 ratio of DNA:PEI (weight:weight). 2–4 h after transfection initiation, bring the culture volume up to 22.5 L in the wave bag by the addition of fresh prewarmed Freestyle 293 medium. The next day, add 2.5 L of a sterile aqueous preparation of Primatone RL hydrolysate to the culture. The final concentration

of Primatone in the culture is 2.5 g/L. Primatone is used to promote cell growth in the absence of serum.

4. 72 h post transfection, clarify the harvest by pumping it out from the WAVE bag through an in situ perfusion filter (~7 μm). Further filter the resulting cell-free harvest through a 0.2 μm PES filter, collecting the filtrate collected in 2 L PETG bottles, and store at −20 °C. 23–24 L of 0.2 μm-filtered harvest can be obtained in each run (*see* **Note 1**).
5. Pack 1,800 mL of SP Sepharose Fast Flow resin (*see* **Note 2**) into a BPG 140/500 column according to the manufacturer's recommendations (*see* **Note 3**). If a Watson/Marlow 620U peristaltic pump is utilized, 80 rpm can be used to sufficiently pack the resin. There should not be a change in back pressure as the column is packed. Maintain the packing and operating pressure at or below 0.7 mPa.
6. Pack the heparin column with 300 mL heparin Sepharose FF resin in an XK 50 column at 40 mL/min (linear flow rate 98 cm/h) with a maximum pressure of 0.35 mPa using a GE Healthcare AKTA Purifier UPC-900 chromatography station.
7. Capture the recombinant C2 protein on an SP Sepharose FF column. On the day before each SP purification run, wash the column with more than 5 column volumes (CV) of MilliQ water to remove the ethanol in the SP Sepharose FF storage buffer.
8. Charge the resin with 4 CV of SP elution buffer and then equilibrate with 5 CV of SP equilibration buffer at 100 mL/min using a GE Healthcare AKTA Purifier UPC-900 chromatography station (*see* **Note 4**).
9. Thaw the conditioned media in a 25 °C water bath. After thawing, adjust the conditioned media pool to pH 6.5 with 0.5 M monobasic sodium phosphate, and check the conductivity (10 mS). Filter the adjusted CM through a sterile 0.8/0.2 μM PES filter prior to loading on the SP Sepharose FF (*see* **Note 5**).
10. If necessary, the adjusted CM can be loaded onto the column overnight. If so, load the adjusted CM onto the column overnight at 24 mL/min (linear flow rate 9.4 cm/h, residence time 75 min). The day after the overnight load, increase the load rate to 100 mL/min (linear flow rate 30 cm/h, residence time 18 min).
11. Maintain a flow rate of 100 mL/min for the wash and elution steps (*see* **Note 6**). Wash the column with a minimum of 5 CV of SP equilibration buffer.
12. Elute the protein with a 0–30 % B (where B was the SP elution buffer) linear gradient over 30 CV (54 L).
13. Collect 2,000 mL fractions in 2 L polypropylene sterile bottles. After collection, store all fractions at 4 °C during analysis.

Clean the column with 100 % SP elution buffer, 1.0 N NaOH, and rinse with MilliQ water. Store the resin in 20 % ethanol at room temperature in between uses.

14. Pool fractions from the SP column containing C2 (10 L total, if process followed to scale) (*see* **Notes 7** and **8**). Concentrate the pool using a Millipore Pellicon-2 mini system (or similar apparatus) to a final volume of 1 L.
15. On the day before each heparin purification run, wash the column with at least 5 CV of MilliQ water followed by equilibration with 10 CV of heparin equilibration buffer (*see* **Note 9**). During the equilibration, load, wash, and elution of C2, run the column at 30 mL/min (linear flow rate 92 cm/h, residence time 10 min). If necessary, the outlet from the column can be disconnected from the AKTA to reduce the pressure on the column.
16. Dilute the 1 L concentrated SP elute with 4 L of heparin equilibration buffer to lower the conductivity to 5.2 mS. Filter the diluted pool using a 0.2 μM PES membrane to remove any precipitated proteins from the load sample.
17. Load the diluted SP pool onto the heparin column, and wash with 5 CV of heparin equilibration buffer.
18. Elute the protein from the column with a linear gradient over 20 CV to 20 % B (where B was heparin elution buffer).
19. Collect 300 mL fractions in 500 mL polypropylene sterile bottles and store at 4 °C during analysis.
20. Clean the column with 100 % heparin elution buffer, 0.1 N NaOH, and rinse with MilliQ water. Store the column in 20 % ethanol at room temperature in between uses.
21. Analyze the fractions by SDS-PAGE silver stain and a BCA protein assay. Select and pool the desired fractions from the heparin column for concentration and buffer exchange (*see* **Note 10**).
22. Concentrate the purified protein fivefold on ice using a Millipore Pellicon-2 mini system with a 10,000 MWCO Pellicon-2 mini membrane. Then buffer exchange the purified C2 into C2 storage buffer using the Pellicon system. Buffer exchange with five exchanges of equal volume and one chase of 200 mL to collect the sample from the tubing.
23. After the buffer exchange, further concentrate the protein with a Vivaspin 20 10,000 MWCO concentrator by centrifuging at 3,000 × *g* at 4 °C in a Sorvall Legend RT centrifuge with a Heraeus Sorvall 75006445 swinging bucket rotor until the final concentration was determined to be greater than 5 mg/mL by a BCA protein assay.
24. Sterile filter the purified protein in a Biosafety cabinet, aliquot into siliconized sterile tubes, and store at −80 °C.

3.2 BCA Protein Assay

1. The BCA protein assay was performed following the manufacturer's recommendations. Pre-diluted BSA protein assay standards are used to generate the standard curve for the analysis.

3.3 SDS-PAGE Silver Stain and GelCode Blue Analysis of C2

1. Prepare all protein samples for gel analysis in microcentrifuge tubes. The loading volume of the samples can vary depending on the well size of the SDS-PAGE gels used. If precision plus marker is used as the molecular weight standard, load 2 or 7.5 μL.
2. Mix 0.5 or 2.0 μg of total protein with 1/6 loading volume of 6X sample buffer and 1/10 loading volume of 1 M DTT and bring to the final volume with MilliQ water. Heat the samples at 37 °C for 15 min prior to loading immediately onto the gel.
3. Run SDS-PAGE gels at 200 V for 50 min.
4. For gel staining use either the Owl Silver Stain Kit or the GelCode Blue Staining Kit (*see* **Note 11**).

3.4 ELISA Analysis of C2

1. Use a 96-well Nunc Immuno plate for the C2 ELISA. Coat the wells with 100 μL of 1 μg/mL anti-human complement component C2 in ELISA coating buffer. Seal the plate and incubate overnight at RT. The next morning wash the plate three times with ELISA wash buffer. Wash for each step of the ELISA by filling each of the wells completely to the top with ELISA wash buffer, pour the buffer off, and tap the plate dry. Remove the TMB reagent from the refrigerator at this time to get to room temperature by the time of its use.
2. Add 300 μL of ELISA blocking buffer to each well. Seal the plate and incubate for 1 h at 37 °C. While the plate is blocking, prepare the standard and sample dilutions in ELISA blocking buffer. To generate the standard curve of C2 include serial dilutions from 200 to 3 ng/mL. At the end of the blocking incubation, remove the blocking buffer and tap the plate dry on a paper towel.
3. Add 100 μL of the diluted standards and unknowns to wells of the plate in duplicate. Seal the plate and incubate in a Jitterbug with shaking at speed at 5 and 25 °C for 2 h. At the end of the incubation wash the plate three times with ELISA wash buffer.
4. Add 100 μL of 1 μg/mL of mouse monoclonal to C2 in ELISA blocking buffer to each well. Seal the plate and incubate for 1 h at 37 °C. After the incubation wash the plate three times with ELISA wash buffer and tap the plate dry.
5. Add 100 μL of 100 ng/mL of anti-mouse HRP conjugate in ELISA blocking buffer to each well. Seal the plate and incubate for 1 h at 37 °C. After the incubation wash the plate three times with ELISA wash buffer and tap the plate dry.
6. Prepare the TMB reagent by mixing nine part Reagent A to one part Reagent B just before use as per manufacturer's

directions. Add 100 μL of the complete TMB reagent to each well. Seal the plate and incubate for 20 min at 37 °C. At the end of the incubation, remove the plate from the incubator, and add 100 μL of ELISA stop buffer to stop the reaction.

7. Read the plate at 450 nm on a Molecular Devices plate reader equipped with SoftMax Pro software.
8. *See* **Note 12** for the details to the commercial ELISA reagents.

3.5 SEC HPLC Analysis of Recombinant C2

1. Analyze samples (5 μg) of the purified protein on size-exclusion chromatography (SEC) column with 25 mM sodium phosphate, pH 6.5 and 500 mM sodium chloride in MilliQ water as the mobile phase at 0.15 mL/min.
2. Quantify the chromatogram using Exponential Skim Integration of the Empower software to account for any carbohydrate modifications on the protein (*see* **Note 13**).

3.6 Reverse-Phase Analysis of Recombinant C2 Protocol

1. Analyze samples (5 μg) of the purified protein on a Symmetry 300 C4 column at 0.2 mL/min.
2. Program the gradient to run from 0 to 100 % B gradient in 40 min. Mobile phase A buffer: 0.1 % TFA in MilliQ water and mobile phase B buffer: 0.085 % TFA in 95 % acetonitrile.
3. Quantify the chromatogram using Exponential Skim Integration of the Empower software to account for any carbohydrate modifications on the protein (*see* **Note 14**).

3.7 SEC MALS Protocol

1. Analyze the molecular weight and hydrodynamic radius of the major peak seen on SEC for C2 using a multi-angle static and dynamic light scattering system from Wyatt Technologies in conjunction with the SEC method described above with the following modifications.
2. Increase the pH of the light scattering mobile phase buffer to pH 7.0. Increase the flow rate throughout the column run to 0.3 mL/min.
3. Dilute the C2 one to ten in light scattering mobile phase buffer, and load 10 μg onto the column (*see* **Note 15**).

3.8 Recombinant Human C2 Activity in Affinity-Depleted C2-Deficient Serum

1. Reconstitution of the classical and lectin complement pathways by C2 is shown in vitro using the Alpco Total Complement 3-pathway ELISA (Alpco). This procedure utilized commercially available, affinity-depleted C2-deficient serum combined with rhC2 to provide all of the proteins needed for the complement cascade to occur.
2. Remove the number of wells required to assay the samples and bring them to room temperature.
3. Reconstitute all buffers.
4. Partially thaw the pooled human serum stripped of C2 at 37 °C with mixing; once partially thawed move onto ice for the

remainder of the time needed for the serum to thaw. Mix briefly on the vortex prior to use. Dilute the serum 1:100 for use in the assay. Add C2 at various concentrations of rhC2 (0–40 μg/mL of rhC2) and load 100 μL of the sample on the wells.

5. Pour the solution out, and mix each well 3× with 300 μL of wash buffer supplied with the kit.
6. Add 100 μL of the conjugate to the well and incubate for 30 min at room temperature.
7. Repeat the wash step 3×.
8. Add 100 μL of the substrate to each well and incubate at room temperature for 30 min.
9. Read the absorbance at 405 nm on a microplate reader (*see* **Notes 16** and **17**).

4 Notes

1. The product titers in the harvests as estimated by ELISA were 15.7 and 37.2 mg/L in the first and second runs, respectively. The total amount of product in the harvests as estimated by ELISA is 1.2 g.
2. The binding capacity of the SP Sepharose resin for the load sample is experimentally determined during process development to be 0.37 mg C2 by ELISA per mL of SP resin. Therefore the 1,800 mL column utilized would bind 660 mg C2. Two identical large-scale purification runs are performed with the starting loads containing 550 mg of recombinant C2 in conditioned media as measured by the ELISA. The first column run of the SP column resulted in 53 % step recovery of C2 evaluated by the C2 ELISA as shown in Table 1. The second run of the same column resulted in 46 % recovery of C2.
3. The desired flow rate for the SP Sepharose purification step is at the maximum flow rate of the AKTA purification system. It is recommended to pack the resin above the desired flow rate of the column operation. Thus, a peristaltic pump is utilized to pack the column in order to pack at 130–200 % of the process flow rate as recommended by the manufacturer.
4. The flow rates used for the SP Sepharose FF column are within the specifications established during the purification process development.
5. Filtration of the pH adjusted 1× CM is done with a PES filter capsule with a 0.8 μm prefilter before the 0.2 μm filter to minimize clogging.
6. Even after the filtration of the 1× CM it is necessary to disconnect the outlet valve of the column from the AKTA purifier to maintain the column pressure under the recommended

Table 1
Protein recovery from the purification process of rhC2 is shown in Table 1. The total C2 recovered from each step of the purification was measured by ELISA as described. Total protein recovery for each purification step was evaluated by measuring with a BCA assay

	mL	Elisa μg/mL	Total μg by ELISA	Step recovery (%)	Total recovery (%)	BCA μg/mL	Total μg by BCA	Step recovery (%)	Total recovery (%)
C2									
CM	23,000	22.4	515,200			964	22,172,000		
SP pool concentrated	1,000	275	275,000	53.30	53.30	237	237,000	10.60	10.60
C2-R1.19 Nov 07	20.5	6,391	131,016	47.64	25.40	5,780	112,340	47.40	0.51

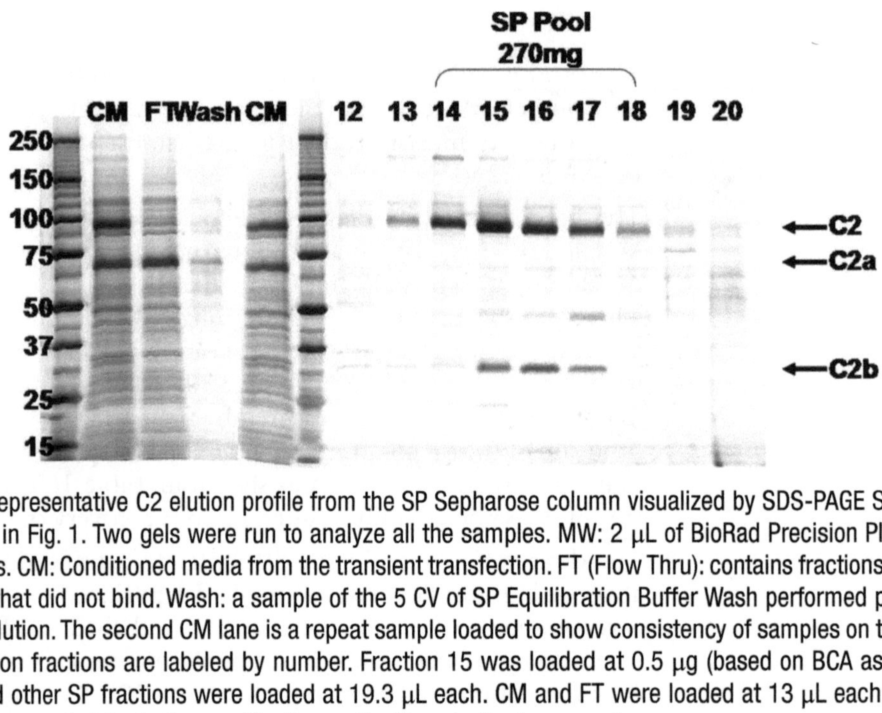

Fig. 1 A representative C2 elution profile from the SP Sepharose column visualized by SDS-PAGE Silver Stain is shown in Fig. 1. Two gels were run to analyze all the samples. MW: 2 μL of BioRad Precision Plus Protein Standards. CM: Conditioned media from the transient transfection. FT (Flow Thru): contains fractions represent proteins that did not bind. Wash: a sample of the 5 CV of SP Equilibration Buffer Wash performed prior to the column elution. The second CM lane is a repeat sample loaded to show consistency of samples on the second gel. Elution fractions are labeled by number. Fraction 15 was loaded at 0.5 μg (based on BCA assay) while Wash and other SP fractions were loaded at 19.3 μL each. CM and FT were loaded at 13 μL each. Fractions 14–18 were pooled for further purification on the Heparin Sepharose column

0.7 mPa with the desired 100 mL/min flow rate. Since the flow cell is off-line from the computer, the total protein content of each fraction is analyzed by a BCA protein assay.

7. Endogenous proteases in the cells clip the full-length C2 protein into its two components C2a and C2b. Capture of the full-length C2 protein and the C2b (inactive form) is complete on the SP Sepharose. The C2a (active form) does not bind to the column and is removed at this step (Fig. 1). The Primatone used during the cell culture also does not bind to the SP Sepharose.

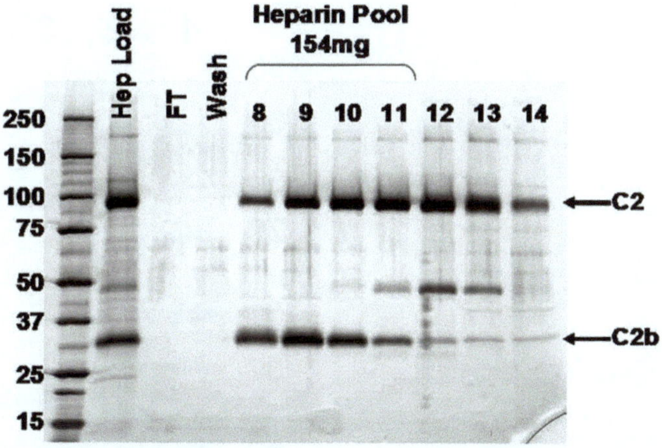

Fig. 2 SDS–PAGE Silver stain analysis of the heparin column fractions are shown in Fig. 2. The molecular weight marker contains 2 μL of BioRad Precision Plus Protein Standards. Hep Load is the pooled SP fractions after preparation for the heparin column. FT (Flow Thru) fractions represent proteins that did not bind to the column. Wash is a sample from the 5 CV of Heparin Equilibration Buffer wash after load. Elution fractions from the salt gradient are labeled by number. Load and Fractions 9–12 were loaded at 0.5 μg (based on BCA assay) while FT, Wash, and Fractions 8, 13–14 were loaded at 19.3 μL each. Fractions 8–11 were pooled for final concentration

8. During process development it was determined that no C2 came off of the column during a 1 M NaCl strip or a 1 N NaOH strip of the SP Sepharose column. SDS-PAGE western blot analysis with an anti-C2 antibody did not show any full-length C2 in the flow-through fraction either. However, there is a prominent C2a band in the flow-through fraction which accounts for the ~50 % C2 recovery by ELISA from the SP Sepharose step (Table 1). Analyze the fractions from the SP column by SDS-PAGE silver staining, ELISA, and a BCA protein assay.
9. The heparin column used for this process is packed on the AKTA purifier system with the outlet valve disconnected. A binding capacity of 1 mg of total protein by BCA assay per mL of heparin resin is used.
10. The long wash during the heparin column step is utilized to ensure complete removal of the EDTA which is in the buffers from the SP Sepharose capture of the recombinant C2. There is no C2 observed in a 1 M NaCl strip or a 0.1 N NaOH strip of the column, but there are minor impurity bands seen on a stained SDS-PAGE gel (*see* Fig. 2).

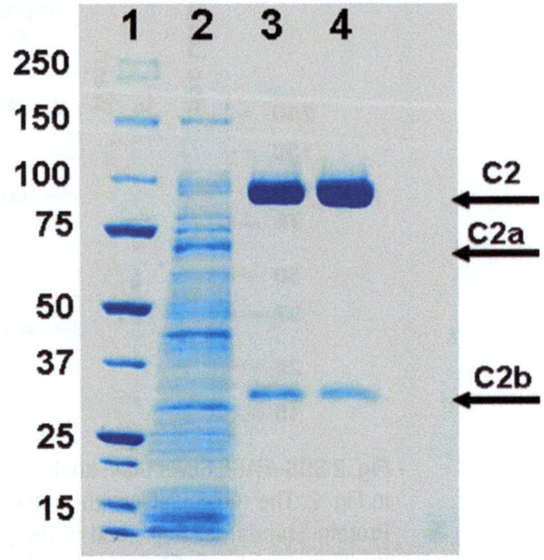

Fig. 3 SDS–PAGE Coomassie stain analysis of the complete purification process. The molecular weight marker contains 7.5 μL of BioRad Precision Plus Protein Standards. Lane 1 is CM, lane 2 is the SP pool, and lane 3 is the final product after Heparin, UF/DF, and filtration. CM (lane 1) is loaded at 13 μL of the starting CM. Lane 2 (SP Pool) of R2 is loaded at 1.0 μg. All other lanes were loaded at 2.0 μg (based on the BCA protein assay)

11. The rhC2 size is estimated to be 100 kDa by SDS-PAGE analysis (Fig. 3). The small contaminant at approximately 30 kDa was C2b (confirmed by western blotting—data not shown) which co-purifies with full-length C2 by this method. The N-terminal sequence of the purified product was verified by Edman degradation at the Mayo Proteomics Research Center, Mayo Clinic College of Medicine in Rochester, MN.
12. Primary antibody for the ELISA is purchased from R&D Systems (Catalog #AP1536). The C2 protein standard for curve generation is purchased from EMD Biosciences (Catalog #204882). The secondary antibody is purchased from Abcam (Catalog #050-08). The detection antibody is purchased from Promega (Catalog #W4021).
13. The purity of full-length rhC2 by SEC on an HPLC yielded 96 % pure (*see* Fig. 4a).
14. The purity of full-length rhC2 by reverse-phase HPLC measured 90 % pure (data not shown).

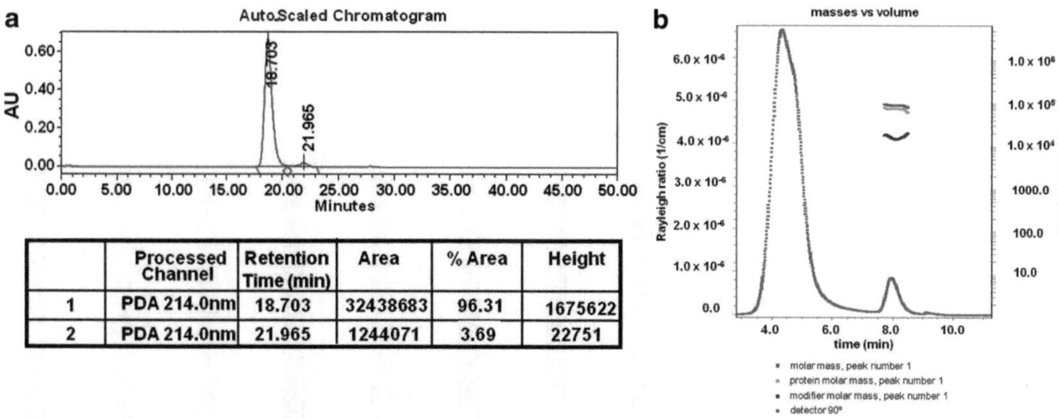

	Processed Channel	Retention Time (min)	Area	% Area	Height
1	PDA 214.0nm	18.703	32438683	96.31	1675622
2	PDA 214.0nm	21.965	1244071	3.69	22751

Fig. 4 SEC Analysis of rhC2. (**a**) The purified rhC2 was 96 % pure by SEC-HPLC. (**b**) SEC-MALS analysis shows the total mass of the purified rhC2 as well as the total protein mass. The modified mass is the measured weight of the posttranslational modifications on the rhC2

15. The weight average molar mass (M_w) of the full-length C2 including glycosylation was determined to be 92,400 g/mol (*see* Fig. 4b). The molar mass of the protein constituent alone was 75,900 g/mol. The difference between the two measurements gives the carbohydrate content of the protein measured at 16,400 g/mol. Carbohydrate modification of the protein was expected by producing the rhC2 in a mammalian system [3].
16. The specific reconstitution of the classical and lectin complement pathways when rhC2 is added to the C2-depleted serum is shown in Fig. 5. The data shows that the alternative pathway, which is independent of C2, is activated in C2-depleted serum regardless of the presence of rhC2. Conversely, the classical and lectin pathways are not activated in the absence of the rhC2.
17. Titration of the assay with increasing amounts of rhC2 clearly shows that an rhC2 concentration of 3 μg/mL restored the classical pathway activity to >50 % above background. Complete activation of the classical and the lectin complement pathways was observed at 12 μg/mL of rhC2. An irrelevant protein (a transferrin fusion protein) with similar MW was used as negative control. This protein did not activate the complement pathway (*see* Fig. 5).

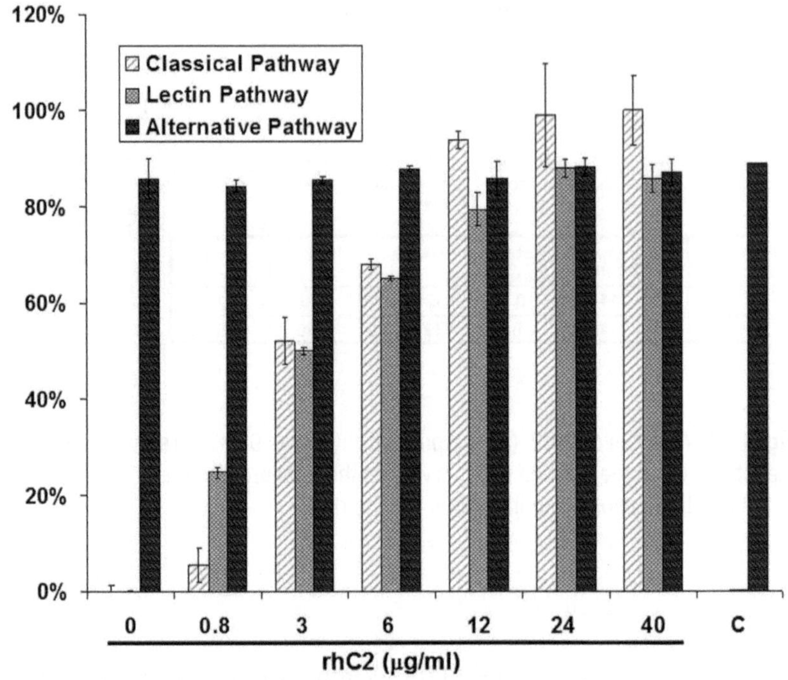

Fig. 5 Reconstitution of complement activity was measured using a complement activation ELISA by adding rhC2 in C2 affinity depleted human serum. The dose response of rhC2 in serum shows activation of the classical pathway at a concentration as low as 3 μg/ml. An irrelevant protein (C) was run as a negative control to confirm specificity of the assay to rhC2. Data represent the mean ± SD of three independent experiments

References

1. Walport MJ (2001) Complement first of two parts. N Engl J Med 344(14):1058–1066
2. Agnello V (1978) Complement deficiency states. Medicine (Baltimore) 57(1):1–23
3. Tomana M, Niemann M, Garner C et al (1985) Carbohydrate composition of the second, third and fifth components and factors B and D of human complement. Mol Immunol 22(2): 107–111
4. Bentley DR (1986) Primary structure of human complement component C2. Homology to two unrelated protein families. Biochem J 239(2):339–345
5. Krishnan V, Xu Y, Macon K et al (2007) The crystal structure of C2a, the catalytic fragment of classical pathway C3 and C5 convertase of human complement. J Mol Biol 367(1): 224–233
6. Nagasawa S, Stroud RM (1977) Cleavage of C2 by C1s into the antigenically distinct fragments C2a and C2b: demonstration of binding of C2b to C4b. Proc Natl Acad Sci U S A 74(7):2998–3001
7. Milder FJ, Raaijmakers HC, Vandeputte MD et al (2006) Structure of complement component C2A: implications for convertase formation and substrate binding. Structure 14(10): 1587–1597
8. Pangburn MK, Rawal N (2002) Structure and function of complement C5 convertase enzymes. Biochem Soc Trans 30(Pt 6):1006–1010
9. Martini PG, Cook LC, Alderucci S et al (2010) Recombinant human complement component C2 produced in a human cell line restores the classical complement pathway activity in-vitro: an alternative treatment for C2 deficiency diseases. BMC Immunol 11:43
10. Kerr MA, Porter RR (1978) The purification and properties of the second component of human complement. Biochem J 171(1): 99–107
11. Hammer CH, Wirtz GH, Renfer L et al (1981) Large scale isolation of functionally active components of the human complement system. J Biol Chem 256(8):3995–4006
12. Thielens NM, Villiers MB, Reboul A et al (1982) Human complement subcomponent C2: purification and proteolytic cleavage in fluid phase by C1s, C1r2-C1s2 and C1. FEBS Lett 141(1):19–24

Chapter 6

Purification and Characterization of Human and Mouse Complement C3

Marieta M. Ruseva and Meike Heurich

Abstract

Complement component C3 is the most abundant complement protein in plasma, central to all three complement activation pathways and essential to complement amplification. Thus, it is one of the most extensively studied complement proteins. This chapter describes the purification of C3 from human and mouse plasma using protein precipitation, followed by classical ion exchange chromatography and gel filtration. The biochemical and functional characteristics of the purified C3 are typically assessed by sodium dodecyl sulfate-polyacrylamide gel electrophoresis and hemolysis assays. The hemolysis assay is a standard technique to assess complement activity monitoring the lysis of red blood cells.

Key words C3, Complement system, Ion exchange chromatography, Hemolysis

1 Introduction

C3 is a central component of the complement cascade. Human complement C3 has a molecular weight (MW) of 185 kDa, containing two disulfide-linked chains comprising an α-chain (MW 110 kDa, 992 amino acids (aa)) and β-chain (MW 75 kDa, 645 aa) [1]. Mouse complement α-chain has a MW of 110 kDa (993 aa) and β-chain of MW 65–70 kDa (642 aa) [2–4], the β-chain of mouse C3 being 9 kDa smaller than that of human C3 [5]. C3 plasma concentration in human is ~1–1.5 mg/ml and mouse ~0.3–0.4 mg/ml. Human C3 is located on chromosome 19: 6,677,846–6,720,662 and mouse C3 is on chromosome 17: 57,203,973–57,228,136, showing 79 and 77 % identity at the nucleotide and amino acid level, respectively [1].

C3 and its activation or breakdown fragments ($C3_{H2O}$, C3b, C3a, iC3b, C3dg) associate with various molecules forming complexes, mediating activation, amplification, and modulating regulation of the complement system. C3 spontaneously auto-activates in

Mihaela Gadjeva (ed.), *The Complement System: Methods and Protocols*, Methods in Molecular Biology, vol. 1100,
DOI 10.1007/978-1-62703-724-2_6, © Springer Science+Business Media New York 2014

aqueous solution due to an internal thioester bond that is susceptible to hydrolysis. Hydrolysis of the internal thioester bond in C3 is denoted by $C3_{H2O}$. C3 autoactivation ($C3_{H2O}$) is marked by major conformational changes within the molecule, enabling it to interact with factor B (see below) [6]. Continuous low-rate cleavage of C3 into C3b is further mediated by plasma proteases [7].

$C3_{H2O}$ as well as the C3 activation product C3b form complexes with factor B (in the presence of factor D, Mg^{2+}) to generate the C3 (C3bBb) and C5 (C3bBbC3b) cleaving enzyme complexes (termed convertases). The C3 convertase, through a positive feedback loop, cleaves more C3 into anaphylatoxin C3a and C3b, thus enabling rapid complement amplification.

These convertases will spontaneously decay, but this process is enhanced by regulatory molecules such as CD55 (also termed "decay-accelerating factor") [8–11] and factor H [12–14]. C3b is proteolytically cleaved by factor I in the presence of fluid-phase cofactors such as factor H and C4bp and membrane-bound cofactors like MCP (CD46) and CR1 (CD35), whereas the latter also acts as cofactor for the cleavage of iC3b into C3dg [14–17].

In rodents, a regulator termed Crry has both cofactor and decay-accelerating activity for the rodent convertases [18, 19].

Although the breakdown fragments of C3b, iC3b, and C3dg can no longer generate a convertase and promote further cleavage of C3, they mediate biological functions by interacting with cellular receptors ("complement receptors") that include CR1 (CD35), CR2 (CD21), CR3 (CD11b/CD18), CR4 (CD11c/CD18), and CRIg (VSIg4) [15, 20] on effector cells, mediating clearance of pathogens and dying cells and modulating the adaptive immune response.

This chapter describes the purification and analysis of human and mouse C3 from plasma using ion exchange and size exclusion chromatography, sodium dodecyl sulfate-polyacrylamide gel electrophoresis (SDS-PAGE), and hemolytic assays. The purification of a number of complement components from plasma has been described earlier [21]. The purification steps explained here are derived from these methods. Even though specific anti-C3 antibodies are available for a number of species, there is no immunoaffinity technique to date that yields functional active C3, since C3 hydrolyzes upon elution in both low- and high-pH solutions. Therefore, classical chromatography-based methods are commonly being used for C3 purification as these can be performed at (near-) physiological pH while varying ionic strength only, resulting in a good yield of purified, active C3. The buffer conditions can be easily adapted for purification of C3 from a broad range of species. Good separation is usually achieved by crude enrichment of the sample with the protein of interest using protein precipitation to separate high-molecular-weight compounds such as fibrinogen and γ-globulins before the first chromatography step. Combination of anion and cation exchange chromatography is often used to obtain a higher degree of protein purity. Ion exchange methods separate proteins based upon difference in charge. Anion exchange columns (such as DEAE or Source Q) bind negatively charged proteins, while cation exchange columns (such as Mono S) bind positively charged proteins. The adsorption of the protein to an ion exchange matrix depends on the net charge of the protein, which is dependent on the pH of the buffer phase. By adjusting the pH, the protein is negatively charged if $pH > $ isoelectric point (pI) and positively charged if $pH < pI$. The pI (isoelectric point = pH at which a protein carries no net charge) of a specific protein depends on its functional groups and amino acid composition. The pI of human C3 was determined as ~5.9 [22] and mouse C3 pI ~ 6.0 [23]. Thus, ion exchange chromatography can be specifically optimized for a target molecule to allow for optimal resolution from contaminants and elution at specific ionic strength. The protein will bind to the ion exchanger matrix when it carries a net charge opposite to that of the ion exchanger. Such binding is reversible at high concentration of salt solution (e.g., sodium chloride (NaCl)), and the proteins bound to the anion or cation exchanger are displaced by the chloride ion (Cl^-) or sodium ion (Na^+), respectively. By changing the ionic strength using a linear salt gradient the proteins bound to the ion exchange matrix are eluted differentially according to their net charge at a set pH.

One of the standard techniques in complement research is the hemolysis assay. Complement activation can be directly monitored through the complement-mediated lysis of red blood cells (RBCs). RBCs can be "sensitized" to complement attack using a species-specific antibody. Sheep RBCs coated with anti-sheep erythrocyte antibody (hemolysin) have traditionally been used to assay the activity of the complement classical pathway in human serum. Rabbit RBCs spontaneously activate the human alternative complement pathway and in the absence of Ca^{2+} can be used to exclusively study the alternative pathway. Rabbit RBCs lack membrane-bound regulators such as DAF, CR1, or CD59. Antibody-"sensitized" rabbit RBCs are also used to study mouse complement [24–26]. To determine the activity of C3, purified C3 is added back to C3-depleted serum to physiological concentration (human or mouse). C3-depleted sera can be obtained via two methods, one by chemically mediated C3 inactivation (hydrolysis) using chaotropic reagents (C3-depleted serum also known as R3) or by immunoaffinity chromatography-based removal of C3 [27]. Serum from gene-targeted C3-deficient mice can be used to assess functional activity of mouse C3.

C3 activity can be assayed as a measure of CH50 (classical pathway, 50 % hemolytic activity) or AH50 (alternative pathway,

50 % hemolytic activity). Highly purified C3 (removed hydrolyzed and aggregated C3) can be further studied in specific hemolysis assays designed to assay a specific interaction, such as C3 convertase formation, decay acceleration by DAF or fH, or fH cofactor activity [28]. In the context of this chapter, hemolysis assays are used for quality control purified C3 to determine the degree of active (non-hydrolyzed) C3 in a sample.

2 Materials

2.1 Plasma

All human blood products are potentially hazardous; treat any sample according to health and safety standards.

2.2 Chromatography Reagents and Equipment

All purification procedures are performed with freshly prepared and sterile filtered (0.2 μm) buffer solutions and plasma.

1. DEAE/Source Q—anion exchange buffers.

   Buffer A: 10 mM Potassium phosphate (KH_2PO_4), 5 mM ethylenediaminetetraacetic acid disodium salt (EDTA), 1 mM benzamidine, pH 7.8 in dH_2O (*see* **Note 1**).

   Buffer B: 10 mM Potassium phosphate (KH_2PO_4), 5 mM EDTA, 1 mM benzamidine, 1 M sodium chloride (NaCl), pH 7.8 in dH_2O.
2. Mono S/Source S—cation exchange buffers

   Buffer A: 50 mM Sodium phosphate (NaH_2PO_4) for human C3 and 20 mM NaH_2PO_4 for mouse C3, pH 6 in dH_2O.

   Buffer B: 50 mM Sodium phosphate (NaH_2PO_4) for human C3, 20 mM NaH_2PO_4 for mouse C3, 1 M sodium chloride (NaCl), pH 6 in dH_2O.
3. SD200—size exclusion/gel filtration buffers.

   Buffer A (isocratic elution): Phosphate-buffered saline (PBS), pH 7 for storage or complement fixation diluent (CFD) for use in functional hemolysis assays.
4. HiPrep DEAE FF 16/10 (20 ml column volume, CV), weak anion exchanger, running flow rate: 2 ml/min, column pressure limit: 0.3 MPa. Column binding capacity: ~100 mg protein (see Note 2).
5. Mono S 5/50 GL (1 ml column volume), strong cation exchanger, running flow rate: 1 ml/min, column pressure limit: 4 MPa. Column binding capacity: ~10 mg protein (*see* **Note 3**).
6. Superdex 200 (SD200) 10/300 GL (24 ml column volume), Spherical composite of cross-linked agarose and dextran,

running flow rate: 0.5 ml/min, column pressure limit: 1 MPa, MW separation range: 10–600 kDa. Recommended injection capacity: <2 % of column volume.

7. Source 15Q (20 ml column volume), strong anion exchanger, running flow rate: 2 ml/min, column pressure limit: 1.2 MPa. Column binding capacity: 100 mg protein.
8. Fast protein liquid chromatography (FPLC) or protein purifier system (e.g., Akta Systems).
9. Other equipment: 50 ml Superloop, 100–500 μl loop (see Note 4), centrifuge (e.g., Sorvall®Legend RT), pH meter, UV spectrophotometer, magnetic stirrer, concentrators, −80 °C freezer for storage, 10–30 kDa molecular weight cutoff dialysis tubing, syringes, syringe filters (0.2 μm), and vacuum filter unit.

2.3 SDS-PAGE Reagents and Equipment

1. 10 % Acrylamide gels.
2. Reducing gel loading buffer: 1 M Tris, 10 % (v/v) glycerol, 2 % (w/v) SDS, 0.01 % bromophenol blue, 100 mM dithiothreitol (DTT), pH 6.8 in dH2O.
3. Gel tank and voltage apparatus.
4. Pre-stained protein marker, e.g., broad range 7–175 kDa (New England BioLabs).
5. Gel running buffer: 25 mM Tris, 191 mM glycine, 1 % (w/v) SDS in dH2O.
6. Coomassie Blue stain: 0.2 % (w/v) Coomassie Blue R250 in 45 % (v/v) methanol, 10 % (v/v) acetic acid in dH2O.
7. Destaining buffer: 20 % (v/v) Methanol, 8 % (v/v) acetic acid in dH2O.
8. A platform rocker is used for agitation of gels in solution.

2.4 Hemolysis Assay Reagents and Equipment

1. Flat and round-bottom 96-well plate.
2. Sheep and rabbit blood/Alsever's (whole blood with final concentration of Alsever's solution of 50 %).
3. Amboceptor/hemolysin, anti-sheep erythrocyte antibody.
4. Mouse anti-rabbit erythrocyte polyclonal serum [24].
5. Complement fixation diluent, CFD (4 mM sodium barbitone, 145 mM NaCl, 0.83 mM $MgCl_2$, 0.25 mM $CaCl_2$, pH 7.2).
6. C3-depleted human serum.
7. C3-deficient mouse serum.
8. Microplate reader with 415 ± 10 nm filter.

3 Methods

3.1 C3 Purification from Human Plasma

3.1.1 Collection of Plasma

1. Add 5 mM EDTA and 1 mM benzamidine immediately to fresh blood.
2. Centrifuge the blood at 2,602 × *g* for 15 min at 4 °C to separate plasma from cell pellet.
3. Remove plasma supernatant carefully (cell pellet is very loose) and filter using a 0.2 μm sterile filter; always store on ice (*see* **Notes 5** and **6**).

3.1.2 Na_2SO_4 Precipitation

The purpose of this step is to remove high-molecular-weight compounds from the plasma prior to protein purification.

1. Measure the volume of plasma, and add 10 % (w/v) Na_2SO_4 (anhydrous) as powdered salt crystals (e.g., 200 ml plasma, add 20 g Na2SO4) slowly to the protein solution while stirring (magnetic stirrer); leave to stir at 4 °C for 2 h.
2. Spin the precipitate using a Sorvall Ultracentrifuge (26,892 × g, break1, 30 min, 4 °C). Remove supernatant, and measure volume.
3. Transfer supernatant into dialysis tubing (see Notes 6 and 7) and dialyze into 5 l DEAE buffer A. Buffer exchange with fresh 5 l after 2 h; for best result, dialyze overnight at 4 °C.
4. Measure dialysate volume, determine A280 (see Note 8), and measure conductivity to verify completion of dialysis (if conductivity meter is available, see Note 9). If solution is cloudy or precipitate, remove precipitates by centrifugation at 2,602 × g for 15 min at 4 °C.
5. Filter dialysate through a 0.2 μm filter prior to purification. Keep the sample on ice.

3.1.3 Anion Exchange Chromatography

The purpose of this step is to remove major contaminants and isolate C3 (*see* **Note 10**).

1. *Preparing the column*: The DEAE column is commonly stored in 20 % ethanol; therefore, equilibrate the column first into H_2O for 2 column volumes at a flow rate of 1 ml/min and maximum pressure of 0.3 MPa, and then equilibrate for 2 column volumes in running buffer A at a flow rate of 2 ml/min.
2. Equilibrate with running buffer A for 1 column volume at a flow rate of 2 ml/min and maximum pressure of 0.3 MPa.
3. Inject the dialysate (Subheading 3.1.2) via a Superloop, or when the injection volume exceeds 50 ml, use direct sample loading using a system-integrated sample pump system. Set injection volume to 50–100 ml (within protein binding capacity of the column), and collect the run-through.

4. Wash column with buffer A for 4 column volumes to remove any unbound protein.
5. Elute bound proteins with a linear gradient from 0 to 35 % buffer B over 15 column volumes. Monitor the eluent at 280 nm (*see* **Note 11**).
6. Clean the column with 3 column volumes of 100 % elution buffer B.
7. Re-equilibrate by washing with 3 column volumes of buffer A. Collect 4 ml fractions throughout gradient elution (*see* **Notes 12** and **13**).
8. Analyze fractions across the gradient using SDS-PAGE (Subheading 3.3) and hemolysis assay (Subheading 3.4).
9. Pool the C3-containing fractions, and determine A_{280} (*see* Fig.1a; **Note 14**).
10. Dialyze pooled fractions into 2 l Mono S buffer A for 2 h at 4 °C (*see* **Note 15**).

3.1.4 Cation Exchange Chromatography

The purpose of this step is to remove hydrolyzed C3 ($C3_{H2O}$).

1. *Preparing the column*: The Mono S column is commonly stored in 20 % ethanol, equilibrate the column in H_2O for 5 column volumes at a flow rate of 0.5 ml/min and maximum pressure limit of 4 MPa, and then equilibrate for 5 column volumes in Mono S running buffer A at a flow rate of 1 ml/min.
2. Equilibrate with running buffer A for 5 column volumes at a flow rate 1 ml/min and maximum pressure of 4 MPa.
3. Inject DEAE dialysate (Subheading 3.1.3) via 50 ml Superloop.
4. Wash column in buffer A for 10 column volumes.
5. Elute proteins with a linear gradient from 0 to 50 % buffer B over 30 column volumes. Monitor the eluent at 280 nm.
6. Clean the column with 5 column volumes of elution buffer B.
7. Re-equilibrate by washing with buffer A for 5 column volumes (see Note 13).
8. Collect 2 ml fractions throughout the gradient elution.
9. Analyze fractions across major peak(s) using SDS-PAGE (Subheading 3.3) and hemolysis assay (Subheading 3.4), and upon C3 confirmation, pool peak center fractions (Fig 1b). Determine A_{280} (*see* **Note 16**).

3.1.5 Gel Filtration/Size Exclusion Chromatography

The purpose of this step is to remove C3 aggregates.

1. *Preparing the column*: Column is commonly stored in 20 % ethanol; therefore, equilibrate the column in H_2O for 1 column volume at a flow rate of 0.25 ml/min, and then

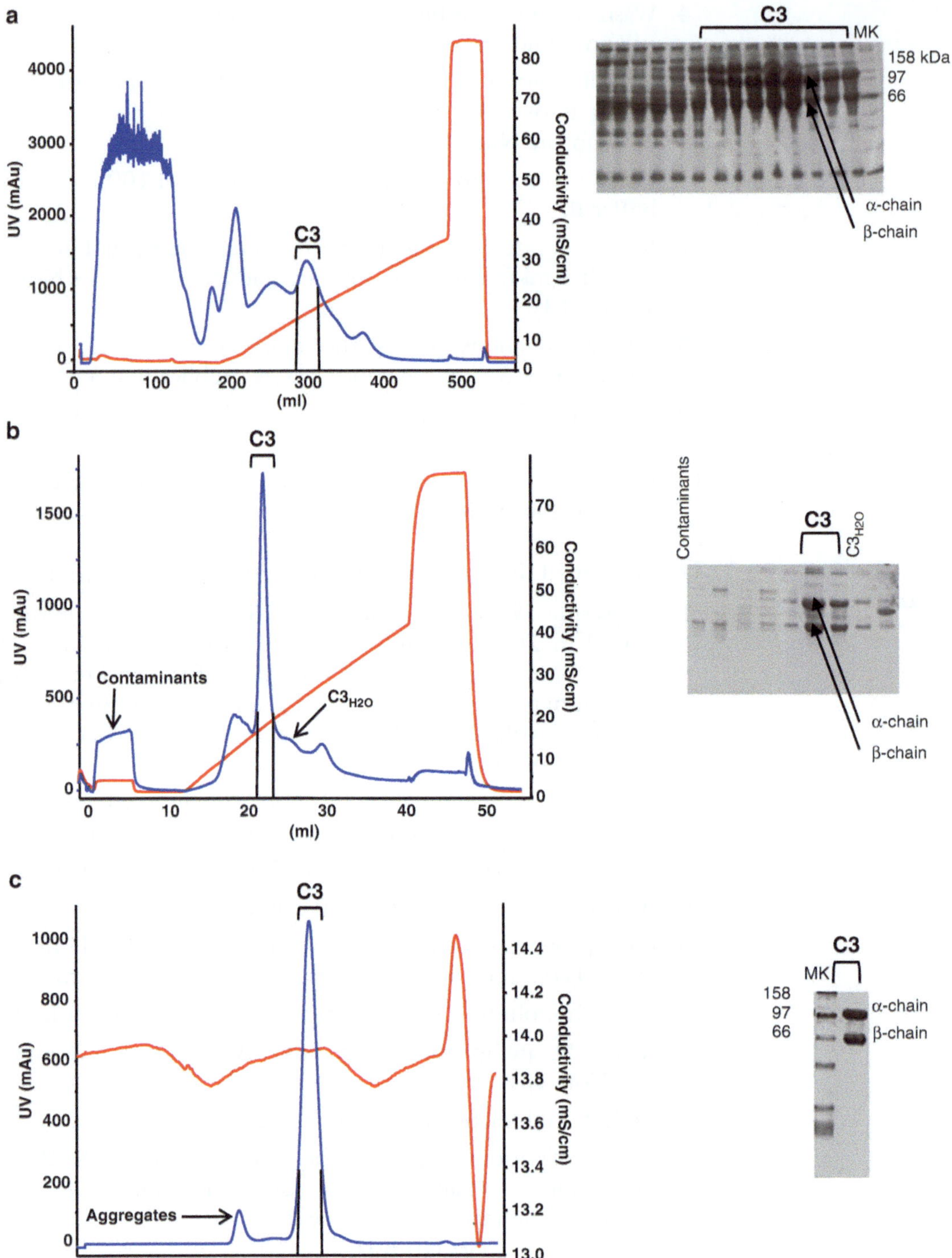

Fig. 1 Purification of human C3: (**a**) Anion exchange chromatography—C3 is isolated via a linear gradient from 0 to 35 % buffer B (10 mM potassium phosphate (KH_2PO_4), 5 mM EDTA, 1 mM benzamidine, 1 M sodium chloride (NaCl), pH 7.8 in dH_2O) over 15 column volumes, monitored as a change in conductivity (*red line*). C3 fractions are pooled as indicated (*horizontal black lines*) and confirmed on a reduced 10 % SDS-PAGE gel (*insert*) using Coomassie staining. C3 α- and β-chain are indicated with *arrows*. (**b**) Cation exchange

equilibrate 1 column volume in running buffer at a flow rate of 0.5 ml/min and maximum pressure of 1 MPa.

2. Equilibrate the column with running buffer A for 1 column volume at a flow rate of 0.5 ml/min and maximum pressure of 1 MPa.
3. Inject 100–500 μl sample manually via a 100–500 μl loop (see Note 17).
4. Elute proteins with isocratic elution in buffer A for 1.5 column volumes. Collect 0.5 ml fractions throughout (see Note 13).
5. Visualize C3 in peak fractions by SDS-PAGE (Fig. 1d; Subheading 3.3). Pool the peak center C3 fractions, and determine A_{280}. Use sample immediately in functional assays.

3.2 C3 Purification from Mouse Plasma

3.2.1 Collection of Plasma

1. Collect mouse blood into a tube containing 10 mM EDTA.
2. Centrifuge the blood at 12,470 × *g* for 15 min using a bench-top centrifuge.
3. Remove the plasma supernatant. Keep at −80 °C for long-term storage (*see* **Note 5**).

3.2.2 PEG 4000 Precipitation

1. Stir the mouse EDTA-plasma and add 20 % (w/v) PEG 4000 dissolved in Source Q buffer A dropwise to achieve a 4 % PEG cut (*see* **Note 18**). Stir for 1 h at 4 °C.
2. Centrifuge PEG cut at 16,900 × g for 15 min at 4 °C.
3. Discard the pellet.
4. Add a measured amount of 20 % PEG solution to the supernatant while stirring to achieve a final 15 % cut (see Note 18). Stir the mixture for 1 h at 4 °C.
5. Centrifuge the mixture at 16,900 × g for 15 min at 4 °C.
6. Discard the supernatant.
7. Resuspend the pellet to the original plasma volume in Source Q buffer A (for mouse C3).

Fig. 1 (continued) chromatography—pooled C3 fractions (**a**) are separated from contaminants (run-through) and $C3_{H2O}$ (indicated by *arrow*) on a linear gradient from 0 to 50 % buffer B (50 mM sodium phosphate (NaH_2PO_4), 1 M sodium chloride (NaCl), pH 6 in dH_2O, monitored as a change in conductivity (*red line*). C3 fractions are pooled as indicated (*horizontal black lines*) and confirmed on a reduced 10 % SDS-PAGE gel (insert) using Coomassie staining. C3 α- and β-Chain are indicated with *arrows*. (**c**) Gel filtration chromatography—pooled C3 fractions (**b**) are separated from C3 aggregates (indicated by *arrow*) using isocratic elution. C3 fractions of the peak center are pooled as indicated (*horizontal black lines*) and confirmed on a reduced 10 % SDS-PAGE gel (*insert*) using Coomassie staining. C3 α- and β-chain are indicated with *arrows*

3.2.3 Anion Exchange Chromatography

Prepare Source Q column as described for DEAE column.

1. Equilibrate with Source Q buffer A for 1 column volume at a flow rate of 2 ml/min and maximum pressure of 1.2 MPa.
2. Inject the sample using a 50 ml Superloop (see Note 8).
3. Wash the column with buffer A for 4 column volumes.
4. Elute the proteins with a linear gradient from 0 to 50 % Source Q buffer B over 15 column volumes at a flow rate of 2 ml/min. Collect 3 ml fractions, and monitor the eluent at 280 nm (see Note 12).
5. Clean the column with 100 % of Source Q buffer B over 3 column volumes.
6. Re-equilibrate with 3 column volumes of buffer A (see Note 13).
7. Identify the fractions containing C3 by SDS-PAGE (Subheading 3.3) and classical pathway hemolysis assay (Subheading 3.4). Pool the fractions containing C3 (Fig. 2a–c), and dialyze the sample in 2 l of Mono S buffer for 1 h at 4 °C (*see* **Notes 6** and 7).

3.2.4 Cation Exchange Chromatography

Prepare the Mono S column as described before.

1. Equilibrate with running buffer A for 5 column volumes at a flow rate of 1 ml/min and maximum pressure of 4 MPa.
2. Inject dialysate (Subheading 3.2.3, step 2) via a 50 ml Superloop (see Note 8).
3. Wash column in buffer A for 10 column volumes.
4. Elute proteins with a linear gradient from 0 to 50 % buffer B over 30 column volumes. Monitor the eluent at 280 nm. Collect 1 ml fractions throughout the gradient elution.
5. Clean the column with buffer B over 4 column volumes.

Fig. 2 (continued) Fractions positive for C3 on SDS-PAGE and adjacent fractions were analyzed on hemolysis assay. ***RbEA*** are incubated with C3-deficient mouse serum, and fraction samples are added. Fractions from C6 to C11 (*bold*) are able to restore complement activity of the C3-deficient serum and were processed further. (**d**) Chromatogram of the cation exchange of mouse C3. Source Q fractions C6–C11 are pooled, dialyzed against 20 mM NaP04 pH 6.0 buffer, and loaded onto Mono S column. The proteins are separated using an increasing salt gradient, monitored as a change in percentage elution buffer (buffer B; *red*). (**e**) SDS-PAGE analysis of the Mono S fractions. The elution fractions are loaded along with a protein sample before being loaded on the column (pre-Mono S) from 10 % gel under reducing conditions. The protein is visualized by staining with Coomassie Blue. The fraction number is shown above each lane. Fractions A13–A15 show typical C3 profile. α- and β-Chains are indicated with *arrows*. (**f**) *Hemolytic activity of Mono S fractions*. Fractions positive for C3 on SDS-PAGE and adjacent fractions are analyzed in hemolysis assay. ***RbEA*** are incubated with C3-deficient mouse serum and fraction samples. Fractions from A13 to A15 (*bold*) are able to restore complement activity of the C3-deficient serum. Dialyze C3-containing fractions against PBS and store at −80 °C until needed

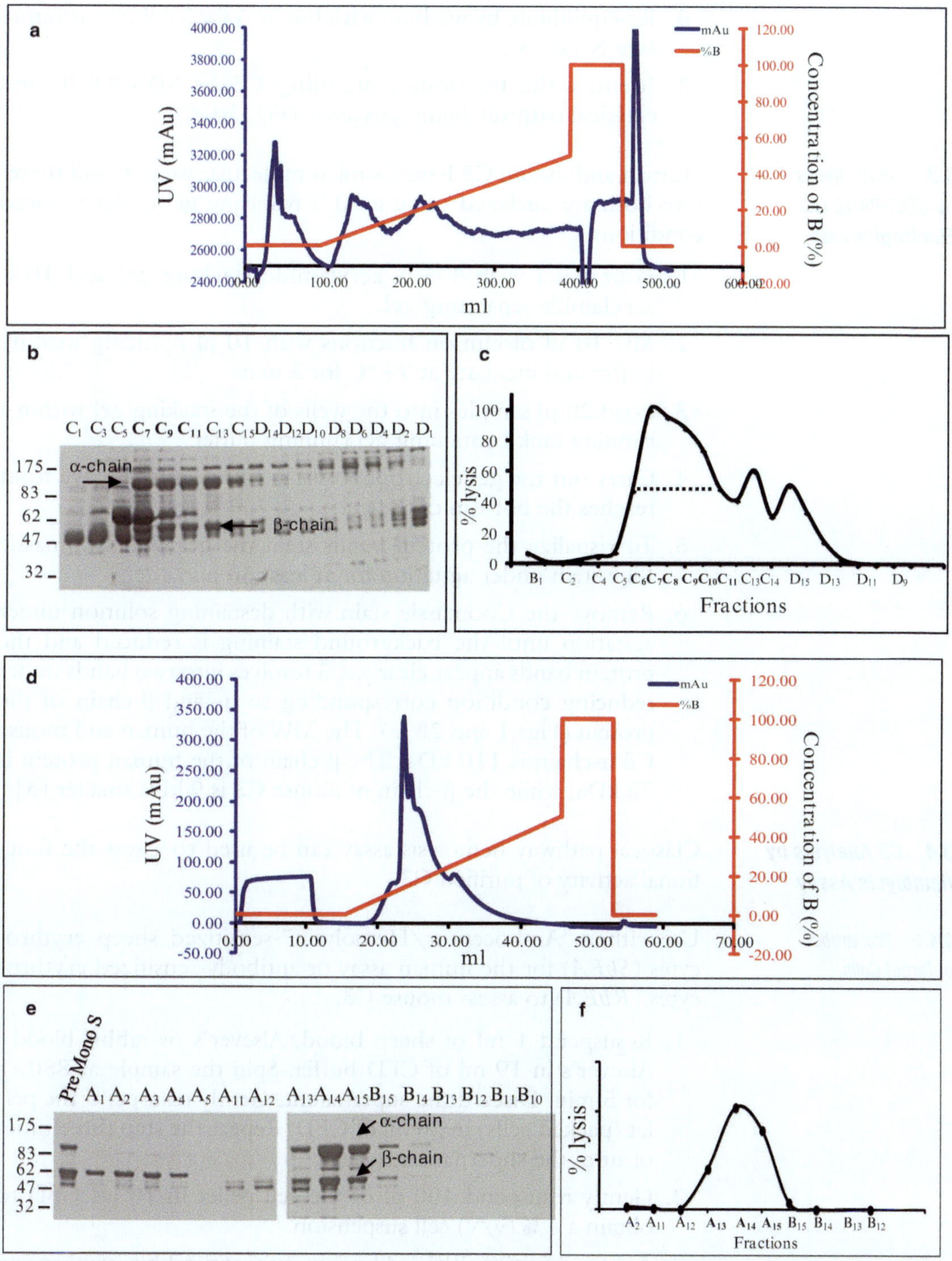

Fig. 2 Purification of mouse C3. (**a**) Chromatogram of the anion exchange of mouse C3. The product from the 15 % cut of mouse plasma is loaded onto Source Q column. The proteins are separated using an increasing salt gradient, monitored as a change in percentage elution buffer (buffer B; *red*). (**b**) SDS-PAGE analysis of the Source Q fractions. The elution fractions are loaded on 10 % gel under reducing conditions. The protein is visualized by staining with Coomassie Blue. The fraction number is shown above each lane. Fractions C7–C11 show typical C3 profile. α- and β-chains are indicated with *arrows*. (**c**) Hemolytic activity of Source Q fractions.

6. Re-equilibrate by washing with buffer A for 5 column volumes (see Note 13).
7. Identify the fractions containing C3 by SDS-PAGE and classical pathway hemolysis assay (Fig. 2d–f).

3.3 C3 Analysis by SDS-PAGE Gel Electrophoresis

Human and mouse C3 have a similar molecular weight, and therefore both are analyzed using a 10 % resolving gel under reduced conditions.

1. Pour a gel with 4–5 % acrylamide stacking gel and 10 % acrylamide separating gel.
2. Mix 10 μl of elution fractions with 10 μl reducing loading buffer and incubate at 99 °C for 2 min.
3. Load 20 μl samples into the wells of the stacking gel within a running tank containing gel running buffer.
4. Carry out the gel electrophoresis at 200 V until the dye front reaches the bottom of the gel.
5. To visualize the protein bands stain the gel with Coomassie Blue stain under agitation for at least 30 min.
6. Remove the Coomassie stain with destaining solution under agitation until the background staining is reduced and the protein bands appear clearly. C3 resolves into two bands under reducing condition corresponding to α- and β-chain of the protein (Figs.1 and 2b, e). The MW of the human and mouse C3 α-chain is 110 kDa. The β-chain of the human protein is 75 kDa, while the β-chain of mouse C3 is 9 kDa smaller [5].

3.4 C3 Analysis by Hemolysis Assay

Classical pathway hemolysis assay can be used to assess the functional activity of purified C3.

3.4.1 Preparation of Target Cells

Use either "Amboceptor/Hemolysin"-sensitized sheep erythrocytes (***ShEA***) for the human assay or antibody-sensitized erythrocytes (***RbEA***) to assess mouse C3.

1. Resuspend 1 ml of sheep blood/Alsever's or rabbit blood/Alsever's in 19 ml of CFD buffer. Spin the sample at 850 × *g* for 5 min. Discard the supernatant. Gently resuspend the pellet (packed cells) in 20 ml of CFD. Repeat the step three times or until the supernatant is clear.
2. Gently resuspend 400 μl of the cell pellet in 10 ml CFD to obtain a 4 % (v/v) cell suspension.
3. A) To sensitize RbE, dilute mouse anti-rabbit erythrocyte antiserum 1/500 in 10 ml preheated (37 °C) CFD (*see* **Note 19**), add to 10 ml 4 % cell suspension, and incubate for 30 min at room temperature under agitation. B) To sensitize ShE, add 5 μl Amboceptor/Hemolysin to 10 ml preheated (37 °C) CFD (*see* **Note 19**). Mix the Amboceptor solution (10 ml)

with 4 % ShE cell suspension (10 ml) and incubate at 37 °C for 30 min.

4. Wash the sensitized cells (***ShEA*** or ***RbEA***) in CFD by centrifugation at 850 × g for 5 min.
5. Resuspend the ***ShEA*** or ***RbEA*** pellet in CFD (20 ml) to 2 % final cell suspension.

3.4.2 Activity of Human C3

1. Thaw one aliquot of C3-depleted serum swiftly at 37 °C and store on ice.
2. Dilute C3-depleted (neat) serum 1/50 in CFD by adding 1 μl C3-depleted serum in 50 μl CFD.
3. Add 50 μl of the 1/50 diluted serum into each well of a round-bottom microtitre plate (4.8 ml of 1/50 diluted serum is required per 96-well plate).
4. Add 20 μl of each elution fraction to be screened to each well containing C3-depleted serum, then add 30 μl CFD, and then add 50 μl ***ShEA***. The total volume should be 150 μl per microtitre well.
5. In separate wells on the same plate add 50 μl ***ShEA*** to 100 μl 0.01 % Triton in dH2O as 100 % lysis positive control. For 0 % lysis negative control, add 50 μl ***ShEA*** to 100 μl CFD.
6. Cover plate with a plastic film seal, mix briefly on plate shaker, and incubate at 37 °C for 30–45 min. Check progress of cell lysis visually at regular time intervals (every 5–10 min).
7. Centrifuge plate at 423 × *g* for 3 min, to separate cells from supernatant (*see* **Note 20**).
8. Remove 100 μl supernatant from each well using a (multichannel) pipette (carefully not to disturb cell pellet) and transfer directly into a flat-bottom 96-well plate.
9. Read absorbance values at 415 nm (hemoglobin release), and calculate percentage lysis as follows (*see* **Note 21**):

$$\%\ lysis = 100 \times \left(Test_{A415} - 0\%_{A415}\right) / \left(100\%_{A415} - 0\%_{A415}\right)$$

3.4.3 Activity of Mouse C3

1. Add 50 μl ***RbEA*** to 22 % (final) C3-deficient mouse serum (45 μl), and then add 5 μl of each elution fraction in a round-bottom 96-well plate (*see* **Note 22**).
2. In a separate well mix ***RbEA*** (50 μl) with 50 μl of 0.01 % Triton (v/v) for 100 % lysis positive control. For 0 % lysis negative control, add 50 μl ***RbEA*** to 50 μl CFD.
3. Cover the plate with a plastic film seal. Shake plate briefly on plate shaker and incubate for 30 min at 37 °C.
4. Spin the plate at 423 × g for 5 min (see Note 20).

5. Transfer 80 μl supernatant from each well into a flat-bottom 96-well plate without disturbing the cell pellet.
6. Measure absorbance at 415 nm, and calculate percentage lysis as described for human C3.

4 Notes

1. It is crucial for classical chromatography methods to determine the pH of the buffers accurately using a three-digit pH meter.
2. Alternatively use HiPrep Q FF 16/10 or Source 15Q.
3. For scale-up use Source 15S.
4. Large sample volumes can be injected over the column using an automated purification system via an integrated sample pump or a 50 ml Superloop. Small sample volumes can be injected using a 100–500 μl loop.
5. Using freshly isolated plasma will increase the final C3 yield. If necessary, EDTA-plasma can be stored at −80 °C until further use. Avoid repeated freeze-thawing to avoid spontaneous hydrolysis of the C3 intramolecular thioester bond [29].
6. We have observed that we yield more active protein when performing all separation steps in the cold (4 °C) and as swift as possible. Precipitation, centrifugation, dialysis, and chromatography should be performed at 4 °C. Alternatively, handle the plasma, protein precipitates, and C3 preparations on ice, whenever possible.
7. Leave extra space in dialysis tubing as volume expands (approximately 30 %) inside the dialyzing tube due to high salt content.
8. Determine A_{280} to estimate total protein content prior to ion exchange chromatography to adjust the injection volume. Do not exceed the binding capacity of the column.
9. Use a conductivity meter (if available) to determine sufficient dialysis into low-ionic-strength buffers. Final conductivity of the sample solution should be equal to the conductivity of the running buffer A of the next purification step.
10. The plasma protein plasminogen is easily activated to plasmin in vitro, which is capable of cleaving C3 into activation fragment C3b, decreasing the yield of purified, active C3. For this purpose, one can include a purification step before the protein precipitation step, removing plasminogen from EDTA-plasma using a lysine-Sepharose column.
11. Benzamidine by itself gives a high absorbance at 280 nm; monitor the eluent at 290 nm (if available).

12. Collect fractions from the autosampler unit, keep on ice, and screen and process as swiftly as possible to reduce C3 degradation.
13. When finished with purification prepare the column for storage. Wash with 5 column volumes of double-distilled H_2O followed by 5 column volumes of 20 % ethanol. Store in 20 % ethanol at 4 °C.
14. At this stage of the separation, the buffer and salt concentration of the pooled C3 fractions is suitable for storage at −80 °C.
15. Sample/dialysis solution ratio should be approximately 1/100 (v/v). Dialysis needs to be as brief as possible (do not exceed 2 h) as we have observed protein precipitation and a drop in C3 yield with prolonged dialysis. We recommend using spin dialyzers at this stage for volumes <50 ml.
16. Active C3 peak should elute just before the $C3_{H2O}$ peak on the gradient (Fig.1b).
17. Choose an injection volume that is less than 2 % of the column volume for good peak resolution. To do so, concentrate the sample before the gel filtration step. Concentration tenfold higher than the desired final protein concentration is recommended.
18. To calculate how much PEG solution is required to achieve the desired percentage concentration of PEG in the plasma sample use the following equation:

    X ml PEG solution $= ((C_f - C_s) \times V)/(C_{stock} - C_f)$, where

    C_f—final PEG concentration

    C_s—start PEG concentration

    C_{stock}—concentration of the stock solution (e.g., 20 %)

    V—plasma volume
19. Use the maximum concentration of the antibody, which does not cause cell agglutination. The dilution factor is usually established in preliminary experiments and could vary between preparations and batches. The working dilution range established in our laboratory was 1:250–1:1,000 for the mouse anti-rabbit erythrocyte antiserum and 1:2,000–1:4,000 for the Amboceptor.
20. A round cell pellet of non-lysed cells should be seen at the bottom of the round-bottom plate in the absence of C3.
21. Cell lysis in fractions obtained from the beginning of the elution gradient where the conductivity is below 5 Ms/cm might be due to low-ionic-strength buffer effect rather than C3 activity.
22. Use fresh serum (if possible) from male mice when performing classical pathway hemolysis assays. Repeated freezing-thawing markedly reduces mouse complement activity [30].

Acknowledgments

The methods and protocols described in this chapter were derived and optimized in the laboratory of Dr. Claire L Harris and Prof. B Paul Morgan (School of Medicine, Cardiff University, United Kingdom).

References

1. de Bruijn MH, Fey GH (1985) Human complement component C3: cDNA coding sequence and derived primary structure. Proc Natl Acad Sci U S A 82:708–712
2. Lundwall A, Wetsel RA, Domdey H et al (1984) Structure of murine complement component C3. I. Nucleotide sequence of cloned complementary and genomic DNA coding for the beta chain. J Biol Chem 259:13851–13856
3. Wetsel RA, Lundwall A, Davidson F et al (1984) Structure of murine complement component C3. II. Nucleotide sequence of cloned complementary DNA coding for the alpha chain. J Biol Chem 259:13857–13862
4. Wetsel R (1995) Structure, function and cellular expression of complement anaphylatoxin receptors. Curr Opin Immunol 7:48–53
5. Nonaka M, Natsuume-Sakai S, Kaidoh T et al (1980) Characterization of allotypic determinants of murine complement C3. J Immunol 125:2025–2030
6. Pangburn MK, Schreiber RD, Müller-Eberhard HJ (1981) Formation of the initial C3 convertase of the alternative complement pathway. Acquisition of C3b-like activities by spontaneous hydrolysis of the putative thioester in native C3. J Exp Med 154:856–867
7. Amara U, Rittirsch D, Flierl M et al (2008) Interaction between the coagulation and complement system. Adv Exp Med Biol 632:71–79
8. Brodbeck W, Mold C, Atkinson J et al (2000) Cooperation between decay-accelerating factor and membrane cofactor protein in protecting cells from autologous complement attack. J Immunol 165:3999–4006
9. Lublin DM, Atkinson JP (1989) Decay-accelerating factor: biochemistry, molecular biology, and function. Annu Rev Immunol 7:35–58
10. Nicholson-Weller A, Wang C (1994) Structure and function of decay accelerating factor CD55. J Lab Clin Med 123:485–491
11. Nicholson-Weller A, Burge J, Fearon DT et al (1982) Isolation of a human erythrocyte membrane glycoprotein with decay-accelerating activity for C3 convertases of the complement system. J Immunol 129:184–189
12. Pangburn MK, Schreiber RD, Muller-Eberhard HJ (1977) Human complement C3b inactivator: isolation, characterization, and demonstration of an absolute requirement for the serum protein beta1H for cleavage of C3b and C4b in solution. J Exp Med 146:257–270
13. Weiler JM, Daha MR, Austen KF et al (1976) Control of the amplification convertase of complement by the plasma protein beta1H. Proc Natl Acad Sci U S A 73:3268–3272
14. Morgan BP, Harris CL (1999) Complement regulatory proteins. Academic, San Diego, London
15. Fearon D (1980) Identification of the membrane glycoprotein that is the C3b receptor of the human erythrocyte, polymorphonuclear leukocyte, B lymphocyte, and monocyte. J Exp Med 152:20–30
16. Ross G, Medof M (1985) Membrane complement receptors specific for bound fragments of C3. Adv Immunol 37:217–267
17. Ross G, Lambris J, Cain J et al (1982) Generation of three different fragments of bound C3 with purified factor I or serum. I. Requirements for factor H vs. CR1 cofactor activity. J Immunol 129:2051–2060
18. Foley S, Li B, Dehoff M et al (1993) Mouse Crry/p65 is a regulator of the alternative pathway of complement activation. Eur J Immunol 23:1381–1384
19. Kim YU, Kinoshita T, Molina H et al (1995) Mouse complement regulatory protein Crry/p65 uses the specific mechanisms of both human decay-accelerating factor and membrane cofactor protein. J Exp Med 181:151–159
20. van Lookeren Campagne M, Wiesmann C, Brown EJ (2007) Macrophage complement receptors and pathogen clearance. Cell Microbiol 9:2095–2102
21. Harrison R (1996) Purification, assay, characterization of complement proteins from plasma in handbook of experimental immunology. In: Leonore A. Herzenberg (ed) Cell surface and messenger molecules of the immune system, Donald M. Weir/co-editors, vol 2, 5th edn, Caroline Blackwell. edn, Blackwell Science, Cambridge
22. Koch C, Skjødt K, Laursen I (1985) A simple immunoblotting method after separation of

proteins in agarose gel. J Immunol Methods 84:271–278
23. Natsuume-Sakai S, Moriwaki K, Amano S et al (1979) Allotypes of C3 in laboratory and wild mouse distinguished by alloantisera. J Immunol 123:216–221
24. Ruseva MM, Hughes TR, Donev RM et al (2009) Crry deficiency in complement sufficient mice: C3 consumption occurs without associated renal injury. Mol Immunol 46:803–811
25. Morgan BP (2000) Complement methods and protocols. Humana, New York
26. van Dijk H, Rademaker PM, Willers JM (1980) Estimation of classical pathway of mouse complement activity by use of sensitized rabbit erythrocytes. J Immunol Methods 39: 257–268
27. Morgan BP (2000) Measurement of complement hemolytic activity, generation of complement-depleted sera, and production of hemolytic intermediates. Methods Mol Biol 150:61–71
28. Heurich M, Martínez-Barricarte R, Francis NJ et al (2011) Common polymorphisms in C3, factor B, and factor H collaborate to determine systemic complement activity and disease risk. Proc Natl Acad Sci U S A 108:8761–8766
29. Isenman DE, Kells DI, Cooper NR et al (1981) Nucleophilic modification of human complement protein C3: correlation of conformational changes with acquisition of C3b-like functional properties. Biochemistry 20:4458–4467
30. Lachmann PJ (2010) Preparing serum for functional complement assays. J Immunol Methods 352:195–197

Chapter 7

Purification of Human Complement Protein C5

Lars Sottrup-Jensen and Gregers Rom Andersen

Abstract

Complement C5 is cleaved by proteolysis in the terminal phase of complement activation generating the pro-inflammatory C5a and membrane attack complex nucleator C5b. Whereas purification of its paralogues C3 and C4 from plasma is relatively straightforward, C5 purification is more complicated due to the lower amounts present and overlaps with the much more abundant C3 during several chromatographic steps. Here we describe our procedure for purifying homogenous, monodisperse, and crystallizable C5.

Key words Ion exchange, Hydrophobic interaction, Gel filtration, Hydroxyapatite, Crystallization, Complement C3, Complement C5

1 Introduction

The C5 protein is a member of the complement system which contains approx. 50 plasma and membrane proteins [1]. C5 is structurally related to the complement proteins C3 and C4 and to the tetrameric plasma proteinase inhibitor α_2-macroglobulin [2]. C5 is a two-chain molecule containing a 115 kDa α-chain and a 75 kDa β-chain [3]. The three-dimensional structure of isolated C5 or in complex with the bacterial protein inhibitor SSL7 and cobra venom factor has been determined recently [4–6].

When activated by the $(C3b)_2Bb$ or the C3bC4bC2a complex C5 is converted to C5b. This occurs by cleaving off the C5a fragment which is the N-terminal 74 residues of the α-chain [7]. The anaphylatoxin C5a is a potent pro-inflammatory mediator that signals through the anaphylatoxin receptors C5aR and C5L2 expressed on a variety of immune and nonimmune cells [8]. C5b forms the focal point for assembly of the membrane attack complex. C6, C7, and C8 are first added sequentially to C5b followed by multiple copies of C9 to create an annular structure which is partially inserted in the membrane of a target cell. This leads to osmotic disturbances resulting in the death of the target cell [9].

Mihaela Gadjeva (ed.), *The Complement System: Methods and Protocols*, Methods in Molecular Biology, vol. 1100, DOI 10.1007/978-1-62703-724-2_7, © Springer Science+Business Media New York 2014

Several procedures exist for purification of human C5. In refs. 3, 10 chromatography on hydroxyapatite is used for the separation of C5 from the closely related C3. A large-scale procedure which also allows purification of several other complement proteins has been given [11]. Hydrophobic interaction chromatography for separation of C5 from C3 has also been used [12].

2 Materials

Outdated human plasma must be obtained from individual donors. The blood is anticoagulated by citrate/phosphate/dextrose. Individual plasma portions are 250–330 ml in volume. Water should have a specific conductivity of less than 0.055 μS cm^{-1} $(18\ M\Omega{\cdot}cm)^{-1}$ (*see* **Note 1**).

1. Buffer A: 20 mM Tris–HCl, 20 mM NaCl, 5 mM EDTA, 2 mM benzamidine (BZA), pH 7.7 (*see* **Note 2**).
2. Buffer B: KH_2PO_4, 100 mM KCl, 25 mM ε-aminocaproic acid, pH 7.4, 200 μg/l pancreatic trypsin inhibitor (PTI) adjusted to pH 7.4 with KOH.
3. Buffer C: 20 mM HepesNaOH, 100 mM NaCl, pH 7.5. Buffer C may also be made up from Tris–HCl.
4. Buffer C high salt: 20 mM HepesNaOH, 1 M NaCl, pH 7.5. This buffer may also be made up from Tris–HCl.
5. Buffer D: 20 mM Tris–HCl, pH 7.5.
6. Buffer D high salt: 20 mM Tris–HCl, 1 M Na_2SO_4, pH 7.5.
7. A solution of 50 % polyethylene glycol (PEG) is made from 1 kg PEG 6000 (Merck) and 1 l of water.
8. Resins: The resins DEAE Sepharose fast flow, Sephacryl S-300, MonoQ column (prepacked column 1×10 cm), Source 15PHE, and Bio-gel HT Gel Hydroxyapatite.

Do not add providers for the reagents or the resins—this is a publisher's requirement.

3 Methods

Please write the methods as commands in a present tense.

1. Outdated human plasma (approx. 300 ml) from two donors is thawed and kept separate. Dilute plasma with an equal volume of Buffer A.
2. Add PTI to 1 mg/l.
3. Add 50 % PEG solution dropwise to each plasma sample while keeping on ice with stirring. A total of 0.041 volume 50 % PEG is used to achieve a final PEG concentration of 2 %. Stir for 15 min.

4. Centrifuge at 2,600 × *g* (please convert the rpm to g) for 15 min 4 °C.

The volume of the supernatants is measured and with stirring on ice 0.11 volume of 50 % PEG is added dropwise. After all PEG solution has been added the suspensions are stirred for 10 min and centrifuged at 2,600 × *g* for 15 min (*see* **Note 3**).

Each precipitate is treated with 100 ml ice-cold Buffer A containing 10 mM BZA and 1 mg/ml PTI. It requires stirring for approx. 90 min on ice to dissolve the sticky precipitate (*see* **Note 4**).

The slightly unclear solutions are then pumped onto a 2.5 cm × 45 cm column packed with DEAE Sepharose fast flow and equilibrated with Buffer A. The column is operated in a cold room, and the flow rate is 150 ml/h. After loading the first portion of the solubilized 2–7 % PEG precipitate from the first portion of plasma, elution is continued with 50 ml Buffer A. Then the second portion is loaded, and finally the column is washed with 500 ml Buffer A (*see* **Note 5**).

The plasma proteins are eluted from the column using a 0–0.3 M linear gradient of NaCl in Buffer A (two times 750 ml in gradient jars or with a gradient pump). The flow rate is approx. 70 ml/h (*see* **Note 6**).

When approx. 1,200 ml effluent has been collected the column may be stripped with 1 M NaCl in Buffer A (300 ml) and re-equilibrated with Buffer A (500 ml). Figure 1 shows a typical

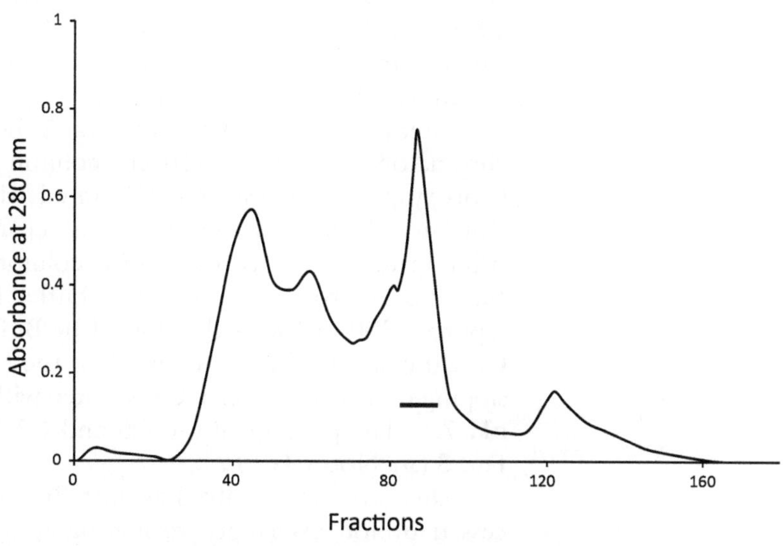

Fig. 1 Separation of the solubilized 2–7 % PEG precipitate of human plasma on a 2.5 cm × 45 cm column of DEAE Sepharose fast flow. The chromatogram shows the elution profile after loading the sample (2× 100 ml) and washing with Buffer A. The start of the gradient of NaCl is at fraction 1. At fraction 170 the column can be eluted with Buffer A containing 1 M NaCl (200 ml, and equilibrated with Buffer A (500 ml; elution profile not shown)). The light path of the UV 280 nm monitor was 2 mm. The fraction size is 8.5 ml. Fractions 84–93 (*bar*) containing the major part of C5 and C3 are pooled. The separation is done at 4–6 °C

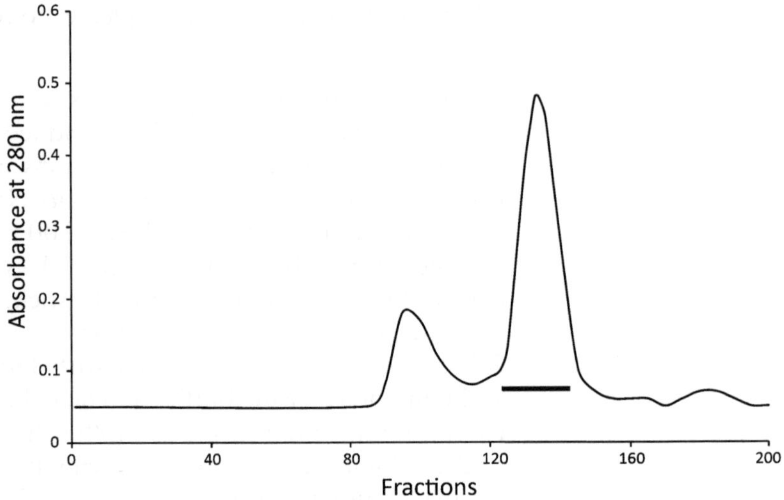

Fig. 2 Separation of the pool from DEAE Sepharose fast flow containing C5 and C3 (Fig. 1) on a 5 cm × 100 cm column of Sephacryl S-300 equilibrated and eluted with Buffer B. The flow rate is 70 ml/h, and the fraction size is 10 ml. The light path of the UV 280 nm monitor is 2 mm. Fractions 127–143 are pooled (*bar*). The separation is done at 4–6 °C

elution profile of the 2–7 % PEG fraction on DEAE Sepharose fast flow (*see* **Notes 7** and **8**).

The C3/C5 containing fractions are pooled as shown in Fig. 1, and the pool is next subjected to gel filtration chromatography on a 5 cm×100 cm column of Sephacryl S-300 as shown in Fig. 2. The column is operated in the cold room and is equilibrated and eluted with Buffer B (*see* **Note 9**).

After pooling as indicated in Fig. 2 the material is subjected to chromatography on a 5×10 cm column of hydroxyapatite. The hydroxyapatite column is equilibrated with the Buffer B. Upon elution with different buffers C5 is separated from C3 (Fig. 3). After loading the hydroxyapatite column it is first eluted with Buffer B (approx. 100 ml). Then buffer B containing 2 M NaCl (approx. 300 ml) is used followed by Buffer B (approx. 100 ml). C5 elutes with other proteins when the concentration of NaCl is sloping back towards zero. C3 is eluted with 150 mM K-phosphate, pH 7.4. The pooling of the C5 and C3 fractions is indicated on Fig. 3 (*see* **Notes 10–12**).

After overnight dialysis against Buffer C the C5 pool is processed by ion exchange chromatography on a MonoQ column (1 cm × 10 cm) operated at room temperature as shown in Fig. 4. The column is equilibrated with Buffer C. A linear gradient to 25 % of Buffer C containing additional 900 mM NaCl (1 M in total) in 20 min is used to elute C5 at a flow rate of 2 ml/min. After the gradient a 1-min step with 75 % high-salt Buffer C is used to elute some tightly bound proteins before equilibration with

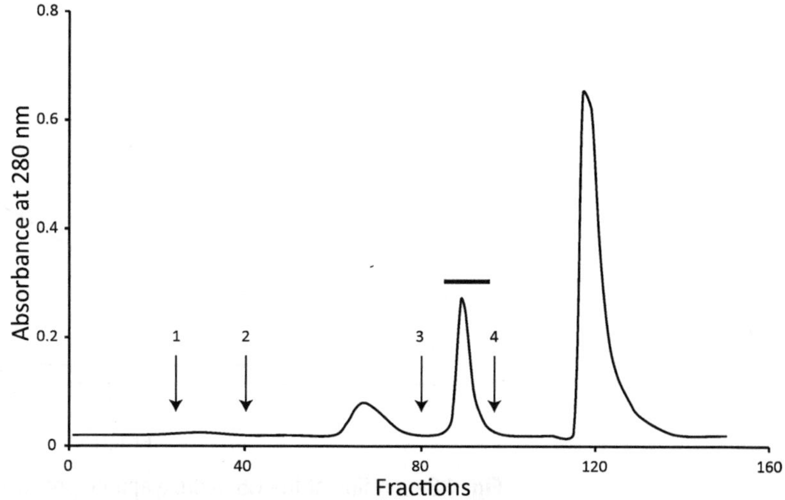

Fig. 3 Separation of the Sephacryl S-300 pool (Fig. 2) on a 5 cm × 10 cm column of hydroxyapatite. The column is equilibrated with Buffer B. After loading the sample the column is washed with Buffer B (*arrow 1*). Then Buffer B containing 2 M NaCl is introduced (*arrow 2*) followed by Buffer B (*arrow 3*). C5 elutes with other proteins in fractions 86–99 (*bar*) when the high NaCl concentration steeply decreases. C3 is eluted by 150 mM K-phosphate, pH 7.4 (*arrow 4*). The flow rate is 120 ml/h, and the fraction size is 10 ml. The light path of the UV 280 nm monitor is 2 mm. The separation is done at 4–6 °C

Buffer C. Due to the relatively high amount of protein present in the C5 pool several MonoQ runs are performed and the C5-containing fractions combined (*see* **Note 13**).

The final purification step for C5 is chromatography on a column of Source 15PHE (1 cm × 10 cm) at room temperature (Fig. 5). The C5 pool is made 0.5 M in Na_2SO_4 by addition of an equal volume of 1 M Na_2SO_4 in water. The column is equilibrated with 50 % high-salt Buffer D. After sample loading the column is eluted with 50 % high-salt Buffer D for a few minutes, and then a linear gradient to Buffer D in 20 min is employed. The flow rate is 2 ml/min. C5 is strongly bound to the column and elutes just before the concentration of Na_2SO_4 reaches zero. Several runs are made, and the fractions are combined (*see* **Notes 14–16**).

The yield of human C5 is 5–20 mg based on $E_{1\%280nm} = 1.08$ (approx. 11–45 %) from approx. 600 ml of human plasma. The yield of C3 is 300–400 mg based on $E_{1\%280\ nm} = 0.97$ (45–60 %). A single MonoQ step starting from the hydroxyapatite C3 pool will yield pure C3. C5 is dialyzed against Buffer C, concentrated on a Centricon device to approx. 1 mg/ml, divided in 1 ml portions, and flash frozen in liquid nitrogen. C3 is also flash frozen by pumping the solution such that drops fall into a beaker with liquid nitrogen. C5 and C3 are stored at −80 °C (*see* **Notes 17** and **18**).

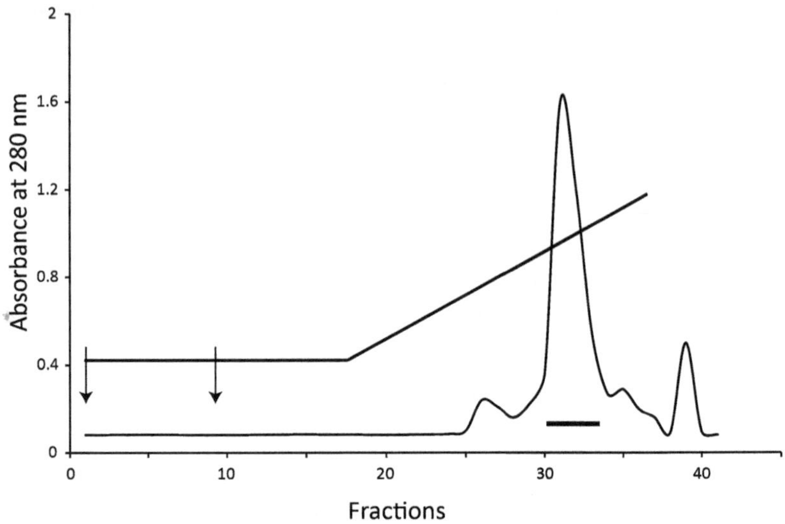

Fig. 4 Separation of the C5 hydroxyapatite pool (Fig. 3) on a 1 cm × 10 cm (8 ml) column of MonoQ equilibrated with Buffer C. Two 8 ml portions of the pooled material, dialyzed overnight against Buffer C, are sequentially loaded onto the column through an 18 ml sample loop (*arrows*). The column is eluted with a 20-min linear gradient of NaCl from Buffer C to 25 % high-salt Buffer C (100–325 mM). Upon loading the second 8 ml portion gradient elution is initiated. As the solvent passes through the sample coil the gradient is delayed by approx. 9 min as indicated. At the end of the gradient elution the column is stripped for 1 min with Buffer C with 700 mM NaCl before equilibration with the starting buffer. The flow rate is 2 ml/min, and the fraction size is 2 ml. The separation is done at room temperature. The light path of the UV 280 nm monitor is 10 mm

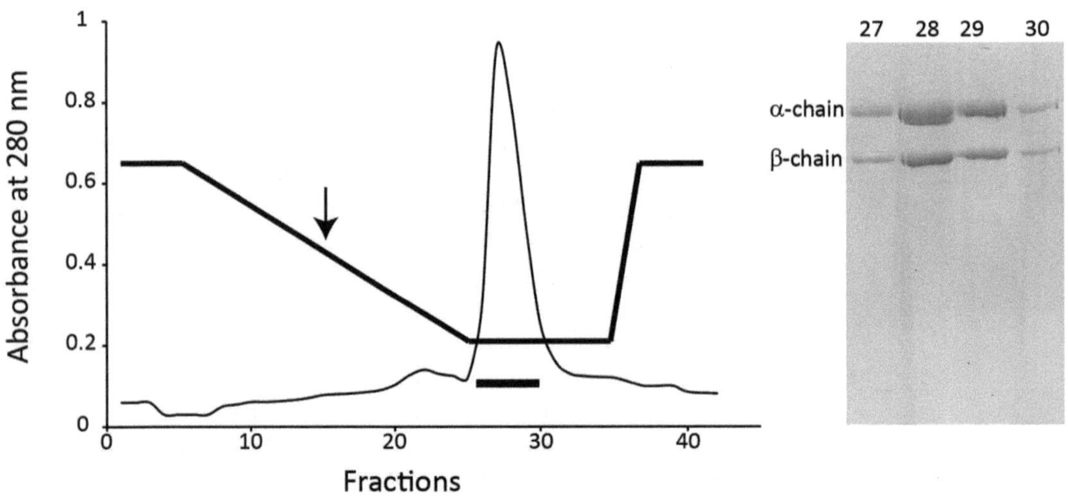

Fig. 5 *Left panel*: Separation of the C5 MonoQ pool (Fig. 4) on a 1 cm × 10 cm (8 ml) column with Source 15PHE. The column is equilibrated with 50 % high-salt Buffer D. A 4 ml portion of the C5 MonoQ pool is mixed with 4 ml high-salt Buffer D and injected. Gradient elution (from 0.5 to 0 M Na_2SO_4 in 20 min) is initiated in fraction 5 (sample coil is not inserted in flow path). The shape of the gradient at the column inlet is indicated. The actual gradient at the outlet of the column will be displaced approx. four fractions to the right as the column volume is 8 ml. The flow rate is 2 ml/min, and the fraction size is 2 ml. The separation is done at room temperature. The light path of the UV 280 nm monitor is 10 mm. The *vertical arrow* halfway through the gradient indicates the peak position of C3. *Right panel*: SDS-PAGE analysis of fractions 27–30 of the Source 15PHE separation of C5

4 Notes

1. Fresh plasma is preferred. Outdated plasma is normally easily available from blood banks.
2. A 2 mM solution of BZA has an absorbance of approx. 0.8 at 280 nm with a light path of 10 mm. It may be difficult to zero adjust the UV monitor for such a solution. In that case its concentration must be decreased. The two 2–7 % PEG fractions must be separately loaded with a Buffer A wash in between to minimize the risk of complement activation. If a low yield of C5 is obtained this may be due to accidental complement activation, either in the plasma samples or during processing.
3. Previous protocols have used 5–12 % PEG fractionation of plasma [3, 11]. This is advantageous if it is of interest to isolate other complement proteins. The 2–7 % PEG fraction used here contains most of C5 and C3 of plasma. It considerably lowers the protein load in the DEAE Sepharose fast flow step, facilitating the subsequent purification steps.
4. PTI is used to suppress the activity of trypsin-like enzymes such as plasmin and kallikrein. Phenylmethanesulfonyl fluoride (PMSF) at 1 mM may be used as a general serine proteinase inhibitor. However, PMSF is hydrolyzed relatively rapidly in aqueous solution and must be added from a 50 mM stock solution in absolute ethanol or propanol just before use.
5. Upon repeated use the top layer of the DEAE Sephacel fast flow column may become clogged. In that case the top 2 cm of the column bed must be replaced by fresh material.
6. The flow rate is set so that approx. 1,200 ml effluent passes through the column in 18 h (approx. 70 ml/h). Fractions of 8–10 ml are collected. When starting the gradient elution late on a working day C5 and C3 will have eluted from the DEAE Sephacel fast flow column during the night. Hence, analysis of the eluate can be started in the morning of the next day.
7. As the protein concentration is relatively high it is best to use a 280 nm UV monitor with a 2 mm flow cell. Alternatively, the wavelength may be set at 295 or 254 nm if a 10 mm flow cell is used. C5 elutes close to C3. It peaks a few fractions before C3 as determined from an ELISA assay.
8. C3 is located in the eluate by reducing SDS-PAGE as the characteristic 70 and 115 kDa bands from its β- and α-chains, respectively, are readily seen. C5 has the same band pattern with a slightly larger β-chain, but it is not seen easily due to the large amount of C3 relative to C5.
9. C3 and C5 co-elute on Sephacryl S-300 but are separated from several proteins of higher and lower molecular weight. SDS-PAGE may be used to monitor the protein pattern.

10. In ref. 3 2 M KCl was used to elute C5. However, it was suggested that the eluted C5 might not be fully active, and NaCl was proposed as an alternative to KCl.
11. The mechanism of separation of C5 and C3 on hydroxyapatite is not known. A hydroxyapatite column can be used maximally three times as unknown changes in the material take place during a run. After back equilibration with Buffer B it is important to stir up the material and let it settle again. Otherwise the column bed develops cracks resulting in uneven flow paths and broad elution peaks.
12. C5 constitutes approx. 10–60 % of the protein in the C5 pool, while C3 constitutes >90 % of the protein in the C3 pool. For unknown reasons part of the C3 present may occasionally elute in the C5 fractions. However, as described in **Note 15** most of the C5 present may actually be recovered free from C3. SDS-PAGE analysis will be guiding in the pooling of C5 and eventually C3.
13. C5 elutes a few fractions before C3 on MonoQ. It makes no difference whether HepesNaOH or Tris–HCl is used as buffer. In case C3 contaminates the C5 pool from the hydroxyapatite step much C5 can be rescued in the MonoQ step. SDS-PAGE analysis will be useful for pooling the effluent. A Source 15 Q will work nearly as well as the MonoQ column, but on Source 15 Q C3 and C5 will bind weaker and elute somewhat earlier.
14. In the present elution conditions several proteins in the hydroxyapatite C5 pool are strongly adsorbed to Source 15PHE. The column must therefore regularly be rinsed with 8 M urea to remove these proteins. The flow direction should be reversed during this process.
15. Source 15PHE gives excellent separation of C5 and C3. C3 has less surface hydrophobicity than C5 and elutes approx. midway in the decreasing gradient of Na_2SO_4. If the hydroxyapatite step results in a C5 pool which is heavily contaminated with C3 (with much more than 40–50 A280 units in the pool) then it can be loaded on a larger 2.5 cm × 10 cm column of Source 15PHE. The pool is made 0.5 M in Na_2SO_4, and the column is eluted for approx. 120 min at a flow rate of 2 ml/min with a gradient from 50 % high-salt Buffer D to Buffer D (0.5–0 M Na_2SO_4). This should be followed by a MonoQ step. In the MonoQ and Source 15PHE steps no proteinase inhibitors are used. In only one case it has been found that the C5 preparation was partially degraded.
16. Upon continuation of elution with 0 M Na_2SO_4 for 10 min a large peak may appear. SDS-PAGE reveals that it is of very high molecular weight. This material may be observed in cases

where the yield of C5 is relatively low. Perhaps it consists of C3b aggregates (partly covalent) resulting from accidental complement activation in the plasma samples as bands corresponding to the C3 β-chain are visible along with weaker bands corresponding to the α-chain.

17. C5 is stable for months when stored at −80 °C. Upon thawing C3 a fraction of the molecules undergoes thiol ester cleavage giving a mixture of C3 and C3-H_2O. The extent of this can be judged using cation exchange chromatography on MonoS at pH 6 according to ref. 13.
18. This preparation protocol has been used for more than 20 preparations of C5. The yield of C5 in most preparations has been 10–15 mg. In a few preparations the yield has been 20 mg. In several preparations the yield has been only 5 mg. The cause of this low yield is not known but may be due to variable handling of plasma pools prior to usage for purification.

Acknowledgement

We thank Lene Kristensen for excellent technical assistance. This work was supported by the Novo-Nordisk Foundation, the Lundbeck Foundation, and the Danish Natural Science Research Council.

References

1. Ricklin D, Hajishengallis G, Yang K, Lambris JD (2010) Complement: a key system for immune surveillance and homeostasis. Nat Immunol 11:785–797
2. Sottrup-Jensen L (1987) α_2-Macroglobulin and related thiol ester plasma proteins. In: Putnam FW (2. ed), vol. 5. The plasma proteins, p 192–291. Putnam, F.W. ed, Academic Press Orlando Florida 32887, USA
3. Tack BF, Morris SC, Prahl JW (1979) Fifth component of human complement: purification from plasma and polypeptide chain structure. Biochemistry 18:1490–1497
4. Fredslund F, Laursen NS, Roversi P, Jenner L, Oliveira CL, Pedersen JS, Nunn MA, Lea SM, Discipio R, Sottrup-Jensen L, Andersen GR (2008) Structure of and influence of a tick complement inhibitor on human complement component 5. Nat Immunol 9:753–760
5. Laursen NS, Andersen KR, Braren I, Spillner E, Sottrup-Jensen L, Andersen GR (2011) Substrate recognition by complement convertases revealed in the C5-cobra venom factor complex. EMBO J 30:606–616
6. Laursen NS, Gordon N, Hermans S, Lorenz N, Jackson N, Wines B, Spillner E, Christensen JB, Jensen M, Fredslund F, Bjerre M, Sottrup-Jensen L, Fraser JD, Andersen GR (2010) Structural basis for inhibition of complement C5 by the SSL7 protein from Staphylococcus aureus. Proc Natl Acad Sci U S A 107: 3681–3686
7. Pangburn MK, Rawal N (2002) Structure and function of complement C5 convertase enzymes. Biochem Soc Trans 30:1006–1010
8. Klos A, Tenner AJ, Johswich KO, Ager RR, Reis ES, Kohl J (2009) The role of the anaphylatoxins in health and disease. Mol Immunol 46:2753–2766
9. Tegla CA, Cudrici C, Patel S, Trippe R 3rd, Rus V, Niculescu F, Rus H (2011) Membrane attack by complement: the assembly and biology of terminal complement complexes. Immunol Res 51:45–60
10. Nilsson UR, Tomar RH, Taylor FB Jr (1972) Additional studies on human C5: development of a modified purification method and characterization of the purified product by polyacrylamide gel electrophoresis. Immunochemistry 9:709–723
11. Hammer CH, Wirtz GH, Renfer L, Gresham HD, Tack BF (1981) Large scale isolation of

functionally active components of the human complement system. J Biol Chem 256: 3995–4006
12. Kunkel SL, Kreutzer DL, Goralnick S, Ward PA (1980) Purification of the third and fifth components of human complement: application of hydrophobic chromatography. J Immunol Methods 35:337–351
13. Pangburn MK (1988) Alternative pathway of complement. Methods Enzymol 162: 639–653

Chapter 8

Quantification of Complement C5b-9 Binding to Cells by Flow Cytometry

Oren Moskovich and Zvi Fishelson

Abstract

Interaction of the complement system, directly or indirectly (e.g., via antibodies), with cells activates the early and late complement components and culminates in the deposition of a membrane-spanning C5b-9 complex on the cell surface. At a high copy number, this C5b-9 will activate cell death, whereas at a low copy number, it will transmit various signals into cells. Quantification of C5b-9 deposition is useful for assessments of the capacity of cells and antibodies to activate complement. By using an antibody that identifies a novel antigen of the C5b-9 complex, the amount of C5b-9 complexes on cells can be quantified by flow cytometry. The detailed protocol is described in this chapter.

Key words Complement, C5b-9, Flow cytometry

1 Introduction

The complement system can be activated via the classical, lectin, or alternative pathways that initiate activation of the terminal pathway and generation of the membrane attack complex (MAC), a heteropolymeric protein complex containing the complement proteins C5b, C6, C7, C8, and C9 (C5b-9) [1, 2]. C5b-9 assembly proceeds through distinct phases of intermediate complexes: C5b-7, C5b-8, and C5b-9. These complexes have also been named terminal complement complexes (TCCs) [3]. When a C9 molecule binds to the C8 α-chain in either membrane-bound C5b-8 or SC5b-8 formed in solution, C9 rapidly interacts with C5b-8 and transforms from a U-shaped into an elongated C9 [4]. The C5b-8,9 complex then assembles several C9 molecules to form C5b-8,9n through C9–C9 interaction [5, 6]. When the number of C9 molecules per membrane-attached C5b-8 exceeds 12, they form a cylinder-shaped transmembrane structure [7–9]. The C5b-9 complex has an annular ring structure with estimated external diameter of 20 nm, internal diameter of 5 nm, and a height of 15 nm [5, 7]. Assembly-related structural changes during MAC assembly

Mihaela Gadjeva (ed.), *The Complement System: Methods and Protocols*, Methods in Molecular Biology, vol. 1100, DOI 10.1007/978-1-62703-724-2_8,

produce antigenic neoepitopes that can be detected by specific monoclonal antibodies [3]. Not all C5b-9 complexes successfully penetrate the plasma membrane, and some remain superficially attached to the cell surface. In addition, SC5b-9 complexes formed in solution upon inactivation of C5b-7, C5b-8, and C5b-9 by S-protein (Vitronectin) [10] tend to adhere to neighboring cells. Unlike the membrane-inserted complexes, surface-attached C5b-9 complexes are sensitive to digestion by trypsin [11]. Even though the increase in number of C9 molecules per C5b-9 yields larger C5b-9 channels, the channel size has only a small influence on the rate of cell death of nucleated cells [12]. Loss of ATP and of mitochondrial membrane potential and increase in intracellular calcium level occur early after C5b-9 deposition [13, 14]. Studies have shown that deposition of toxic doses of the C5b-9 complex induces primarily plasma membrane perforation and necrotic cell death, but there were also reports of apoptotic consequences of C5b-9 binding to cells [15–17]. The necrotic cell death activated by the C5b-9 complexes partly depends on a signaling cascade involving JNK and Bid [18, 19]. In contrast, deposition of sublytic doses of C5b-9 may induce numerous stimulatory signals and biological responses in various cells [20]. Cells protect themselves from complement-dependent cytotoxicity by multiple evasion strategies, including a blockade of C5b-9 assembly by the membrane complement regulatory protein CD59 [21]. Rapid elimination of the lytic C5b-9 from the cell surface is also a major defense mechanism. Removal of the C5b-9 by endocytosis or exo-vesiculation was described in several normal cell types and tumor cells [22–24].

Complement activation occurs in numerous diseases and has been implicated in pathogenesis in many of them. The presence of C5b-9 deposits in human tissues indicates in situ complement activation [25] and can be measured by immunofluorescence, histochemistry, or immunoenzymatic methods as described before [26]. Several sensitive ELISA assays that detect SC5b-9 in plasma have also been described [27–30]. When considering the relevance to disease of C5b-9 deposits in tissue or SC5b-9 in plasma, one should also consider the nonlytic, potentially stimulatory, effects of C5b-9 and the futile deposition of C5b-9 on cells. In this chapter, we describe a flow cytometry method to quantify in vitro C5b-9 deposition on cells. This method is useful, for example, for analysis of the capacity of monoclonal antibodies to activate CDC and the ability of novel reagents to sensitize cells to CDC.

2 Materials

1. Cell culture medium appropriate for optimal, sterile growth of cells.
2. Sterile tissue culture plates.

3. Tubes: 12 mm × 75 mm glass tubes; 50 ml capped plastic tubes.
4. Refrigerated centrifuge with a swing out rotor and holders for 12 mm × 75 mm and 50 ml tubes.
5. Shaking water bath set at 37 °C.
6. Phosphate-buffered saline (PBS).
7. Cell counter (e.g., hemocytometer), Trypan blue stain, and a light microscope.
8. A complement-fixing antibody (polyclonal or monoclonal) directed to an antigen on the target cells.
9. Normal human serum (NHS), as a source for complement (prepared from healthy individuals). Limit blood clotting time to 30 min at room temperature plus 60 min on ice (for clot shrinking), collect serum after centrifugation at 500 × *g* for 10 min, and freeze in aliquots at −70 °C until used.
10. Heat-inactivated serum (HIS) as control. Warm NHS to 56 °C for 30 min to inactivate complement activity.
11. Mouse monoclonal antibody directed to a neoepitope on C5b-9, such as clone aE11 (Diatec Monoclonals AS, Oslo, Norway; Hycult biotechnology b.v., Uden, The Netherlands). For other similar antibodies *see* **Note 1**.
12. FITC-conjugated goat anti-mouse IgG (e.g., Jackson Immunoresearch Labs, West Grove, PA, USA).
13. Trypsin-TPCK-treated from bovine pancreas (Sigma, St. Louis, MO, USA).
14. Flow cytometer tubes.
15. Flow cytometer (e.g., BD Biosciences, San Jose, CA, USA).

3 Methods

1. Keep cells growing in culture in logarithmic phase and collect them for an experiment when they are at about 70 % confluence. Basal cell death should be well below 10 %.
2. If cells are adherent, remove them from plate with trypsin/EDTA into 50 ml plastic tubes, and after washing with cell culture medium, let them recover in cell culture medium for 60 min at 37 °C. If cells are non-adherent, just collect them into 50 ml plastic tubes.
3. Wash cells twice by centrifugation (10 min at 200 × *g*) with PBS and suspend them in 1 ml PBS.
4. Count the cells and bring to 20×10^6/ml in PBS.
5. Divide 1×10^6 cells (50 μl) in 12 mm × 75 mm tubes.
6. Add to the tubes 50 μl of an antibody directed to the target cell antigen (diluted in PBS to a non-lytic concentration,

see **Note 2**) and incubate for 30 min on ice; shake the cells every ~5 min.

7. Add 100 μl NHS or HIS (final: 50 %) and incubate for 10–20 min at 37 °C (time required for maximal specific deposition of C5b-9 on cells). Shake the cells every ~3 min.
8. Add 1 ml of cold PBS (to stop the reaction), and wash the cells three times with PBS by centrifugation (10 min at 200 × *g*).
9. *Optional*: In order to remove the surface-attached C5b-9, treat the cells with 100 μg/ml trypsin in PBS (or with PBS as control) for 20 min at 25 °C. Wash the cells two times with PBS by centrifugation. *See* **Notes 3** and **4.**
10. Add to cells in pellet 100 μl of mouse monoclonal antibody directed to C5b-9 (e.g., aE11) (diluted in PBS according to the manufacturer's recommendation) and incubate for 30 min at 4 °C. Shake the tubes every 5 min. *See* **Note 1**.
11. Wash the cells three times with PBS by centrifugation (10 min at 200 × *g*).
12. Add to cells in pellet 100 μl of FITC-conjugated goat anti-mouse IgG antibody (diluted 1:100 in PBS) and incubate for 30 min at 4 °C. Shake the tubes every 5 min (*see* **Note 5**).
13. Wash the cells three times with PBS by centrifugation (10 min at 200 × *g*).
14. Add to cells in pellet 400 μl PBS and transfer them to FACS tubes.
15. Analyze the cells in a fluorescence-activated cell sorter, and determine values of mean fluorescence intensity (MFI) by using a flow cytometry software such as WinMDI or FlowJo (*see* **Note 6**).

4 Notes

1. Besides aE11, several other anti-C5b-9 antibodies have been developed [30]. Their efficacy in the C5b-9 flow cytometry assay described here needs to be examined.
2. Before setting up the C5b-9 deposition assay, perform a cytotoxicity assay with serially diluted anti-target cell antibody and a fixed concentration of NHS (50 %). The protocol (Subheading 3, **steps 1–7**) should be performed exactly as described above with one modification: in Subheading 3, **step 7**, the cells should be incubated with NHS at 37 °C for 60 min (for maximal cytotoxicity). Next, wash the cells, and determine the percentage of cell death by any one of the following methods: Trypan blue inclusion, propidium iodide inclusion, LDH release, G6PD release, MTT, WST, etc. For the

Trypan blue assay, mix the cells in pellet after Subheading 3, **step 7** gently with Trypan blue (final: 0.2 % in PBS), remove a sample into a hemocytometer, and determine under the microscope the percent of dead (blue) cells. For the C5b-9 deposition assay choose an antibody dilution that would yield around 10–20 % cell death (sublysis).

3. For a rough estimation of the quantity of C5b-9 fully inserted into the membrane versus loosely attached C5b-9, compare the MFI of the C5b-9 on cells treated with trypsin (Subheading 3, **step 9**) (loosely attached C5b-9 is sensitive to trypsin) with that of untreated cells (total C5b-9, both inserted and loosely attached C5b-9).
4. Within minutes after C5b-9 deposition, the cells begin to internalize it via caveolin/dynamin-mediated endocytosis [31]. For a rough estimation of the quantity of C5b-9 deposited on the cell surface versus C5b-9 inside the cells (following its endocytosis), compare the MFI of C5b-9 profile on fixed and permeabilized cells (labeling both surface and intracellular C5b-9) versus that of untreated cells (labeling only surface C5b-9). Fix the cells after Subheading 3, **step 8** with paraformaldehyde (1 %, 15 min), permeabilize with saponin (1 mg/ml, 20 min), and block with fetal bovine serum (10 %). Continue the protocol from Subheading 3, **step 10** as described above.
5. Remember to include as negative controls cells labeled with the FITC-tagged secondary antibody but without the anti-C5b-9 antibody. Subtract the MFI of the negative controls from MFI of all other experimental groups.
6. As an alternative to C5b-9 labeling with an antibody, you may label the purified C9 (Quidel or CompTech) with an AlexaFluor dye (Molecular Probes) and add the labeled C9 into C9-depleted human serum (Quidel, CompTech, Sigma-Aldrich, others). Thus C5b-9 is generated with a fluorescently labeled C9, and Methods labeling Subheading 3, **steps 10–14** are not required [23]. Cells labeled with the C9-AlexaFluor dye can also be studied under a confocal microscope for tracing of the C5b-9 inside viable cells [31].

References

1. Walport MJ (2001) Complement. Second of two parts. N Engl J Med 344:1140–1144
2. Muller-Eberhard HJ (1986) The membrane attack complex of complement. Annu Rev Immunol 4:503–528
3. Mollnes TE, Harboe M (1987) Immunohistochemical detection of the membrane and fluid-phase terminal complement complexes C5b-9(m) and SC5b-9. Consequences for interpretation and terminology. Scand J Immunol 26:381–386
4. DiScipio RG, Berlin C (1999) The architectural transition of human complement component C9 to poly(C9). Mol Immunol 36:575–585
5. Podack ER, Tschopp J (1982) Polymerization of the ninth component of complement (C9): formation of poly(C9) with a tubular ultrastructure resembling the membrane attack complex of complement. Proc Natl Acad Sci U S A 79:574–578
6. Tschopp J, Podack ER, Muller-Eberhard HJ (1985) The membrane attack complex of

complement: C5b-8 complex as accelerator of C9 polymerization. J Immunol 134:495–499
7. Whitlow MB, Ramm LE, Mayer MM (1985) Penetration of C8 and C9 in the C5b-9 complex across the erythrocyte membrane into the cytoplasmic space. J Biol Chem 260: 998–1005
8. Ramm LE, Whitlow MB, Mayer MM (1982) Size of the transmembrane channels produced by complement proteins C5b-8. J Immunol 129:1143–1146
9. Ramm LE, Whitlow MB, Mayer MM (1982) Transmembrane channel formation by complement: functional analysis of the number of C5b6, C7, C8, and C9 molecules required for a single channel. Proc Natl Acad Sci U S A 79:4751–4755
10. Preissner KP, Podack ER, Muller-Eberhard HJ (1989) SC5b-7, SC5b-8 and SC5b-9 complexes of complement: ultrastructure and localization of the S-protein (vitronectin) within the macromolecules. Eur J Immunol 19:69–75
11. Bhakdi S, Tranum-Jensen J, Klump O (1980) The terminal membrane C5b-9 complex of human complement. Evidence for the existence of multiple protease-resistant polypeptides that form the trans-membrane complement channel. J Immunol 124:2451–2457
12. Kim SH, Carney DF, Hammer CH, Shin ML (1987) Nucleated cell killing by complement: effects of C5b-9 channel size and extracellular Ca2+ on the lytic process. J Immunol 138:1530–1536
13. Papadimitriou JC, Ramm LE, Drachenberg CB, Trump BF, Shin ML (1991) Quantitative analysis of adenine nucleotides during the prelytic phase of cell death mediated by C5b-9. J Immunol 147:212–217
14. Morgan BP, Luzio JP, Campbell AK (1986) Intracellular Ca2+ and cell injury: a paradoxical role of Ca2+ in complement membrane attack. Cell Calcium 7:399–411
15. Cragg MS, Howatt WJ, Bloodworth L, Anderson VA, Morgan BP, Glennie MJ (2000) Complement mediated cell death is associated with DNA fragmentation. Cell Death Differ 7:48–58
16. Fishelson Z, Attali G, Mevorach D (2001) Complement and apoptosis. Mol Immunol 38:207–219
17. Nauta, A. J., M. R. Daha, O. Tijsma, B. van de Water, F. Tedesco, and A. Roos (2002) The membrane attack complex of complement induces caspase activation and apoptosis. Eur J Immunol 32:783–792
18. Gancz D, Donin N, Fishelson Z (2009) Involvement of the c-jun N-terminal kinases JNK1 and JNK2 in complement-mediated cell death. Mol Immunol 47:310–317
19. Ziporen L, Donin N, Shmushkovich T, Gross A, Fishelson Z (2009) Programmed necrotic cell death induced by complement involves a Bid-dependent pathway. J Immunol 182: 515–521
20. Bohana-Kashtan O, Ziporen L, Donin N, Kraus S, Fishelson Z (2004) Cell signals transduced by complement. Mol Immunol 41:583–597
21. Gancz D, Fishelson Z (2009) Cancer resistance to complement-dependent cytotoxicity (CDC): problem-oriented research and development. Mol Immunol 46:2794–2800
22. Morgan BP, Dankert JR, Esser AF (1987) Recovery of human neutrophils from complement attack: removal of the membrane attack complex by endocytosis and exocytosis. J Immunol 138:246–253
23. Moskovich O, Fishelson Z (2007) Live cell imaging of outward and inward vesiculation induced by the complement c5b-9 complex. J Biol Chem 282:29977–29986
24. Pilzer D, Gasser O, Moskovich O, Schifferli JA, Fishelson Z (2005) Emission of membrane vesicles: roles in complement resistance, immunity and cancer. Springer Semin Immunopathol 27:375–387
25. Dalmasso AP, Falk RJ, Raij L (1989) The pathobiology of the terminal complement complexes. Complement Inflamm 6:36–48
26. Vakeva A, Meri S (2000) Complement deposition in tissues. Methods Mol Biol 150: 113–121
27. Accardo-Palumbo A, Triolo G, Casiglia D, Salli L, Giardina E, Triolo G (1993) Two-site ELISA for quantification of the terminal C5b-9 complement complex in plasma. Use of monoclonal and polyclonal antibodies against a neoantigen of the complex. J Immunol Methods 163:169–172
28. Hugo F, Kramer S, Bhakdi S (1987) Sensitive ELISA for quantitating the terminal membrane C5b-9 and fluid-phase SC5b-9 complex of human complement. J Immunol Methods 99:243–251
29. Matsell DG, Roy S III, Tamerius JD, Morrow PR, Kolb WP, Wyatt RJ (1991) Plasma terminal complement complexes in acute poststreptococcal glomerulonephritis. Am J Kidney Dis 17:311–316
30. Wurzner R (2000) Immunochemical measurement of complement components and activation products. Methods Mol Biol 150: 103–112
31. Moskovich O, Herzog LO, Ehrlich M, Fishelson Z (2012) Caveolin-1 and dynamin-2 are essential for removal of the complement C5b-9 complex via endocytosis. J Biol Chem 287:19904–19915

Chapter 9

Challenges and Opportunities in Fractionation of Recombinant Human Mannan-Binding Lectin

Thomas Vorup-Jensen

Abstract

Mannan-binding lectin is an oligomeric protein of the innate immune system. Both natural MBL as well as recombinant protein is a heterogeneous composition of oligomers containing from two up to at least eight structural units. Recombinant synthesis in mammalian cell lines often leads to a composition containing small oligomers not abundant in MBL from natural sources such as human plasma. Here, two procedures for fractionation of MBL oligomers are described. In one case, affinity chromatography is employed to enrich the abundance of large MBL oligomers to produce a composition of oligomers resembling natural MBL. In a second case, large-volume ion exchange chromatography is employed to separate these oligomers into fractions with an enhanced size homogeneity. Finally, a well-established procedure for estimating the MBL protein concentration is detailed.

Key words Mannan-binding lectin, Size fractionation, Recombinant synthesis, Lectin affinity chromatography

1 Introduction

Mannan-binding lectin (MBL, sometimes also referred to as mannose-binding lectin or mannan- or mannose-binding protein, MBP) belongs to the group of soluble lectins named collectins [1].

The MBL polypeptide contains an N-terminal segment of 21 residues with 3 cysteines, followed by collagen-like Gly-Xaa-Yaa repeats, which is interrupted by a Gly-Gln-Gly sequence, followed by a second collagen-like region. This collagen-like region is joined at the C terminus to a short neck region and the carbohydrate-recognition domain (CRD) [2]. Structural work on this part of the molecule has nicely explained how coordination bonds between hydroxyls in carbohydrates and a Ca^{2+} ion, chelated in the CRD, confer together with side chain in the CRD a binding selectivity for certain hexoses such as mannose and *N*-acetyl glucosamine while others such as galactose are essentially not bound [3, 4]. The collagenous regions form a structural unit of three MBL monomers

Mihaela Gadjeva (ed.), *The Complement System: Methods and Protocols*, Methods in Molecular Biology, vol. 1100, DOI 10.1007/978-1-62703-724-2_9, © Springer Science+Business Media New York 2014

(MBL_3), which are organized into higher order oligomers through interchain disulfide bridge formation [5].

Both in natural as well as in preparations of recombinant MBL the composition of oligomers is highly heterogeneous [6–8]. A recent study [8] used atomic force microscopy to directly image single oligomers and found the oligomers in a size range spanning from some with two MBL_3 units ($2 \times MBL_3$) to others with at least eight units ($8 \times MBL_3$). The functional role of this oligomerization in the physiology of the immune system is not clear. Experimental enquiry has suggested that complex formation with the MBL-associated serine proteases (MASP) differed between the oligomers in such a way that MASP-1 was predominantly found in complexes with smaller MBL_3 oligomers while MASP-2 and MASP-3 were found in complex with the larger oligomers [9]. With regard to their ligand binding, an initial analysis made by use of a surface plasmon resonance biosensor reported near-identical binding constants for $3 \times MBL_3$ and $4 \times MBL_3$ [10], in contrast to the expectation that the difference in polyvalency of these oligomers would enhance the avidity for ligands. More recently, Gjelstrup et al. demonstrated a clear correlation between oligomer size, and hence polyvalency, and avidity [11].

In the case of recombinant synthesis and functional studies concerning the binding to ligand, the ability to separate the MBL_3 oligomers has played a significant role [7, 12]. Attempts to synthesize recombinant human (rh)MBL in transfected mammalian cell lines produce in general a composition of oligomers, which are strikingly different compared to natural MBL. Vorup-Jensen et al. [7] showed, however, that a composition of recombinant oligomers more similar to natural MBL can be obtained by fractionation using affinity chromatography. Specifically, when unfractionated supernatant from transfected cells was analyzed by SDS-PAGE and Western blotting low-molecular-weight oligomeric species were found, which had no apparent equivalents in normal human serum [7]. Similarly, when analyzed under non-denaturing conditions, some preparations of recombinant MBL contain oligomers smaller than their natural counterparts [7]. Affinity chromatography-fractionated rhMBL, prepared according to the procedure described in Subheading 3.1 below, showed a profile more similar to natural MBL. The procedure has attracted interest mainly because it was demonstrated to permit synthesis of pharmaceutical-grade recombinant MBL [12–14]. In hindsight, it is now possible to conclude that the recent findings by Gjelstrup et al. on the crucial role of polyvalency in MBL ligand binding [11] are also reflected in the findings by Vorup-Jensen et al. [7]. The ability to exclude the binding by small MBL_3 oligomers to surfaces sparsely coated with ligand certainly speaks to the role of polyvalency and avidity in target recognition by this molecule.

Insight into the role of MBL_3 oligomerization has mainly been found in studies fractionating natural or $rhMBL_3$ oligomers by ion exchange chromatography. This procedure was apparently instigated by Lu et al. [6] who separated the MBL_3 oligomers for structural studies by rotary-shadowing electron microscopy. Dahl et al. [9], using a similar procedure, addressed the complex formation with MASPs. To date, no studies have reported a fractionation of human natural or recombinant MBL_3 oligomers to reasonable purity. Both the reports by Teillet et al. [10], Dahl et al. [9], and, more recently, Gjelstrup et al. [11] reached certain levels of fractionation, in particular of the smaller MBL_3 oligomers [10, 11]. However, it would seem tenuous at this point to claim that these procedures produce size-homogenous preparations. Indeed, as reported by Gjelstrup et al., analysis with small-angle X-ray analysis suggested that none of the fractions prepared according to a method described also in this chapter (in Subheading 3.2) achieved a size homogeneity better than providing an abundance of the dominating oligomeric species of approximately 90 % [11]. This should be compared with the situation for rat recombinant MBL-A, where fractionation apparently delivers a better fraction [15]. The reason for this discrepancy remains enigmatic but may be influenced by species differences in the size distribution of the oligomers.

In understanding the biology of any component of the immune system, robust quantitative analyses are paramount. The MBL concentration in human plasma differs between healthy individuals with as much as 1,000-fold from concentrations in ng per ml to several μg per ml [1]. Quantification was initially carried out by enzyme-linked immunosorbent assays (ELISA) [16], but more recently assay methodologies based on time-resolved fluorometry have been applied [17, 18]. As is well known, due to the enzymatic amplification ELISA is an extremely sensitive mean of detection. However, both intra-assay and inter-assay variation is often considerable, probably in consequence of difficulties in reproducing the exact conditions that regulate the readout, typically color formation from the enzymatic cleavage of a chromogen. By contrast, the use of fluorescently tagged proteins for detection, e.g., fluorescently tagged streptavidin, yields a largely invariant signal with very low intra-assay variation and a remarkable reproducibility also recorded in the low inter-assay variation. When antibodies are used for antigen detection, the methodology has been named time-resolved immunofluorometry assay (TRIFMA) [17, 18]. The robustness of TRIFMA is not only the case with MBL measurements but also for several other plasma protein species [19–22]. One recent example from our laboratory includes measurements on shed β_2 (CD18) integrins [23], which were reproducibly measured with essentially the same type of assay as used for MBL. The concentration of shed CD18 rarely exceeds the femto molar level, and the ability in this situation of the TRIFMA to achieve acceptable inter-assay coefficients of variation recommends more broader application of this methodology. In case of MBL, the TRIFMA methodology has now been employed in a large number of studies correlating the MBL plasma or serum concentration with human diseases [24]. The assay is, of course, also applicable as part of the attempt to fractionate MBL, e.g., as a method for following the elution profile in gel-permeation chromatography or in other means of chromatographic characterization.

Below, two procedures for fractionation of MBL_3 oligomers by affinity and ion exchange chromatography are detailed. Means of the detection and quantification of MBL by use of a TRIFMA is also described.

2 Materials

All buffers and solutions are made with ultrapure water prepared by purifying deionized water to attain a resistivity of 18 MΩ cm at 25 °C. Analytical grade reagents were obtained from major commercial providers such as Sigma-Aldrich or Merck K.G. Buffers were stored at 4 °C until use when the liquid was left to equilibrate to room temperature and degassed under air suction prior to chromatography. Running and washing buffers were typically supplemented with 10 mM NaN_3 to preserve sterility (*see* **Note 1**).

2.1 Preparation of Affinity Chromatography Matrix

1. Fractogel TSK HW-75 beads (*see* **Note 2**).
2. Activation buffer: 50 ml of 0.5 M Na_2CO_3, pH 11, mixed with 10 ml divinyl sulfone.
3. D-mannose.
4. Blocking buffer: 0.1 M ethanolamine, pH 9.0.
5. Tris-buffered saline (TBS): 10 mM Tris–HCl, 140 mM NaCl, pH 7.4.

2.2 Affinity Chromatography of MBL_3 Oligomers

1. Rinsing buffer: 0.1 M glycine, pH 3.0.
2. Supernatant from cultured cells expressing human recombinant MBL.
3. Running buffer: TBS with 2 mM CaCl2.
4. Elution buffer: TBS with 5 mM EDTA.
5. Liquid chromatography column with a total volume of ~6 ml or larger.

2.3 Ion Exchange Chromatography-Based Separation of MBL_3 Oligomers

1. 2 mg rhMBL (*see* **Note 3**).
2. MonoQ HR 5/5 ion exchange chromatography column (*see* **Note 4**).

3. Buffer A: 10 mM $CaCl_2$, 50 mM NaCl, 20 mM Tris–Cl, pH 8.2.
4. Buffer B: 10 mM $CaCl_2$, 500 mM NaCl, 20 mM Tris–Cl, pH 8.2.
5. Spin concentrator columns with M_r cutoff at 30,000.

2.4 Biotinylation of Antibodies

1. PBS: 137 mM NaCl, 2.5 mM KH_2PO_4, 6.9 mM $K_2HPO_4 \cdot 3H_2O$, pH 7.4.
2. Dialysis chamber with Mr cutoff at 10,000.
3. (+)-Biotin N-hydroxysuccinimide ester.
4. Dimethylsulfoxide (DMSO).
5. TBS (as described in Subheading 2.1, **item 5**).

2.5 Assay for MBL Quantification

1. 96-well microtiter plates (*see* **Note 5**).
2. Plastic boxes, with sealable lids and sufficiently large to contain several 96-well plates and wetted paper towels. This setup serves to reduce evaporation from the liquid-containing plate wells.
3. Murine monoclonal (m) antibody (Ab) to human MBL, e.g., clone 131-1, either in its native state for use as capture mAb or in a biotinylated state for signal development (*see* **Note 6**).
4. PBS (as described in Subheading 2.4, **item 1**).
5. Human serum albumin (HSA).
6. TBS (as described in Subheading 2.1, **item 5**).
7. TBS/Tw: TBS with 0.05 % (v/v) Tween-20.
8. Eu^{3+}-conjugated streptavidin (*see* **Note 7**).
9. Human IgG (*see* **Note 8**): The IgG was heat-aggregated by incubation of TBS with 10 mg/ml IgG at 63 °C for 30 min.
10. Bovine IgG (*see* **Note 9**).
11. Enhancement solution: A volume of 5.7 ml of glacial acetic acid is mixed with 0.1 M potassium hydrogen phthalate to obtain a pH value of 3.2. The total volume is adjusted to 1 l with demineralized water. From a stock solution with 15 μM 2-naphthoyltrifluoroacetate and 50 μM tri-o-octylphosphine oxide, 2 μl is mixed with the acetic acidic/potassium hydrogen phthalate buffer immediately before use.
12. Assay binding buffer (*see* **Note 10**): 100 μg/ml heat-aggregated IgG, 10 mg/ml BSA, 0.05 % (v/v) Tween-20, 10 mM EDTA, 0.5 M NaCl, 20 mM Tris–Cl, pH 7.4.
13. Biotinylated Ab binding buffer (*see* **Note 11**): TBS/Tw, 1 mM $CaCl_2$, 1 mM $MgCl_2$, and 100 μg/ml bovine IgG.

3 Methods

All procedures can be carried out at room temperature (RT) without apparent signs of MBL degradation.

3.1 Fractionation of MBL_3 Oligomers by Affinity Chromatography

Culture supernatant from mammalian cells producing rhMBL usually contains a heterogeneous composition of MBL oligomers with regard to the size of the oligomers. The method below instructs how to prepare a matrix for purification of recombinant human MBL in such a way that small oligomers, i.e., 1–2 × MBL_3 as judged from SDS-PAGE analysis, are excluded from the purified oligomers, which contain 3–8 × MBL_3.

1. Prepare the affinity chromatography matrix by activating 50 ml of beads with 50 ml 0.5 M Na_2CO_3, pH 11, and 10 ml of divinyl sulfone. Leave with agitation for 1.5 h at ambient temperature. Collect the beads in a semidry state on a glass filter with gentle air suction and wash once in H_2O and once in 0.5 M Na_2CO_3, pH 11. Then, resuspend the beads in 0.5 M Na_2CO_3, pH 11 and add D-mannose to a final concentration of 10 % (w/v), followed by incubation with agitation for ~16 h at ambient temperature. Following a rinse in H_2O, block residual reactive divinyl sulfone groups by incubation in 0.1 M ethanolamine, pH 9.0. Finally, rinse in H_2O, and store in TBS.
2. The chromatography is initiated by packing a volume of 5 ml of beads into a suitable column (*see* **Note 12**) by gravitational settlement. Clean the beads by gradually transferring 15 ml of 0.1 M glycine, pH 3.0 to the packed column followed by equilibration in running buffer with 0.05 % (v/v) Tween-20.
3. Immediately prior to the chromatography, clear the MBL oligomer-containing supernatant for cellular debris and precipitated constituents by centrifugation in 50-ml tubes at 5,000 × g. Carefully remove the supernatant (~280 ml) (*see* **Note 13**) from the tubes and dilute with 280 ml of running buffer to stabilize the pH. Siphon the diluted supernatant over the column. To avoid the matrix running dry, place a part of the tube connecting the supernatant reservoir below the level of the column, this way permitting gravitational trapping of the last part of the supernatant. Washing is carried out by passing 75 ml of running buffer over the column in a similar way.
4. The elution is carried out by adding manually 500 μl of elution buffer to the column and collecting the fraction by gravitation. The procedure should be repeated adding a total volume of elution buffer to the column, i.e., corresponding to ~1.5–2 column volumes.
5. The concentration of rhMBL in the fraction is determined as described below by TRIFMA. Pool fractions with suitable high concentrations of rhMBL.

3.2 Ion Exchange Chromatography-Based Separation of MBL_3 Oligomers

The present procedure was developed by Gjelstrup et al. [11] from several other attempts using ion exchange chromatography for separating MBL_3 oligomers [6, 9, 10]. As also evidenced by these earlier reports, the fractionation is unlikely to lead to chemical purity of the individual oligomers. Nevertheless, both analyses by use of SDS-PAGE [6, 9–11], electron microscopy [6], and small-angle X-ray scattering [11] point to that this type of fractionation separates the smaller and larger oligomers in a systematic manner. As demonstrated by Gjelstrup et al. [11], the functionality of the oligomers found in the fractions with regard to the affinity for mannosylated albumin differed in a way suggesting that the separation was sufficient to provide insight into the ligand-binding properties of the MBL_3 oligomers. The procedure described here requires a handsome amount of rhMBL. However, similar fractionation has been performed earlier on plasma-derived MBL [6].

1. Load 2 mg of rhMBL in 2 ml of Buffer A onto a Mono Q chromatography column connected to an Äkta Fast-performance liquid chromatography equipment (UPC-900, GE Healthcare) with a fraction collector permitting collection in 50-ml tubes (Frac-950, GE Healthcare).
2. With a flow rate of 0.5 ml/min an elution gradient is created in eight steps with 8 % (v/v) Buffer B over an elution volume (Ve) of 30 ml (Step 1, referred to in the following as Fraction I), followed by 18 % (v/v) Buffer B over a volume of 199 ml (Step 2/Fraction II), 20 % (v/v) Buffer B over 39 ml (Step 3), 21.5 % (v/v) Buffer B over 199 ml (Step 4/Fraction III), 24 % (v/v) Buffer B over 38 ml (Step 5/Fraction IV), 26 % (v/v) Buffer over 199 ml (Step 6/Fraction V), 30 % (v/v) Buffer B over 39 ml (Step 7), and 100 % (v/v) Buffer B over 19 ml (Step 8). The gradient steps and the expected elution profile are shown in Fig. 1a.
3. Concentrate Fractions I–V in spin columns. The expected outcome is shown in Fig. 1b as analyzed electrophoresis and appropriate protein staining.

3.3 Biotinylation of Antibodies

Biotinylated antibodies in combination with appropriately labeled streptavidin are an efficient mean of detection. Below, the procedure for biotinylation is described. While it is tempting to couple a high-amount biotin per immunoglobulin molecule, "over-biotinylation" should be avoided as it may damage the reactivity of the antibody.

1. Load the liquid containing the antibody into the dialysis chamber. Transfer the chamber to a beaker with the dialysis buffer and a magnetic stir bar and dialyze against PBS for two intervals of 1 h with change of the dialysis buffer, followed by a final ~16-h dialysis, with gentle stirring of the liquid.

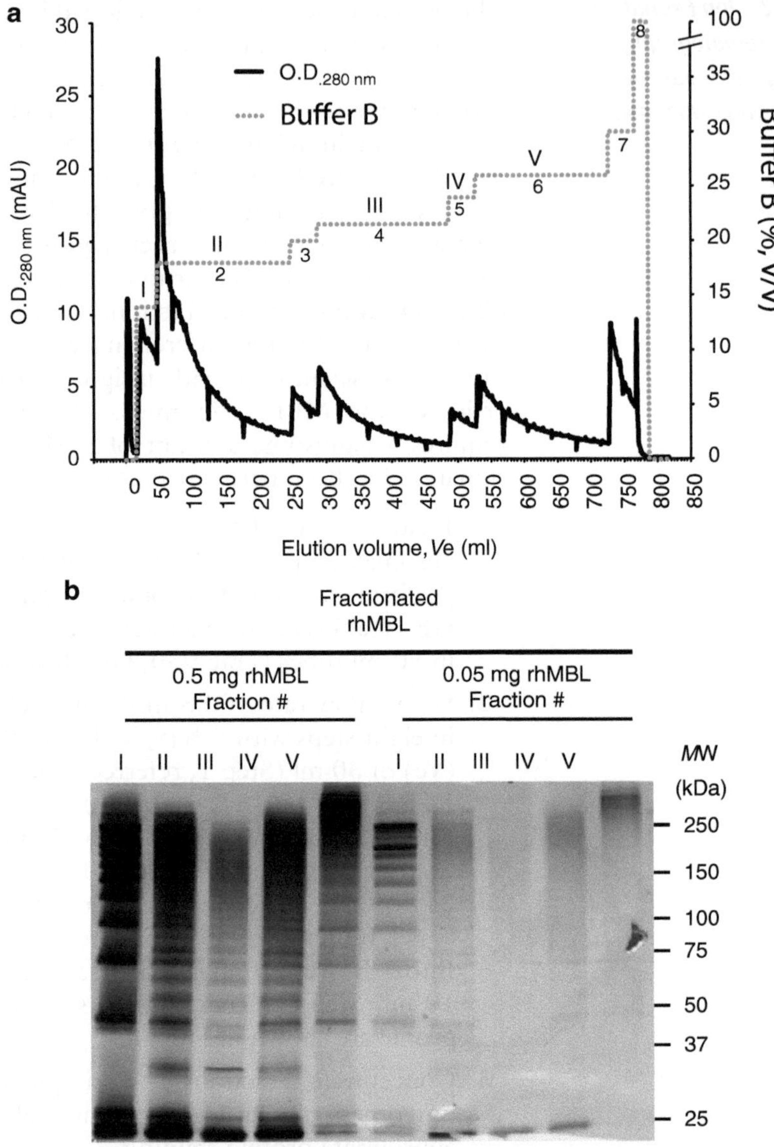

Fig. 1 Fractionation of rhMBL. (**a**) Ion exchange chromatography fractionation of MBL_3 oligomers. rMBL was loaded onto the anion exchange column equilibrated in a low-salt buffer. The bound protein was eluted through increment of the salt concentration in eight steps. These are shown in *Panel A* with *Arabic numerals* and a *dotted line* stating the percentage of the high-salt Buffer B. The elution of protein was monitored by the absorption at O.D.$_{280\ nm}$ indicated with a solid black line. The collected fractions are indicated with Roman numerals *I–V*. (**b**) SDS-PAGE of unfractionated and fractionated rhMBL. The exposed fractions were applied to the gel in amounts of 0.5 and 0.05 mg for each Fraction *I–V* as indicated, followed by *silver staining* of the gel. For details of this analysis, the reader is referred to Gjelstrup et al. [23]. Reproduced with the kind permission by the Editors of *The Journal of Immunology* (color figure online). Copyright 2012. The American Association of Immunologists, Inc

2. Repeat the dialysis with a PBS buffer adjusted to pH 8.5 with 5 % (w/v) Na2CO3.
3. Dissolve biotin N-hydroxysuccinimide ester in DMSO (with a stock concentration of 1 mg/ml), and add it to the dialysate in such an amount that the total weight of biotin N-hydroxysuccinimide ester equals 1/6 of the total protein weight. Let the reaction proceeds for 4 h with agitation of the tube.
4. Dialyze the biotinylated antibody as described in Subheading 3.3, step 1, against TBS.
5. Remove aggregated material by centrifugation at 10,000 × *g* for 30 min.

3.4 Quantification of the MBL Protein Concentration by TRIFMA

The method described below presents a previously described assay for measuring the MBL protein concentration [17, 18]. The methodology is applicable both to native and rhMBL. The typical standard curve was established by serial dilution of a standard serum with a known concentration (in weight units per ml of serum) of MBL.

1. The developing mAb, biotinylated HYB 131-1, or another mAb of choice to MBL is prepared as described in Subheading 3.3 above. Since MBL is a oligomeric molecule it is possible to use the same mAb as capture and developing Ab. Coat the capture mAb into the wells of the 96-well plates at a concentration of 5 μg per ml PBS using a total volume per well of 100 μl. Leave the plates in moisted plastic boxes for ~16 h.
2. Empty the plate wells into a sink (*see* **Note 14**), followed by a more thorough emptying by repeated tapping of the plates on paper towels. Nonspecific binding sites were blocked by incubation of the wells with 200 μl TBS/Tw for 1 h, followed by washing of the wells three times in the same buffer.
3. Apply MBL-containing samples to the wells. These samples may be either human serum or plasma, culture supernatant from transfected cell culture or fractions from the chromatography described in Subheadings 3.1 and 3.2. Since the intra-assay variation usually is small in this type of assay, the sample may be applied in duplicates. Sera and plasmas are typically diluted 100- or 200-fold in assay binding buffer. Other sources may require different degrees of dilution albeit the dynamic range of the TRIFMA is considerably larger than for ELISA. A total of 100 μl should be applied to each well. Incubate the wells for ~16 h at 4 °C and wash three times in TBS/Tw as described above (*see* **Note 14**).
4. Dilute the biotinylated antibody to MBL to 1 μg/ml in biotinylated Ab binding buffer and add in a volume of 100 μl

to each well. Following ~1.5-h incubation in the moist boxes, wash the plates three times as described above (*see* **Note 14**).

5. Dilute the Eu3+-conjugated streptavidin sufficiently, usually in the order of 1,000–16,000-fold, in TBS/Tw with 25 μM EDTA, followed by incubation for ~1.5 h. The wells are washed three times as described above (*see* **Note 14**).
6. Add a volume of 200 μl enhancement solution to each well, followed by vigorous shaking of the plates on a specialized plate shaking device and reading of the signals in a machine equipped for time-resolved fluorometry measurements (*see* **Note 15**).

4 Notes

1. Buffers can also, more widely than indicated here, be supplemented with nonionic detergents such as Tween-20 to prevent protein loss on the plastic surfaces of utensils and tubings.
2. Beads are available from Merck KgaA, Darmstadt, Germany.
3. The source of rhMBL used in our work has mainly been obtained from NatImmune A/S, Copenhagen, Denmark. NatImmune sought to provide clinical-grade preparations of rhMBL for reconstitution therapy in immune-suppressed patients. The license to make such rhMBL was obtained by Enzon Pharmaceuticals, Inc., which, however, ended the production of rhMBL in 2009. Reports on the synthesis of rhMBL from academic groups have been made in the literature recently suggesting other sources of such material [25, 26].
4. The chromatography procedures described are made with the equipment from GE Healthcare, Uppsala, Sweden.
5. Plates such as the Fluorosorp™ (Thermoscientific-Nunc, Kamstrup, Denmark) typically produce an acceptable background level.
6. The antibody is available from BioPorto, Gentofte, Denmark.
7. Available from PerkinElmer, Waltham, MA.
8. We have used Beriglobin™ from ZLB Behring GmbH, Marburg, Germany.
9. We have used bovine IgG from Lampire Biological, Ottsville, PA.
10. The inclusion of aggregated human IgG is a mean of avoiding an influence of human immunoglobulins binding to murine immunoglobulins, notably human rheuma factors. Rheuma

factors are immunoglobulins of several isotypes reacting with IgG. Since rheuma factors are cross-reacting with IgG from several species, the presence of these proteins in human samples may cause a false-positive signal through the binding to and capture of the murine antibodies applied for antigen detection. Other immunoglobulin-reactive antibodies are also found in human plasma [27].

11. Preparations of murine monoclonal Ab contains a significant fraction of bovine immunoglobulins, which are added to the hybridoma cell culture as a consequence of the inclusion of fetal calf serum in the culture medium. The subsequent purification of the murine immunoglobulins through Protein G affinity chromatography consequently leads to co-purification of bovine immunoglobulins as well. Human Ab to bovine proteins are probably a consequence of the dietary intake of bovine meat [28]. Unlike the rheuma factors, these Ab are specific to bovine immunoglobulins and may not be blocked by the addition of IgG from other species. By adding bovine IgG to the biotinylated Ab binding buffer, the capture of biotinylated bovine IgG in the well is prevented, this way avoiding a false contribution to the signal generated by addition of Eu^{3+}-conjugated streptavidin.
12. For example, the Tricorn® series from GE Healthcare.
13. The volume of this material applied to the chromatography must, of course, take into consideration the capacity of the matrix. Interestingly, the described procedure worked for transient expression of an MBL-encoding construct in cells cultivated in serum-free medium. In general, this culture only gave rise to a low concentration (~300 ng/ml) of rhMBL in the medium.
14. Depending on the nature of the samples analyzed and relevant guidelines for handling biological samples, all appropriate measures must be taken to avoid that hazardous material is released from the wells to the surroundings.
15. Equipment for performing this part of the analysis and reading of the TRIFMA signals is available from PerkinElmer. These include the DELFIA® Plateshake and the Victor® plate reader series.

Acknowledgements

I am indebted to Drs. Jens C. Jensenius and Steffen Thiel for introducing me to the biology and chemistry of MBL. This work was financially supported by the Lundbeck Foundation and the Danish Council for Independent Research | Natural Sciences.

References

1. Holmskov U, Thiel S, Jensenius JC (2003) Collections and ficolins: humoral lectins of the innate immune defense. Annu Rev Immunol 21:547–578
2. Ezekowitz RA, Day LE, Herman GA (1988) A human mannose-binding protein is an acute-phase reactant that shares sequence homology with other vertebrate lectins. J Exp Med 167(3):1034–1046
3. Drickamer K (1992) Engineering galactose-binding activity into a C-type mannose-binding protein. Nature 360(6400):183–186
4. Weis WI, Drickamer K, Hendrickson WA (1992) Structure of a C-type mannose-binding protein complexed with an oligosaccharide. Nature 360(6400):127–134
5. Jensen PH, Weilguny D, Matthiesen F, McGuire KA, Shi L, Hojrup P (2005) Characterization of the oligomer structure of recombinant human mannan-binding lectin. J Biol Chem 280(12):11043–11051
6. Lu JH, Thiel S, Wiedemann H, Timpl R, Reid KB (1990) Binding of the pentamer/hexamer forms of mannan-binding protein to zymosan activates the proenzyme C1r2C1s2 complex, of the classical pathway of complement, without involvement of C1q. J Immunol 144(6):2287–2294
7. Vorup-Jensen T, Sorensen ES, Jensen UB, Schwaeble W, Kawasaki T, Ma Y, Uemura K, Wakamiya N, Suzuki Y, Jensen TG, Takahashi K, Ezekowitz RA, Thiel S, Jensenius JC (2001) Recombinant expression of human mannan-binding lectin. Int Immunopharmacol 1(4):677–687
8. Jensenius H, Klein DC, van Hecke M, Oosterkamp TH, Schmidt T, Jensenius JC (2009) Mannan-binding lectin: structure, oligomerization, and flexibility studied by atomic force microscopy. J Mol Biol 391(1):246–259
9. Dahl MR, Thiel S, Matsushita M, Fujita T, Willis AC, Christensen T, Vorup-Jensen T, Jensenius JC (2001) MASP-3 and its association with distinct complexes of the mannan-binding lectin complement activation pathway. Immunity 15(1):127–135
10. Teillet F, Dublet B, Andrieu JP, Gaboriaud C, Arlaud GJ, Thielens NM (2005) The two major oligomeric forms of human mannan-binding lectin: chemical characterization, carbohydrate-binding properties, and interaction with MBL-associated serine proteases. J Immunol 174(5):2870–2877
11. Gjelstrup LC, Kaspersen JD, Behrens MA, Pedersen JS, Thiel S, Kingshott P, Oliveira CL, Thielens NM, Vorup-Jensen T (2012) The role of nanometer-scaled ligand patterns in polyvalent binding by large mannan-binding lectin oligomers. J Immunol 188(3):1292–1306
12. Jensenius JC, Jensen PH, McGuire K, Larsen JL, Thiel S (2003) Recombinant mannan-binding lectin (MBL) for therapy. Biochem Soc Trans 31(Pt 4):763–767
13. Oliveira C, Teixeira JA, Domingues L (2012) Recombinant lectins: an array of tailor-made glycan-interaction biosynthetic tools. Crit Rev Biotechnol
14. Thiel S, Jensenius JC, Jensen TV (2005) Recombinant human mannan-binding lectin. United States of America Patent 6846649
15. Wallis R, Drickamer K (1999) Molecular determinants of oligomer formation and complement fixation in mannose-binding proteins. J Biol Chem 274(6):3580–3589
16. Super M, Thiel S, Lu J, Levinsky RJ, Turner MW (1989) Association of low levels of mannan-binding protein with a common defect of opsonisation. Lancet 2(8674):1236–1239
17. Gadjeva M, Thiel S, Jensenius JC (2004) Assays for the mannan-binding lectin pathway. Curr Protoc Immunol. In: John E Coligan et al (eds) Chapter 13:Unit 13–16
18. Frederiksen PD, Thiel S, Jensen L, Hansen AG, Matthiesen F, Jensenius JC (2006) Quantification of mannan-binding lectin. J Immunol Methods 315(1–2):49–60
19. Degn SE, Thiel S, Nielsen O, Hansen AG, Steffensen R, Jensenius JC (2011) MAp19, the alternative splice product of the MASP2 gene. J Immunol Methods 373(1–2):89–101
20. Bernth-Jensen JM, Moller BK, Jensenius JC, Thiel S (2011) Biological variation of anti-alphaGal-antibodies studied by a novel Time-Resolved ImmunoFluorometric Assay. J Immunol Methods 373(1–2):26–35
21. Degn SE, Jensen L, Gal P, Dobo J, Holmvad SH, Jensenius JC, Thiel S (2010) Biological variations of MASP-3 and MAp44, two splice products of the MASP1 gene involved in regulation of the complement system. J Immunol Methods 361(1–2):37–50
22. Wittenborn T, Thiel S, Jensen L, Nielsen HJ, Jensenius JC (2010) Characteristics and biological variations of M-ficolin, a pattern recognition molecule, in plasma. J Innate Immun 2(2):167–180
23. Gjelstrup LC, Boesen T, Kragstrup TW, Jorgensen A, Klein NJ, Thiel S, Deleuran BW, Vorup-Jensen T (2010) Shedding of large functionally active CD11/CD18 Integrin complexes from leukocyte membranes during synovial inflammation distinguishes three types of arthritis through differential epitope exposure. J Immunol 185(7):4154–4168

24. Thiel S, Frederiksen PD, Jensenius JC (2006) Clinical manifestations of mannan-binding lectin deficiency. Mol Immunol 43(1–2): 86–96
25. Ahn BC, Park JS, Kim D, Park J, Pi J, Yum JS, Jeong Y, Baek K, Moon HM, Yoon J (2012) Overproduction of recombinant human mannose-binding lectin (MBL) in Chinese hamster ovary cells. Protein Expr Purif 88(1):1–6
26. Rajagopalan R, Salvi VP, Jensenius JC, Rawal N (2009) New insights on the structural/functional properties of recombinant human mannan-binding lectin and its variants. Immunol lett 123(2):114–124
27. Degn SE, Andersen SH, Jensen L, Thiel S, Jensenius JC (2011) Assay interference caused by antibodies reacting with rat kappa light-chain in human sera. J Immunol Methods 372(1–2):204–208
28. Husby S, Oxelius VA, Teisner B, Jensenius JC, Svehag SE (1985) Humoral immunity to dietary antigens in healthy adults. Occurrence, isotype and IgG subclass distribution of serum antibodies to protein antigens. Int Arch Allergy Appl Immunol 77(4):416–422

Chapter 10

Genotyping of *FCN* and *MBL2* Polymorphisms Using Pyrosequencing

Lea Munthe-Fog, Hans Ole Madsen, and Peter Garred

Abstract

Pyrosequencing represents one of the most thorough methods used to analyze polymorphisms. One advantage of using pyrosequencing for genotyping is the ability to identify not only single-nucleotide polymorphisms (SNPs) but also tri-allelic variations, insertions and deletions (InDels). In contrast to most other genotyping assays the sequence surrounding the polymorphism provides an internal control making this method highly reliable.

Key words Pyrosequencing, Pyrogram, Genotyping, Polymorphism, PCR

1 Introduction

Pyrosequencing is a method for real-time DNA sequencing for short DNA sequences [1]. In contrast to Sanger sequencing which relies on the termination of the sequence elongation by incorporation of a dideoxynucleotide [2] pyrosequencing is based on the detection of the pyrophosphate released upon the incorporation of a nucleotide. Each nucleotide is added sequentially (dispensation order) enabling the DNA sequence to be determined.

Following an initial polymerase chain reaction (PCR) amplification of the target DNA sequence a sequencing primer is hybridized to the single-stranded PCR amplicon. The actual pyrosequencing is a series of repeated steps that all start by the addition of one of the four deoxynucleotide triphosphates (dNTPs) to the sequencing reaction (Fig. 1). Upon incorporation of the nucleotide by the DNA polymerase (primer elongation) pyrophosphate (PPi) is released triggering a cascade reaction. Adenosine 5′phosphosulfate ATP sulfurylase converts the released PPi to ATP that in turn drives the conversion of luciferin to oxyluciferin generating a visible light which is detected with a camera and seen as a peek in the data output (pyrogram) (Fig. 2). The amount of light

Mihaela Gadjeva (ed.), *The Complement System: Methods and Protocols*, Methods in Molecular Biology, vol. 1100, DOI 10.1007/978-1-62703-724-2_10, © Springer Science+Business Media New York 2014

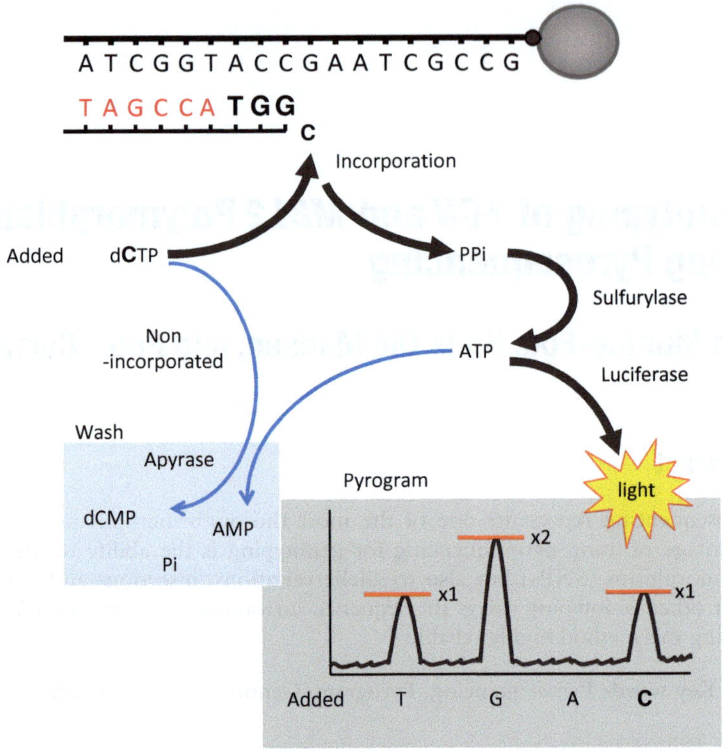

Fig. 1 Overview of the pyrosequencing assay. A biotinylated single-stranded PCR fragment has been caught on a streptavidin-coated sepharose bead, and the pyrosequencing primer (indicated with *red*) has been hybridized to the fragment. The deoxynucleotide triphosphate, dCTP, is then added and incorporated into the sequence by the polymerase. As a result pyrophosphate is released and by sulfurylase converted into ATP. Through a two-step reaction ATP is converted to light by luciferase, which is detected by a highly sensitive camera and seen as a peek in the pyrogram. Between every addition of a nucleotide apyrase removes the unincorporated nucleotides and ATP (wash)

produced is proportional with the amount of ATP generated from the PPi released by the incorporation of the nucleotide during primer elongation. Thus the height of the peak is proportional to the number of nucleotide incorporated into the sequence. The residual nucleotides and ATPs are then degraded by apyrase, and the reaction is restarted with the addition of yet another nucleotide [3].

Fig. 2 (continued) when the substrate is added. On top of each pyrogram the analyzed genotype is shown. The called genotype of each individual is as follows: (**a**) first individual C/C, T/T, and G/G; (**b**) second individual C/C, C/T, and C/C; and (**c**) third individual C/C, C/C, and G/G

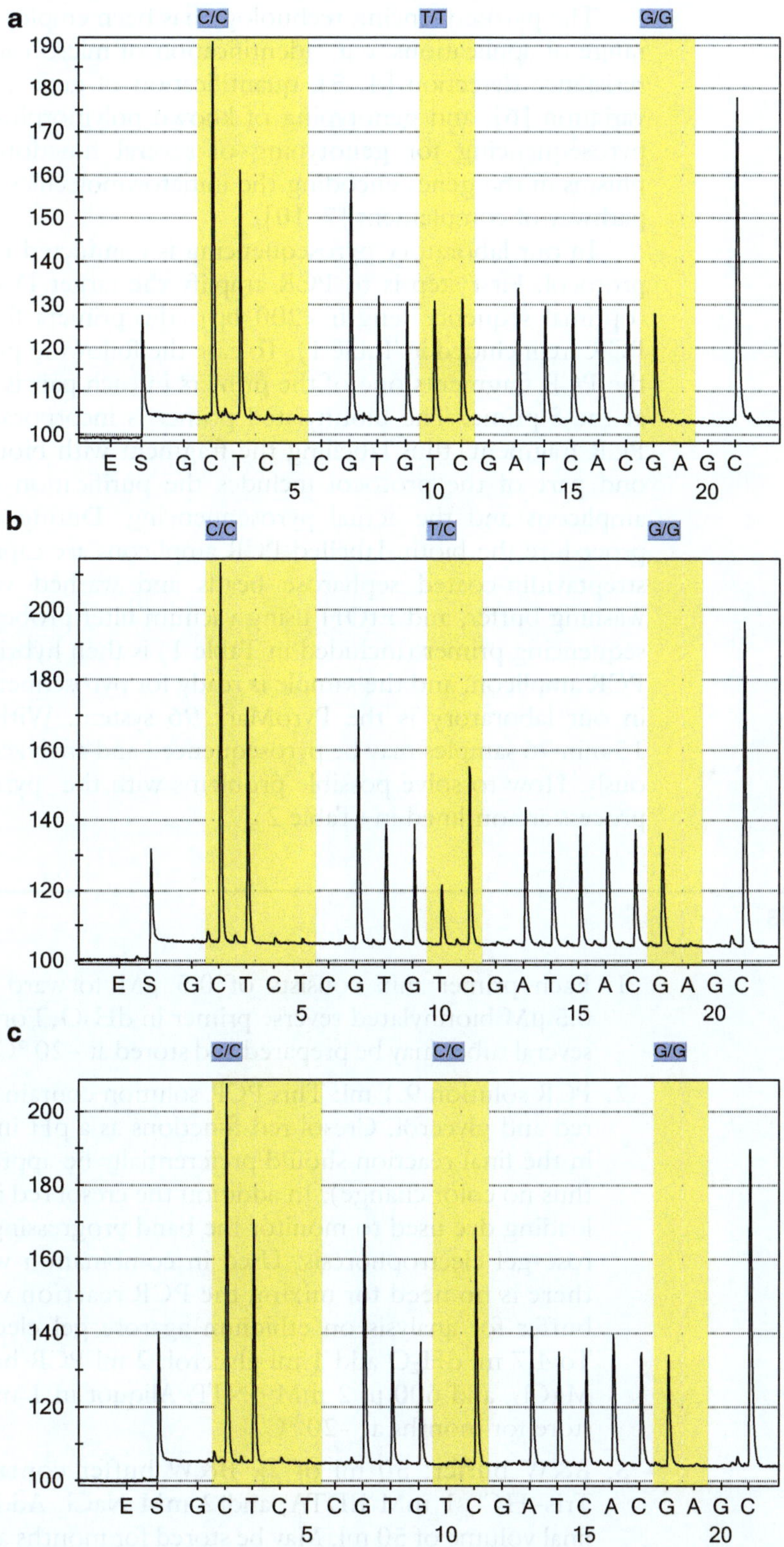

Fig. 2 Pyrogram results from MBL2 D, B, and C variant genotyping of three individuals. The analyzed sequence is T/CCCTTGGTGT/CCATCACG/ACCC. In the bottom of each pyrogram the dispensation order and the resulting peaks are shown. No peak should be seen when only enzyme (E) has been added, whereas a peak should be seen

The pyrosequencing technology has been employed to a wide range of applications, e.g., identification of microbial species and resistance detection [4, 5], quantification of gene copy number variation [6], and genotyping of known polymorphisms. We use pyrosequencing for genotyping of several functional polymorphisms in the genes encoding the initiator molecules of the lectin pathway of complement [7–10].

In our laboratory pyrosequencing is conducted in a two-step protocol. First step is to PCR amplify the target DNA sequence (optimal sequence length <200 bp) (the primers for this initial PCR are included in Table 1). To ease the following purification of the PCR fragments one of the primers in each pair is biotinylated at the 5′prime. The biotinylated primer is incorporated into the PCR fragment, thus labelling the fragment with biotin. The second part of the protocol includes the purification of the PCR amplicons and the actual pyrosequencing. During the washing procedure the biotin-labelled PCR amplicons are captured by the streptavidin-coated sepharose beads and washed with NaOH, washing buffer, and EtOH using vacuum filter probes. The pyrosequencing primer (included in Table 1) is then hybridized to the PCR amplicon, and the sample is ready for pyrosequencing, which in our laboratory is the PyroMark 96 system. Within the next 15 min 96 samples may be pyrosequenced and analyzed simultaneously. How to solve possible problems with the pyrosequencing process are outlined in (Table 2).

2 Materials

1. Each primer mix consists of 0.5 μM forward primer and 0.5 μM biotinylated reverse primer in dH_2O. For large setups several tubes may be prepared and stored at −20 °C for months.
2. PCR solution 9.1 ml: This PCR solution contains both cresol red and glycerol. Cresol red functions as a pH indicator (pH in the final reaction should preferentially be approximately 7, thus no color change). In addition the cresol red is a common loading dye used to monitor the band progressing in the agarose gel electrophoresis. Used in combination with glycerol there is no need for mixing the PCR reaction with loading buffer for analysis on ethidium agarose gel electrophoresis. To 4.7 ml dH_2O add 1 ml glycerol, 2 ml PCR buffer, 600 μl $MgCl_2$, and 600 μl 2 mM dNTP. Aliquot in 1 ml tubes, and store for months at −20 °C.
3. B&W buffer: 50 ml of 2× B&W buffer contains 10 mM Tris–HCl, 1 mM EDTA, and 2 mM NaCl. Add dH_2O to a final volume of 50 ml. May be stored for months at room temperature. For 1× B&W buffer mix 25 ml dH_2O with 25 ml 2× B&W buffer.

Table 1
List of all primers, sequences, and dispensation order in the established genotyping assay

SNP	NCBI ID	PCR primer forward*biotinylated	PCR primer reverse	Sequencing primer	Sequence to analyze	Dispensation order
FCN1-542	rs10120023	ATTTCTCCAGCTGTAACTTTCAA	CCCAAATACTATTTCCATCATATC	CTTGCACCAGCCCCA	TTC/TGGTGGAGTAAATTATTTGAA	ATCAGTGAG
FCN1-144	rs10117466	TCTCGCCTTGTGCCACAGTTTT	TGAGGAGCTCTCTGGACTGG	GAAACATCCTTTGAGATGA	CA/CTCATACCTCTCC	GCAGTCATA
FCN2-986	rs3124952	TGTAGGATGGCTGTGGACTAC	CATTGAAGGAAAATCCGATGG	CCTCGGCATCCCGATGGC	A/GGCAGGTGGCA	CAGTCAGTG
FCN2-602	rs3124953	AGTCCACAGCCATCCTACA	GGCAGTATGTAGAGCAC	GTAGAGCACAGGGGCA	CAT/CGAACAGG	GCATCTGAC
FCN2-4	rs17514136	CATGCCCAGGAAAGAGAGCAG	TGACAGTCGCCATGGGATC	TTTGAAGCAAAGACC	AGAA/GGAGATGG	CAGAGCAGA
FCN2+6359 and *+6424*	rs17549193 rs7851696	CTAGGCAGGTCGCACCTTC	TAATGATGTTACTGCCTGTAAC	CACAGGAGATTCCCTGA GATCTTACCACCGGAAATT	C/TGTTCCACAACAACCAGT GTG/TCTGTGATGTTTCAG	ACTCGTGTCTAGC
MBL2 X/Y	rs7096206	TGGTGTGAGAAAACTCAGGGAAG	GCACGGTCCCATTTGTTCTC	CTGGAAGACTATAAACATGCTT	TCG/CGTGGCAGTGA	GTCGCTGCA
MBL2 D, B and *C*	rs1800450 rs1800451 rs5030737	CCTTCCCTGAGTTTTCTCAC	AACAGCCCAACACGTACCTG	CGTACCTGGTTCCCCCTTTTCT	T/CCCTTGGTGT/CCATCACG/ACCC	GCTCTCGTGTCGATCACGAGC

Table 2
Troubleshooting

Trouble	Likely reason	Solution
Low peaks	Insufficient PCR	Check the fragments of 2 % agarose with EtBr and/or add more PCR product to the pyrosequencing reaction
	Bad sequencing primer stock or dilution of same	Make a new dilution or order a new batch
High background	Insufficient washing	Replace the filters on the vacuum bench station

4. Washing buffer: To 1 l dH_2O add 10 mM Tris–acetate, and adjust pH with a 5 M NaOH solution to pH 7.6. May be stored for months at room temperature.
5. Annealing buffer: To 1 l dH2O add 20 mM Tris–acetate and 5 mM MgAc2. Adjust to pH 7.6 with a 5 M NaOH solution pH 7.6. May be stored for months at room temperature.
6. In our laboratory we use the pyrosequencing machine PSQ 96MA and the PyroMark Vacuum Prep Workstation; however other systems may be used: a mono shaker and a heating cabinet or alternatively a heating block for 96-well PCR plate.

3 Methods

3.1 Initial PCR

1. Mix the following components at room temperature. For each reaction of a total of 24 μl add 10 μl PCR solution, 4.5 μl primer mix (1 μM) to a final concentration of 0.2 μM, 0.4 units Platinum Taq polymerase, and 50 ng DNA. Add dH2O to a total volume of 24 μl.
2. Perform the PCR amplification at the following cycling parameters: 1× (10 min at 95 °C) and 35× (15 s at 94 °C, 60 s at 60 °C, and 45 s at 72 °C).
3. The PCR fragments may be visualized on a 2 % EtBr agarose gel.

3.2 Purification of PCR Amplicons and Annealing of Pyrosequencing Primers

1. Resuspend the streptavidin sepharose beads. Streptavidin sepharose beads precipitate quickly; therefore efficient workflow is recommended. Mix 2 μl beads with 38 μl 1×B&W buffer per reaction, and add 40 μl of the mix to each PCR sample. Seal the plate with caps and vortex vigorously.
2. Incubate the plate on a plate mixer for 5–10 min allowing the biotinylated PCR amplicons to bind to the streptavidin-coated sepharose beads.

In the meantime use the PSQ 96MA software to calculate the amount of consumables needed in the automated sequencing steps, and prepare the master mix for the pyrosequencing reactions.

3. Add 1.6 μl 10 μM sequencing primer with 38.4 μl annealing buffer to each well in a flat-bottom PSQ96 plate.

Set up the PyroMark Vacuum Prep Workstation for purification.

4. Fill the trays with 70 % EtOH, 0.5 M NaOH, and washing buffer.
5. Wash the filters in EtOH for 20 s.

Purification of the PCR products.

6. Vortex the plate with the samples thoroughly, remove the caps, and transfer the plate to the Vacuum Prep Workstation.
7. Lower the vacuum prep tool into the samples, all the way to the bottom of the wells, and aspirate. Ensure that all liquid has been aspirated uniformly across the plate (beads precipitate fast, so this step must be performed within 3 min after the final vortex). The beads are now caught in the filters and ready to be washed.
8. Move the vacuum prep tool through the EtOH, NaOH, and washing buffer, leaving the tool in each tray for approximately 10 s. Drain the residual liquid from the vacuum prep tool by tipping it 90°.
9. Release the vacuum and lower the tool into the well on the PSQ96 plate. Tap gently the tool within the wells to release the beads from the filters. The filters are not to be touched during this process.
10. Lid the plate with an easily removable hard cover and incubate in the heating cabinet in the pyrosequencing cobber plate for 5 min. Allow the plate to cool down before proceeding with the analysis.
11. Load the pyrosequencing cartridge during incubation according to the calculation done in advance, and place the cartridge and the PSQ96 sample plate in the pyrosequencing machine.
12. Start analyzing.
13. Remember to close down the Vacuum Prep Workstation while pyrosequencing: wash the filters with the dH_2O and EtOH and turn off the pump.

4 Note

Follow the protocol provided by the manufacturer when starting up the pyrosequencing machinery and for calculating the consumables needed in the automated steps. In every run individuals with known genotypes for each polymorphism should be analyzed as controls.

References

1. Ronaghi M, Karamohamed S, Pettersson B, Uhlen M, Nyren P (1996) Real-time DNA sequencing using detection of pyrophosphate release. Anal Biochem 242(1):84–89
2. Sanger F, Nicklen S, Coulson AR (1977) DNA sequencing with chain-terminating inhibitors. Proc Natl Acad Sci U S A 74(12):5463–5467
3. Ahmadian A, Ehn M, Hober S (2006) Pyrosequencing: history, biochemistry and future. Clin Chim Acta 363(1–2):83–94
4. Arnold C, Westland L, Mowat G, Underwood A, Magee J, Gharbia S (2005) Single-nucleotide polymorphism-based differentiation and drug resistance detection in Mycobacterium tuberculosis from isolates or directly from sputum. Clin Microbiol Infect 11(2):122–130
5. Amoako KK, Thomas MC, Kong F, Janzen TW, Hahn KR, Shields MJ et al (2012) Rapid detection and antimicrobial resistance gene profiling of Yersinia pestis using pyrosequencing technology. J Microbiol Methods 90(3):228–234
6. Setty P, Gessi M, Waha A, Hammes J, El-Maarri O, Pietsch T et al (2011) Sensitive determination of BRAF copy number in clinical samples by pyrosequencing. Diagn Mol Pathol 20(3):148–157
7. Madsen HO, Satz ML, Hogh B, Svejgaard A, Garred P (1998) Different molecular events result in low protein levels of mannan-binding lectin in populations from southeast Africa and South America. J Immunol 161(6):3169–3175
8. Hummelshoj T, Munthe-Fog L, Madsen HO, Fujita T, Matsushita M, Garred P (2005) Polymorphisms in the FCN2 gene determine serum variation and function of Ficolin-2. Hum Mol Genet 14(12):1651–1658
9. Munthe-Fog L, Hummelshoj T, Honore C, Moller ME, Skjoedt MO, Palsgaard I et al (2012) Variation in FCN1 affects biosynthesis of ficolin-1 and is associated with outcome of systemic inflammation. Genes Immun 13(7):515–522
10. Vengen IT, Madsen HO, Garred P, Platou C, Vatten L, Videm V (2012) Mannose-binding lectin deficiency is associated with myocardial infarction: the HUNT2 study in Norway. PLoS One 7(7):e42113

Chapter 11

Assay for Estimation of the Functional Activity of the Mannan-Binding Lectin Pathway of the Complement System

Troels R. Kjaer and Steffen Thiel

Abstract

Mannan-binding lectin (MBL) is a soluble pattern recognition molecule of the innate immune system. It is found in plasma in complex with MBL-associated serine proteases (MASPs). When MBL recognizes foreign, e.g., the surface of some microorganisms, or altered host surfaces the MASPs are activated and this will in turn lead to the initiation of the complement system, i.e., activation of complement by the MBL pathway. This will end up in increased phagocytosis of the microorganism and killing by insertion of pore structures in the membrane of the microorganisms. Lack of MBL seems significant in specific situations, e.g., in immunocompromised individuals were MBL is important in battling infections and, e.g., in ischemia/reperfusion injuries were MBL can have a negative inflammatory generating, and thus tissue destructive role, as it recognizes epitopes emerging in the ischemic tissue. It may thus be relevant in several situations to test for the presence of the MBL pathway in human sera. Here we describe a functional assay for estimation of MBL pathway activity by detection of complement factor deposition onto microtiter plate wells coated with a physiological relevant ligand for MBL.

Key words Complement, Lectin pathway activity, Mannan-binding lectin, Mannose-binding lectin, MBL, MBL-associated serine protease 2 (MASP-2)

1 Introduction

Mannan-binding lectin (MBL), also known as Mannose-binding lectin, activates the complement system when binding to a fitting pattern of carbohydrates and thus triggers an innate antimicrobial defense mechanism [1]. Such patterns of carbohydrate structures may be presented on the surface of microorganisms or on altered self-surfaces.

In addition there are two other complement pathways. The classical pathway where the recognition molecules C1q recognizes a pattern of antibodies and the alternative pathway which is initiated when the fragment C3b is deposited on a non-inhibitory

Mihaela Gadjeva (ed.), *The Complement System: Methods and Protocols*, Methods in Molecular Biology, vol. 1100, DOI 10.1007/978-1-62703-724-2_11, © Springer Science+Business Media New York 2014

surface. Completion of any of the three complement pathways may eventually lead to death of the incoming microorganism either by lysis or phagocytosis of the microorganism [2].

MBL is a large molecule found in blood as oligomers of a structural unit which itself contain three identical polypeptide chains. Each polypeptide chain contains one carbohydrate recognition domain (CRD) and one structural unit thus contains three CRDs, and an oligomer of four (the predominant type) structural units thus contain 12 CRDs. Each CRD binds with low affinity, but the overall binding strength is high when many of these CRDs bind at the same time. MBL thus binds to microorganisms by recognition of a pattern of certain sugars, e.g., mannose, glucose, L-fucose, and *N*-acetyl-glucosamine [3].

MBL is synthesized in the liver and the final products are released into the plasma where it associates with the MBL-associated serine proteases (MASPs): MASP-1 (MBL-associated serine protease-1), MASP-2 (MBL-associated serine protease-2), and MASP-3 (MBL-associated serine protease-3) as well as two nonenzymatic proteins, MBL-associated protein of 19 kDa (MAp19) and MBL-associated protein of 44 kDa (MAp44) [4]. The MASPs are activated when MBL binds to a fitting pattern of carbohydrates. The function of most of these associated MASPs and MAps remains to be determined, but we believe that the main function of activated MASP-2 is to proteolytically cleave complement components C4 and C2 to generate the C3 convertase C4bC2b.

This protocol describes how to determine the ability of serum or plasma samples to mediate activation of complement factor C4 via the MBL pathway of complement. The described method uses detection with Eu^{3+}-labeled streptavidin in a Time-Resolved Immunofluorometric Assay (TRIFMA). The TRIFMAs are similar to ELISAs with the only difference being the type of labeling of detecting molecules. Instead of enzyme-linked antibodies or streptavidin in ELISAs, Eu^{3+} is used to label antibodies or streptavidin in TRIFMAs. In the ELISAs a colorimetric reaction is detected, whereas in the TRIFMAs fluorescence is determined through time-resolved fluorometry [5]. We find that using this assay in a TRIFMA format provides enhanced sensitivity, a broader dynamic range and improved reproducibility. An ELISA version of the assay is described in detail in Petersen et al. [6].

In the present method a surface of mannan (which is a preparation of carbohydrate structures from the surface of *Saccharomyces cerevisiea*) coated in microtiter wells is used for the binding of MBL/MASP complexes from serum or plasma samples (Fig. 1). Any classical pathway activity, which can also result in C4 activation is inhibited by the high ionic strength buffer used in the assay [6]. Under these conditions the classical pathways is not functional, because the binding of C1q to immune complexes is inhibited.

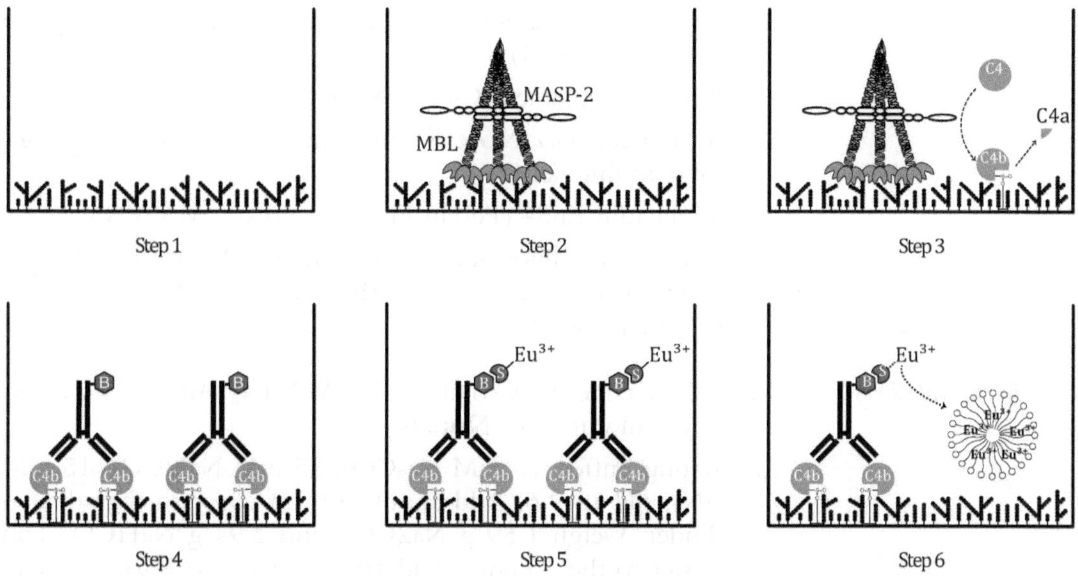

Fig. 1 The different steps in the assay for MBL pathway activity. *Step 1* is the coating with mannan. *Step 2* is the binding of MBL/MASP-2 complexes to the mannan. *Step 3* is the incubation of C4, which is then cleaved and C4b deposited in the wells. *Step 4* is the binding of anti-C4 antibody to the deposited C4 fragment. *Step 5* is the binding of europium-labeled streptavidin to the biotinylated anti-C4 antibody. *Step 6* is the addition of enhancement solution to the wells which is followed by reading by time-resolved fluorometry

Since the activation of C4 by MASP-2 is inhibited by high ionic strength the assay requires subsequent incubation with purified C4 in an isotonic buffer. After incubation at 37 °C with purified human C4, the C4b deposition is detected with biotin-labeled antibodies against C4b and europium-labeled streptavidin.

2 Materials

2.1 Preparation of Serum or Plasma (See Note 1)

1. Serum: Blood from healthy individuals is drawn into serum tubes (e.g., from Terumo) and allowed to coagulate at room temperature for ½ h before centrifugation (2,000 × *g*, 10 min) and removal of serum. Serum aliquots are stored at −80 °C until use.
2. Plasma: Blood from healthy individuals is drawn into citrate, EDTA or Heparin tubes (e.g., from Terumo). The stabilized blood is centrifuged (2,000 × *g*, 10 min) and the plasma is removed. Plasma aliquots are stored at −80 °C until use.

2.2 Assay Components

1. Ninety six-well FluoroNunc microtiter plates (*see* **Note 2**).
2. Mannan.

3. Human serum albumin (HSA) or bovine serum albumin (BSA) (*see* **Note 3**).
4. Human complement C4 (*see* **Note 4**).
5. Biotinylated (*see* **Note 5**) antihuman C4 antibodies (e.g., rabbit antihuman C4).
6. Streptavidin-Eu3+ (Perkin Elmer, Waltham, MA, USA).
7. Time-resolved fluorometer, e.g., Victor™ X4 Multilabel Plate Reader (Perkin Elmer) or PHERAstar Plus (BMG Labtech, Ortenberg, Germany).

2.3 Assay Solutions

1. Sodium azide stock solution: 1.5 M NaN_3. Add 9.75 g NaN_3 to 100 ml water (*see* **Note 6**).
2. Coating buffer: 15 mM Na_2CO_3, 35 mM $NaHCO_3$, 15 mM NaN_3, pH to 9.6. Add about 500 ml water to a graduated cylinder. Weigh 1.59 g Na2CO3 and 2.94 g NaHCO3 and transfer to the cylinder. Add 10 ml NaN3 stock solution and add water to a volume of 900 ml. Mix and adjust pH with (HCl or NaOH). Make up volume to 1 l. Store at RT.
3. Blocking buffer: 1 mg/ml HSA in 10 mM Tris, 145 mM NaCl, 15 mM NaN3, pH 7.4. Dissolve 1.21 g Tris and 8.47 g NaCl in 900 ml water. Add 10 ml NaN3 stock solution and adjust pH (*see* **Note 7**). Add 5 ml HSA (200 mg/ml) and make up to 1 l with water. Store at 4 °C.
4. MBL-binding buffer: 20 mM Tris, 1 M NaCl, 0.05 % (v/v) Triton X-100, 10 mM CaCl2, 15 mM NaN3, 1 mg/ml HSA, pH7.4. Dissolve 2.42 g Tris, 58.44 g NaCl and 1.11 g CaCl2 in 900 ml water. Add 10 ml NaN3 stock solution and adjust pH with HCl. Add 0.5 ml Triton X-100 and 5 ml HSA (200 mg/ml). Make up to 1 l. Store at RT.
5. Washing buffer with Calcium: 10 mM Tris, 145 mM NaCl, 5 mM CaCl2, 15 mM NaN3, 0.05 % (v/v) Tween-20 (TW), 15 mM NaN3, pH 7.4. Dissolve 1.21 g Tris, 8.47 g NaCl, and 0.55 g CaCl2 in 900 ml water. Add 10 ml NaN3 stock solution and 50 ml TW. Adjust pH with HCl. Make up to 1 l. Store at RT.
6. Washing buffer without Calcium: As above, but without the added CaCl2.
7. C4 dilution buffer: 4 mM Barbital, 145 mM NaCl, 2 mM CaCl2, 1 mM MgCl2, pH 7.4. Dissolve 0.37 g barbital, 4.24 g NaCl, 0.11 g CaCl2, 0.05 g MgCl2 in 400 ml water. Adjust pH and make up to 500 ml.
8. Europium dilution buffer: 10 mM Tris, 145 mM NaCl, 0.05 % (v/v) TW, 15 mM NaN_3, 25 μM EDTA, pH 7.4. Dissolve 0.48 g Tris and 3.4 g NaCl in 350 ml water. Add 4 ml NaN_3 stock solution, 17.5 ml TW and 25 μM EDTA (25 μl of a

0.4 M EDTA solution) (*see* **Note 8**). Make up to 400 ml with water. Store at RT.

9. The enhancement solution be made as follows: 0.57 % (v/v) Acetic acid, 1 % (w/v) PEG 6000, 0.1 % (v/v) Triton X-100, 15 μM β-NTA (2-napthoyltrifluoroacetone), 50 μM TOPO (tri-*n*-octylphosphine oxide), pH 3.2. Add 5.7 ml of glacial acetic acid to 900 ml water and adjust pH to 3.2 with potassium hydrogen phthalate (0.1 M in water). Dissolve 10 g PEG 6000 in the solution and add 1 ml Triton X-100. Add 2 ml β-NTA/TOPO solution (*see* **Note 9**) and make up to 1 l with water. The enhancement solution should be stored at 4 °C and kept dark.

3 Methods

3.1 Performing the Assay

Carry out all procedures at RT unless otherwise specified.

1. Coat a FluoroNunc 96-well plate with mannan, 100 μl/well at 10 μg mannan/ml diluted in coating buffer and incubate at RT over night in a moist-chamber (Step 1, Fig. 1) (*see* **Note 10**).
2. Empty the wells and block the wells with 200 μl/well of *blocking buffer*. Incubate 1 h at RT. After incubation, wash the plates three times with *washing buffer with* $CaCl_2$.

   If the plates are to be stored for later use, empty the wells and add 200 μl/well of *washing buffer without* $CaCl_2$ and store them at 4 °C in a moist-chamber.
3. Dilute samples in *MBL-binding buffer*, add the samples to the wells, 100 μl/well, in duplicates, and incubate in a moist-chamber over night at 4 °C (Step 2, Fig. 1). Usually 200-fold sample dilution is adequate. Wash three times with *washing buffer with* $CaCl_2$. To be able to compare the activity of samples a standard curve must be included in the assay. We use a dilution series of a serum with high MBL content (see below in Subheading 3.2), starting at a 1/10 dilution followed by threefold dilutions reaching 1/21,870 as the last dilution. Also include buffer only wells.
4. Add 0.5 μg/ml human C4 diluted in C4 dilution buffer, 100 μl/well (*see* **Note 11**) and incubate 1.5 h at 37 °C (*see* **Note 12**) (Step 3, Fig. 1). Wash three times with washing buffer with CaCl2.
5. Detect deposited C4b fragments with 0.2 μg/ml biotinylated antihuman C4 antibody (*see* **Note 13**) (Step 4, Fig. 1). Dilute the biotinylated antibodies in *washing buffer with* $CaCl_2$ and use 100 μl/well and incubate for 2 h at RT in a moist-chamber. Wash the wells three times with *washing buffer with* $CaCl_2$.
6. Detect the bound biotin anti-C4 with 1 μg/ml Streptavidin-Eu^{3+} (*see* **Note 14**) diluted in europium dilution buffer, 100 μl/well

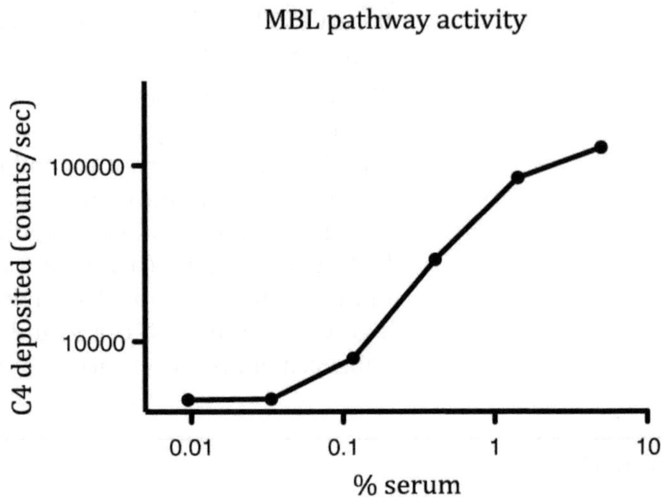

Fig. 2 The appearance of a typical standard curve in the assay. The serum concentration is given on the *x*-axis (log scale) and the signal is given on the *y*-axis (log scale). Here the highest serum concentration used is 1/20 followed by 3.5-fold dilutions. We often also use 1/10 dilution followed by threefold dilutions

(*see* **Note 15**) and incubate for 1 h at RT in a moist-chamber (Step 5, Fig. 1). After incubation wash the plates three times in washing buffer with CaCl2.

7. The europium is released from the Streptavidin and incorporated into micelles after addition of 200 µl/well enhancement solution (Step 6, Fig. 1).
8. Shake the plate on a microplate shaker for 5 min before reading on a fluorometer supporting time-resolved fluorometry (*see* **Note 16**).

3.2 Evaluating the Data

To be able to compare different sera in terms of MBL pathway activity a standard curve is made (as described above). The data obtained from the reading of the assay should be plotted as depicted in Fig. 2. The serum concentration at the *x*-axes (on a log scale) and the results from the time-resolved fluorometry (counts per second) at the *y*-axes (on a log scale). For data analysis and plotting of the data it is convenient to use a graphical software, e.g., Prism, SigmaPlot or Excel. The standard curve should be S-shaped and the curve should contain at least three data sets in the linear range of the S-shaped curve (*see* Fig. 2).

The MBL pathway activity of the standard serum is given the arbitrary value of 1 unit per ml (equal to 1,000 mU/ml). The MBL pathway activity of the other sera that is tested is then read from the standard curve—taking into account that the sera were tested at a 200-fold dilution. The MBL pathway activity of the tested sera is thus given as mU/ml as compared to the standard serum used.

It is advisable to include internal standards as controls in each assay if several assays are performed. We usually use samples of plasma with known high, medium, and low activity. Based on the internal controls the reproducibility of the assays can be determined. The calculated inter assay coefficient of variation (%CV, i.e., the standard deviation divided by the mean and this number multiplied by 100 to get percentage) should be below 20 % for high, and medium internal standards, but may be slightly higher if the low internal standard is close to the lower end of the dilution curve.

The time to perform assay as described is three days. Preparing stocks of pre-coated plates with mannan can considerably shorten the process. The coated plates may be stored at 4 °C for up to 2 months. We use overnight incubations for practical reasons, but the whole assay may easily be performed in two days if desired with pre-coated plates. The incubation with C4 must be for the given time at 37 °C.

If no fluorescence response is seen, possible errors could be: (a) The enhancement buffer in the wells was discarded instead of left in the wells when measured in the fluorometer. (b) The complement factor C4 has been inactivated by incorrect storage (e.g., the freezer is defrosting by itself or the C4 has been thawed and frozen more than once. (c) Ca^{2+} was omitted from the washing buffer, the sample buffer or the C4 dilution buffer. (d) Too much EDTA was present in the europium dilution buffer, i.e., 25 μM and NOT 25 mM is to be used.

As noted in the introduction an ELISA version of the assay is described in detail in Petersen et al. [6]. The only difference in this version is the use of enzyme-labeled streptavidin instead of the europium-labeled streptavidin and the use of a substrate for the enzyme to get a color reaction in the wells which is then read by colorimetry.

The MBL pathway activity closely follows the concentration of MBL in the sera tested. In seldom cases (estimated 1 per 10.000 samples tested in a normal Caucasian population) a low MBL pathway activity in a serum with normal MBL level may be found, due to a deficiency of MASP-2 [7].

4 Notes

1. Both serum and plasma (EDTA, citrate, or heparin) samples may be used, despite the presence of calcium in the sample buffer, since the high NaCl concentration in the sample buffer is inhibiting coagulation. The assays are not influenced by possible variations of other serum factors, e.g., complement factor C4 or C1-inhibitor (which is a promiscuous serine protease inhibitor that also inhibits MASP-2 if presented at physiological salt concentrations).

2. When measuring europium by time-resolved fluorometry in microtiter wells it is important that the plastic of the plates contain very low levels of europium as is the case with FluoroNunc plates (Thermo Scientific, Waltham, MA). The Maxisorb plates from Nunc may contain substantial amounts of europium and may thus give a high background in the assay.
3. HSA can be replaced with BSA if this is more convenient. We use a solution of 200 mg/ml HSA normally used as infusion fluid (10 96 97, CSL Behring, Marburg, Germany). Other sources of HSA may also be used.
4. Complement C4 can easily be purified by conventional laboratory techniques from human plasma as described elsewhere [8]. C4 may also be purchased (A105, CompTech, Tyler, Texas).
5. One milligram IgG from a polyclonal rabbit antihuman C4c Antiserum (A0065, DAKO, Glostrup, Denmark) was dialysed against PBS for 2 h at RT in a tween-20 pre-blocked dialysis tube with a cut-off value of 6–10 kDa. Afterwards the antibody was further dialysed O/N in fresh PBS at RT. Fresh PBS was adjusted to pH 8.5 with 5 % Na_2CO_3, the tube dialysed for 3–4 h at RT and then we open the tube and add 167 μg biotin *N*-hydroxysuccinimide ester (H1759, Sigma-Aldrich) dissolved in dimethyl sulfoxid to the tube content and close the tube again. The dialysis tube was incubated 4 h on a rocking table. Biotin *N*-hydroxysuccinimide ester is very susceptible to hydrolysis and is therefore kept in dimethyl sulfoxid. The dialysis tube was dialysed in TBS O/N at RT, and finally 2× 2 h in TBS/azide at RT.
6. NaN_3 is toxic and should be handled with care. We used 15 mM NaN_3 in the majority of our buffers to prevent fungal and bacterial contamination. NaN_3 does not influence this assay in any way.
7. We prefer to adjust pH prior addition of protein components in our buffer to avoid contaminating future adjusted buffers.
8. The 0.4 M EDTA, pH 7.4 solution is made by adding 76 g EDTA tetrasodium salt dihydrate (ED4SS, Sigma-Aldrich) to 450 ml water. Adjust pH and make up to 500 ml.
9. The β-NTA/TOPO solution is composed of β-NTA (4,4,4 trifluoro-1-(2-naphyl)-1,3-butandion) (343633, Sigma-Aldrich) and TOPO (trioctylphosphine oxide) (223301, Sigma-Aldrich) dissolved in methanol. 0.03993 g β-NTA is dissolved in 10 ml methanol and 0.19333 g TOPO is dissolved in 10 ml methanol. The two solutions are mixed and kept at −80 °C.
10. A plastic box with a lid and a wet paper towel inside is sufficient as a moist-chamber. The plates are incubated in moist-chambers to avoid evaporation of the solutions added to the wells.

11. C4 is thawed on ice. C4 is diluted in *C4 dilution buffer* immediately before use. We advise that C4 is kept in aliquots with only enough protein for a single assay (i.e., one microtiter plate), as C4 subjected to freeze/thaw cycles severely looses its activity. Therefore, do NOT use already thawed C4. Different preparations of purified C4 may differ in activity. It is thus recommended to initially try with a few concentrations (e.g., 1, 0.5, and 0.25 μg/ml) of this before testing many samples.
12. This incubation time is important and should not be shortened or extended unless a less sensitive or a more sensitive assay is wanted, respectively.
13. Anti-C4 antibodies recognizing the small anaphylotoxin fragment C4a will NOT detect the bound C4b fragments.
14. If an ELISA setup is preferred enzyme linked streptavidin can be used instead of Eu^{3+}-labeled streptavidin. This is followed by wash and the relevant substrate solution is added [6].
15. It is important to note that MBL is a calcium-dependent lectin, thus all buffers for dilution and washing contains 5 mM $CaCl_2$, except the ***europium dilution buffer***. This contains 25 μM EDTA which ensures that free Eu^{3+} ions from the Eu^{3+}-coupled streptavidin solution is chelated and prevented from adsorption to, e.g., the microtiter plate, while the EDTA concentration is not enough to dissociate the Eu^{3+} ion from the streptavidin chelator.
16. Fluorometers supporting time-resolved fluorometry, e.g., Victor™ X4 Multilabel Plate Reader (Perkin Elmer) or PHERAstar Plus (BMG Labtech).

References

1. Thiel S (2007) Complement activating soluble pattern recognition molecules with collagen-like regions, mannan-binding lectin, ficolins and associated proteins. Mol Immunol 44(16):3875–3888
2. Ricklin D, Hajishengallis G, Yang K et al (2010) Complement: a key system for immune surveillance and homeostasis. Nat Immunol 11(9): 785–797
3. Holmskov U, Thiel S, Jensenius JC (2003) Collections and ficolins: humoral lectins of the innate immune defense. Annu Rev Immunol 21:547–578
4. Degn SE, Jensenius JC, Thiel S (2011) Disease-causing mutations in genes of the complement system. Am J Hum Genet 88(6):689–705
5. Lovgren T, Hemmilä I, Halonen P (1985) Time-resolved fluoremetry in immunoassay. In: Collins WP (ed) Alternative immunoassays. Wiley, New York, pp 203–217
6. Petersen SV, Thiel S, Jensen L et al (2001) An assay for the mannan-binding lectin pathway of complement activation. J Immunol Methods 257(1–2):107–116
7. Stengaard-Pedersen K, Thiel S, Gadjeva M et al (2003) Inherited deficiency of mannan-binding lectin-associated serine protease 2. N Engl J Med 349(6):554–560
8. Dodds AW (1993) Small-scale preparation of complement components C3 and C4. Methods Enzymol 223:46–61

Chapter 12

Purification, Measurement of Concentration, and Functional Complement Assay of Human Ficolins

Misao Matsushita, David Kilpatrick, Hiroshi Shiraki, Yu Liu, Koichiro Tateishi, Mitsushi Tsujimura, Yuichi Endo, and Teizo Fujita

Abstract

Ficolins constitute a group of lectins involved in innate immunity. L-Ficolin, H-ficolin, and M-ficolin are present in human serum. The human ficolins differ in carbohydrate-binding specificity, but they have in common the ability to recognize the acetyl group. L-Ficolin and H-ficolin are associated with serine proteases termed MASPs (MBL-associated serine proteases) and their truncated proteins, and the complexes (L/H-ficolin–MASP) activate the lectin pathway of complement upon binding to their ligands. Recombinant M-ficolin is also able to form a complex with MASP, resulting in complement activation. L-Ficolin and H-ficolin can be purified as a complex with MASP from serum by utilizing their binding specificities. These ficolin–MASP complexes have an ability to activate C4. Human ficolins are quantified by ELISA using specific antibodies or ligands.

Key words L-Ficolin, H-Ficolin, M-Ficolin, Lectin, MASP, C4 activation

1 Introduction

The ficolins are a group of lectins defined by having a collagen-like domain combined with a fibrinogen-like domain; the basic triplet subunits oligomerize to form higher multimers [1, 2]. They play a crucial role in innate immunity. In humans, there are three types: L-ficolin, H-ficolin, and M-ficolin. L-Ficolin (also called P35, ficolin-2, EBP-37, or hucolin) is present in serum and recognizes the acetyl group moiety present in substances such as *N*-acetyl-D-glucosamine (GlcNAc) [3]. L-Ficolin also recognizes 1,3-β-glucan and galactose [4, 5]. The fibrinogen-like domain is involved in binding. L-Ficolin forms a complex with three types of MBL-associated serine proteases (termed MASP-1, MASP-2, and MASP-3) and two types of their truncated forms, sMAP (MAp19) and MAp44 (MAP-1) [6–13]. Binding of the L-ficolin–MASP complex (i.e. a complex composing of L-ficolin, MASPs and their truncated proteins) to carbohydrates on the surface of pathogens

Mihaela Gadjeva (ed.), *The Complement System: Methods and Protocols*, Methods in Molecular Biology, vol. 1100,
DOI 10.1007/978-1-62703-724-2_12, © Springer Science+Business Media New York 2014

initiates the activation of the lectin pathway of complement [14]. H-Ficolin (also called Hakata antigen, ficolin-3, thermolabile β-2 macroglycoprotein, or thermolabile substance) is present in serum, bile duct, alveolus, and bronchus [15]. H-Ficolin was initially identified in serum as an autoantigen that was recognized by an autoantibody produced in a small minority of patients with systemic lupus erythematosus (SLE) [16, 17]. H-Ficolin recognizes acetyl groups [18]. It has also been shown to bind to a polysaccharide of *Aerococcus viridans* [19] and to certain lipopolysacchades of *Hafnia alvei* [20], although sugar moieties recognized by H-ficolin remain unsolved. The serum H-ficolin forms a complex with MASPs and their truncated proteins like L-ficolin [21]. Upon binding to its ligands, H-ficolin-MASP activates complement. M-Ficolin (also called ficolin-1) is present on membranes of monocytes and granulocytes and in serum [22, 23]. M-Ficolin recognizes GlcNAc, GalNAc, and sialic acid. It remains unknown whether the serum M-ficolin is present complexed with MASP. In vitro experiments using recombinant M-ficolin, however, revealed that it is able to form a complex with MASP, resulting in complement activation upon binding to GlcNAc or the acetyl group [24, 25].

In this chapter, we introduce methods for purification, measurement of concentration, and functional complement assay of L-ficolin and H-ficolin. We also introduce a method for functional complement assay of M-ficolin.

2 Materials

2.1 Purification of L-Ficolin

1. Loading buffer for GlcNAc-agarose affinity chromatography: 50 mM Tris, 200 mM NaCl, 10 mM $CaCl_2$, pH 7.8 (buffer A). Weigh 6.1 g Tris, 11.7 g NaCl and 1.5 g $CaCl_2 \cdot 2H_2O$ and transfer to the cylinder. Add water to a volume of 900 mL. Mix and adjust pH with HCl to 7.8. Make up to 1 L with water. Store at 4 °C.
2. Elution buffer for mannose-binding lectin (MBL) from GlcNAc-agarose: 50 mM Tris, 200 mM NaCl, 10 mM $CaCl_2$, 300 mM mannose pH 7.8 (buffer B). Prepare the same as buffer A except that buffer B contains 54.1 g mannose as well as other solutes.
3. Elution buffer for L-ficolin from GlcNAc-agarose: 50 mM Tris, 200 mM NaCl, 10 mM $CaCl_2$, 300 mM GlcNAc pH 7.8 (buffer C). Prepare the same as buffer A except that buffer C contains 66.4 g GlcNAc as well as other solutes.
4. Loading buffer for Mono Q ion-exchange chromatography: 20 mM Tris, 50 mM NaCl, 10 mM $CaCl_2$, pH 7.8 (buffer D). Weigh 2.4 g Tris, 2.9 g NaCl, and 1.5 g $CaCl_2 \cdot 2H_2O$ and transfer to the cylinder. Add water to a volume of 900 mL.

Mix and adjust pH with HCl to 7.8. Make up to 1 L with water. Store at 4 °C.

5. Elution buffer for Mono Q ion-exchange chromatography: 20 mM Tris, 1 M NaCl, 10 mM $CaCl_2$, pH 7.8 (buffer E). Weigh 2.4 g Tris, 58.4 g NaCl, and 1.5 g $CaCl_2 \cdot 2H_2O$ and transfer to the cylinder. Add water to a volume of 900 mL. Mix and adjust pH with HCl to 7.8. Make up to 1 L with water. Store at 4 °C.

2.2 Assay for Measuring L-Ficolin Concentration

1. Coating buffer: carbonate buffer for coating ELISA plates is made by dissolving, for example, 1.6 g of Na_2CO_3 and 2.9 g $NaHCO_3$ per liter. The pH should be 9.6 at room temperature without further adjustment.
2. Diluent: the standard "Diluent" used throughout the assay consists of 20 mM Tris, 2 mM $CaCl_2$, and 140 mM NaCl adjusted to pH 7.4 with concentrated HCl.
3. Avidin–biotin complex (ABC) reagent is prepared by mixing horseradish peroxidase-conjugated avidin and biotin in Diluent supplemented with 0.05 % Tween-20. After gentle mixing, the ABC reagent is first allowed to stand for 30 min, then used immediately.
4. ABTS reagent: prepare 50 mM sodium citrate/50 mM NaH_2PO_4 (pH 6.3) and titrate it with 50 mM citric acid/50 mM NaH_2PO_4 until the pH is at 5.3. Immediately before use, prepare 10 mg 2,2′-Azino-bis (3-ethylbenzothiazoline-6-sulphonic acid, diammonium salt (ABTS)) in 10 mL of the citrate:phosphate buffer, then dilute 1 in 10 and add H_2O_2 to 0.015 %. For example, 3 mL of 1 mg/mL ABTS, 27 mL of additional buffer, 15 μl of 30 % H_2O_2.
5. Monoclonal antibodies: Mouse monoclonal antibodies (GN1 and GN5) against L-ficolin were generated in Fukushima Medical University, Japan. GN5 is commercially available through Hycult biotechnology, Uden, Netherlands.
6. Biotinylated second (GN5) antibody: GN5 at 1 mg/mL phosphate-buffered saline (Dulbecco A) was mixed for 4 h at room temperature with N-hydroxysuccinimido-biotin at 1 mg/mL dimethyl sulfoxide using 60 μl of the latter/mL of antibody solution. The biotinylated GN5 thus obtained was freed of reactants by extensive dialysis.

2.3 Assay for L-Ficolin-Mediated Complement Activation

1. Carbonate buffer (0.1 M, pH 9.6): Mix 0.1 M $NaHCO_3$ solution and 0.1 M Na_2CO_3 solution (approximately 2:1) to adjust pH to 9.6.
2. TBS: 20 mM Tris, 150 mM NaCl, pH 7.5. Weigh 2.4 g Tris and 8.8 g NaCl and transfer to the cylinder. Add water to a volume of 900 mL. Mix and adjust pH with HCl to 7.5. Make up to 1 L with water. Store at 4 °C.

3. TBST-Ca^{2+}: TBS containing 2 mM $CaCl_2$ and 0.1 % Tween 20. Weigh 2.4 g Tris, 8.8 g NaCl, and 0.3 g $CaCl_2 \cdot 2H_2O$ and transfer to the cylinder. Add water to a volume of 900 mL. Mix and add 5 mL of 10 % Tween 20 solution. Mix and adjust pH with HCl to 7.5. Make up to 1 L with water. Store at 4 °C.
4. 0.1 M citrate buffer pH 4.3: Mix 0.1 M trisodium citrate dehydrate solution and 0.1 M citric acid solution to adjust pH to 4.3 (approximately 1:1).

2.4 Purification of H-Ficolin

1. Monoclonal anti-H-ficolin (4H5) (Hycult biotechnology, Uden, Netherlands).
2. 4H5-Sepharose is prepared by conjugating 4H5 with cyanogen bromide-activated Sepharose 4B according to the manufacturer's instructions.
3. Loading buffer for 4H5-Sepharose affinity chromatography: 50 mM Tris, 200 mM NaCl, 10 mM $CaCl_2$, pH 7.8 (buffer A). Weigh 6.1 g Tris, 11.7 g NaCl, and 1.5 g $CaCl_2 \cdot 2H_2O$ and transfer to the cylinder. Add water to a volume of 900 mL. Mix and adjust pH with HCl to 7.8. Make up to 1 L with water. Store at 4 °C.
4. Elution buffer for H-ficolin from 4H5-Sepharose: 0.1 M glycine–HCl pH 2.2 (buffer B). Weigh 7.5 g glycine and transfer to the cylinder. Add water to a volume of 900 mL. Mix and adjust pH with HCl to 2.2. Make up to 1 L with water. Store at 4 °C.
5. Neutralizing buffer for 4H5-Sepharose affinity chromatography: 1 M Tris–HCl pH 8.2. Weigh 121.1 g Tris and transfer to the cylinder. Add water to a volume of 900 mL. Mix and adjust pH with HCl to 8.2. Make up to 1 L with water. Store at 4 °C.
6. Elution buffer for H-ficolin from Lentil lectin-Sepharose: 50 mM Tris, 200 mM NaCl, 10 mM $CaCl_2$, 0.2 M α-methylmannopyranoside, pH 7.8. Prepare the same buffer as buffer A except that this buffer contains 38.8 g α-methylmannopyranoside per liter.
7. Loading buffer for anti-IgM-Sepharose and Protein A-Sepharose: 20 mM Tris–HCl, 150 mM NaCl, 2 mM $CaCl_2$, pH 7.6 (buffer B). Weigh 2.4 g Tris, 8.7 g NaCl, and 0.3 g $CaCl_2 \cdot 2H_2O$ and transfer to the cylinder. Add water to a volume of 900 mL. Mix and adjust pH with HCl to 7.6. Make up to 1 L with water. Store at 4 °C.

2.5 Assay for Measuring H-Ficolin Concentration

1. *Aerococcus viridans* (a laboratory isolate, Fukuoka Red Cross Blood Center, Chikushino, Japan): This Gram-positive bacterium is grown to mid-log phase in brain heart infusion broth

at 37 °C with aeration. Following centrifugation for 10 min at 10,000 × *g*, the precipitates are washed three times in 10 mM phosphate buffer, pH 7.2 containing 0.15 M NaCl (PBS) and resuspended in PBS.

2. PSA: PSA is an extracellular polysaccharide produced by *A. viridans* and is composed of D-glucose, GlcNAc, D-mannose, and D-xylose. PSA is prepared from the supernatant of the culture medium of *A. viridans* strain. 2×10^{10} *A. viridans* (*see* **Note 1**) is added to 1 L of brain heart infusion broth and incubated at 37 °C for 12 h with aeration. Following centrifugation at 10,000 × *g* for 10 min, the supernatant is mixed with 1/10 volume 3 M sodium acetate (pH 3.5) and subsequently mixed with 2.5-fold volume cold 95 % ethanol. After being left to stand for 30 min at −80 °C, the precipitate is collected by centrifugation, dissolved in 20 mM Tris–HCl buffer, pH 8.0 (TB), and then dialyzed overnight against TB. This dialysate is digested with DNase 1 (10 μg in 20 mM TB) and RNase A (100 μg in 20 mM TB) for 10 min end-over-end at room temperature. The reaction mixture is extracted with equal volume of phenol saturated with 1 M Tris. After being left to stand for 10 min at room temperature, the resultant phenol layer is mixed with double the volume of cold ethanol. After being left to stand for −80 °C for 30 min, the precipitate is collected by centrifugation for 10 min at 10,000 × *g*, and dissolved in 10 mM PB. Subsequently, the solution is applied to a DEAE-Sepharose column (2 cm × 20 cm) equilibrated with PB. After washing the column with 100 mL PB-containing 0.2 M NaCl, the column is eluted with PB-containing 0.3 M NaCl. The fractions with precipitin-line forming activity in 0.7 % agarose gel are collected (*see* **Note 2**) and then concentrated by ethanol precipitation as described above. The pellet is dissolved in PBS, and then applied to a Sephacryl S-400 column (2.4 cm × 40 cm) equilibrated with PBS. Following elution by PBS, the fractions with precipitin-line forming activity are combined, dialyzed against distilled water, and then lyophilized.

2.6 Assay for H-Ficolin-Mediated Complement Activation

1. TBS-Ca^{2+}: 20 mM Tris, 150 mM NaCl, 2 mM $CaCl_2$ pH 7.5. Weigh 2.4 g Tris, 8.8 g NaCl, and 0.3 g $CaCl_2 \cdot 2H_2O$ and transfer to the cylinder. Add water to a volume of 900 mL. Mix and adjust pH with HCl to 7.5. Make up to 1 L with water. Store at 4 °C.
2. TBST-Ca^{2+}: TBS containing 0.1 % Tween 20. Weigh 2.4 g Tris, 8.8 g NaCl, and 0.3 g $CaCl_2 \cdot 2H_2O$ and transfer to the cylinder. Add water to a volume of 900 mL. Mix and add

10 mL of 10 % Tween 20 solution. Mix and adjust pH with HCl to 7.6. Make up to 1 L with water. Store at 4 °C.

3. 0.1 M citrate buffer pH 4.3: Mix 0.1 M trisodium citrate dehydrate solution and 0.1 M citric acid solution to adjust pH to 4.3 (approximately 1:1).

2.7 Assay for M-Ficolin-MASP-Mediated Complement Activation ([24], See Note 3)

1. Recombinant M-ficolin: Prepared by *Drosophila* expression system and affinity purification as reported [24].
2. Human MASP: Human MASP (a mixture of MASP-1, MASP-2, MASP-3, sMAP, and MAp44 in which MASP-1, MASP-2, and MASP-3 are in the proenzyme forms) is obtained from human serum as reported [26]. In brief, the MBL–MASP complex is purified in the presence of protease inhibitors by affinity chromatography on mannan-Sepharose and then anti-MBL-Sepharose. After the MBL-MASP complex is dialyzed against a high ionic strength buffer containing EDTA, the dialysate is passed through an anti-MBL-Sepharose column. MASPs and their truncated proteins are recovered in the unbound fractions, while MBL is retained to the column.
3. 10× Tris-Buffered Saline (TBS) buffer: 500 mM Tris–HCl, 1.5 M NaCl, pH 8.0. Add about 100 mL water to a 2 L graduated cylinder or a glass beaker. Weigh 60.6 g Tris and 87.7 g NaCl, and transfer to the cylinder. Add water to a volume of 900 mL. Mix and adjust pH to 8.0 with HCl. Make up to 1 L with water. Dilute ten times before use.
4. 1 M $CaCl_2$: Dissolve 14.7 g $CaCl_2{\cdot}2H_2O$ in 100 mL water.
5. TBS-Ca^{2+} buffer: 50 mM Tris–HCl, 150 mM NaCl, 5 mM $CaCl_2$, pH 8.0. Add 100 mL 10× TBS buffer and 5 mL 1 M $CaCl_2$ to a 2-L graduated cylinder or a glass beaker. Adjust final volume to 1 L with water.
6. Blocking buffer: TBS-Ca^{2+}-0.1 % BSA buffer, dissolve 0.1 g BSA in 100 mL TBS-Ca^{2+} buffer.
7. TBS-Ca^{2+}-3 % BSA buffer: Dissolve 3 g BSA in 100 mL TBS-Ca^{2+} buffer.
8. TBST-Ca^{2+} buffer: Add 0.5 mL Tween 20 to 1 L TBS-Ca^{2+} buffer.
9. Stop solution: 1 M phosphoric acid.
10. Carbonate coating buffer (0.1 M): Add about 100 mL water to a 2-L graduated cylinder or a glass beaker. Weigh 3.0 g Na_2CO_3 and 6.0 g $NaHCO_3$, and transfer to the cylinder. Add water to a volume of 900 mL. Mix and adjust pH to 9.6 with HCl. Make up to 1 L with water.
11. 10× GlcNAc-BSA stock (250 μg/mL): dissolve 0.25 mg GlcNAc-BSA powder in 1 mL of 0.1 M Na_2CO_3 (pH 9.6). Dilute ten times by 0.1 M Na_2CO_3 before use.

3 Methods

3.1 Purification of L-Ficolin

1. Prepare 1 L pooled human plasma (starting material). Add 1 M $CaCl_2$ to the plasma to a final concentration of 10 mM and incubate for 1 h at 37 °C to allow clotting.
2. Centrifuge the plasma at 10,000 × *g* for 30 min at 4 °C, and save the supernatant as the human serum.
3. Add polyethylene glycol 4000 to the serum to a final concentration of 8 % and incubate for 1 h at 4 °C.
4. Centrifuge the serum at 10,000 × *g* for 30 min at 4 °C. Dissolve the precipitate in 200 mL of GlcNAc-agarose loading buffer (buffer A) (*see* **Note 4**).
5. Apply the solution to the GlcNAc-agarose column previously equilibrated with buffer A.
6. Wash the column with approximately 10 column volumes of buffer A.
7. Elute the bound components with buffer B (*see* **Note 5**).
8. Elute the bound components with GlcNAc-agarose elution buffer for L-ficolin (buffer C).
9. Concentrate the eluate from GlcNAc-agarose with buffer C by centrifugation in (cutoff, 30 kDa) Amicon Ultra to approximately 8 mL.
10. Dialyze the concentrated fraction against loading buffer for Mono Q (buffer D).
11. Apply the dialysate, being passed through a 0.22-μm membrane filter, to Mono Q previously equilibrated with buffer D.
12. Wash the column with buffer D.
13. Elute the bound components with a linear gradient from 50 mM NaCl (100 % buffer D) to 0.5 M NaCl (50 % buffer E). L-Ficolin is eluted as a complex formed with MASPs and their truncated proteins (L-ficolin-MASP) at a concentration between 0.15 M NaCl and 0.2 M NaCl (*see* **Note 6**).

3.2 Assay for Measuring L-Ficolin Concentration

1. Coat ELISA plate overnight at 4 °C with coating antibody (clone GN1) at 1 μg/mL in 50 mM carbonate buffer, pH 9.6 (*see* **Note 7**). A volume of 100 μl/well is used for this and all subsequent steps.
2. Wash wells three times with 0.05 % Tween-20 in Diluent, then block with 1 % BSA in Diluent (100 μl/well) for 2 h at 37 °C before washing again as before.
3. A doubling dilution series up to 1/32 is prepared from a serum of known (and relatively high) L-ficolin concentration (*see* **Note 8**). This series is then diluted a further 1 in 10 in

Diluent to occupy (in duplicate) the top row of the ELISA plate and provide values for a calibration curve.

4. Serum samples of unknown concentration are prepared at 1 in 20 dilution in Diluent and applied to the plate in duplicate (*see* **Note 9**). Diluent alone is put into the final two wells of the plate as a negative control.
5. Incubate plate for 2 h at 37 °C.
6. Wash plate as before, then add biotinylated second antibody (clone GN5) at 5 μg/mL in Diluent containing 0.1 % BSA. Incubate overnight at 4 °C (*see* **Note 10**).
7. Prepare avidin–biotin complex (ABC) reagent and leave for 30 min. Then wash plate as before and add ABC reagent. Incubate for 2 h at 37 °C.
8. Wash with Diluent containing Tween-20 (twice), then again with Diluent without Tween-20 (three times).
9. Add buffered ABTS reagent (*see* **Note 11**) and leave at room temperature in the dark for 30 min.
10. Measure absorbance at 410 nm using an ELISA Reader and calculate results (*see* **Note 12**).

3.3 Assay for L-Ficolin-Mediated Complement Activation

1. Coat a microtiter plate with 10 μg/mL Ac-LDL in carbonate buffer (100 μl/well) for 18 h at 4 °C.
2. Add blocking solution (300 μl/well) to wells and incubate for 2 h at 37 °C.
3. Wash wells three times with TBST-Ca^{2+}.
4. Add L-ficolin-MASP (100 μl/well) diluted with TBST-Ca^{2+} to wells and incubate for 2 h at 4 °C (*see* **Note 13**).
5. Wash wells three times with TBST-Ca^{2+}.
6. Add 10 μg/mL of human C4 in TBST-Ca^{2+} (100 μl/well) to wells.
7. Incubate for 1 h at 37 °C (*see* **Note 14**).
8. Wash wells three times with TBST-Ca^{2+}.
9. Add HRP-conjugated anti-human C4 in TBST-Ca^{2+} (100 μl/well) to wells.
10. Incubate for 1 h at room temperature.
11. Wash wells three times with TBST-Ca^{2+} and then once with TBS.
12. Add 100 μl of a mixture of 0.1 M citrate buffer, 3 % H_2O_2 and ABTS (100:1:1) to wells.
13. Incubate at room temperature.
14. Measure absorbance at 415 nm (*see* Fig. 1, **Note 15**).

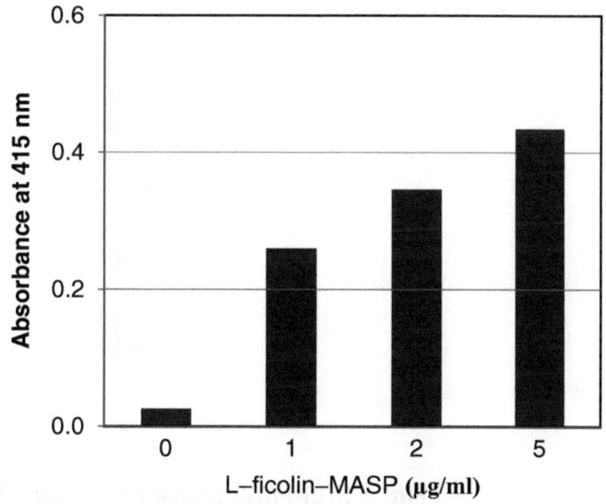

Fig. 1 C4 activation by L-ficolin-MASP bound to Ac-LDL. After L-ficolin-MASP (0, 1, 2, 5 μg/mL) was incubated in the wells coated with Ac-LDL, C4 was added to the wells. After incubation, deposition of C4b onto the wells was determined

3.4 Purification of H-Ficolin

1. Prepare 1 L pooled human plasma (starting material). Add 1 M $CaCl_2$ to the plasma to a final concentration of 10 mM and incubate for 1 h at 37 °C to allow clotting.
2. Centrifuge the plasma at 10,000 × *g* for 30 min at 4 °C, and save the supernatant as the human serum.
3. Add polyethylene glycol 4000 to the serum to a final concentration of 8 % and incubate for 1 h at 4 °C.
4. Centrifuge the serum at 10,000 × *g* for 30 min at 4 °C. Dissolve the precipitate in 200 mL of loading buffer (buffer A).
5. Apply the solution to the 4H5-Sepharose column previously equilibrated with buffer A.
6. Wash the column with approximately 10 column volumes of buffer A.
7. Elute and collect the bound components with 0.1 M glycine–HCl buffer pH 2.2. Neutralize the pH of the eluates with 1 M Tris–HCl pH 8.2 (*see* **Note 16**).
8. Concentrate the eluate from 4H5-Sepharose by centrifugation in (cutoff , 30 kDa) Amicon Ultra to approximately 8 mL.
9. Dialyze the concentrated fraction against loading buffer A.
10. Apply the dialysate to Lentil lectin-Sepharose previously equilibrated with buffer A (*see* **Note 17**).
11. Wash the column with buffer A.
12. Elute the bound components with buffer A containing 0.2 M α-methylmannopyranoside.

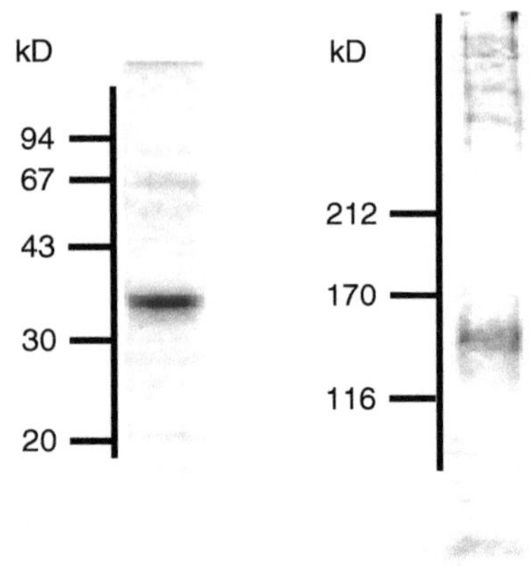

Fig. 2 SDS-PAGE profile of H-ficolin. H-Ficolin purified from human serum was subjected to SDS-PAGE under reducing (*left*, 10 % gel) and nonreducing (*right*, 4 % gel) conditions followed by protein staining with Coomassie brilliant blue R-250. H-Ficolin shows an approximately 34 kDa band under reducing conditions. Under nonreducing conditions, H-ficolin shows a size heterogeneity, indicating various oligomeric forms

13. Concentrate the eluate from Lentil lectin-Sepharose by centrifugation in (cutoff, 30 kDa) Amicon Ultra to approximately 3 mL.
14. Dialyze the concentrated fraction against buffer B.
15. Apply the dialysate to a column packed with a mixture of anti-IgM-Sepharose and Protein A-Sepharose previously equilibrated with buffer A and collect the unbound fractions (Fig. 2, *see* **Note 18**).

3.5 Assay for Measuring H-Ficolin Concentration

1. Prepare the wells of a 96-well microtiter plate coated with PSA or rabbit anti-human H-ficolin antibody. 100 μl of PSA (2 μg/well) or rabbit anti-H-ficolin antibody (500 ng/well) dissolved in 10 mM $NaHCO_3$ buffer, pH 9.6, is added to the wells of the plate and left overnight at 4 °C. Unreacted sites on the solid phase are blocked with PBS containing 1 % BSA at room temperature for 3 h. After washing six times with PBS containing 0.05 % Tween 20 (PBST), diluted serum sample is added to the coated wells and incubated at 37 °C for 1 h. A standard dilution series of pooled donor serum with known concentration of H-ficolin are added to each assay.
2. After washing six times with PBST, the plate is incubated with 100 μl of rabbit anti-H-ficolin antibody or biotinylated anti-H-ficolin antibody diluted in PBS for 1 h at 37 °C. After washing with PBS, the plate is incubated with goat anti-rabbit IgG antibody conjugated with horseradish peroxidase or streptavidin conjugated with horseradish peroxidase for 30 min at 37 °C.

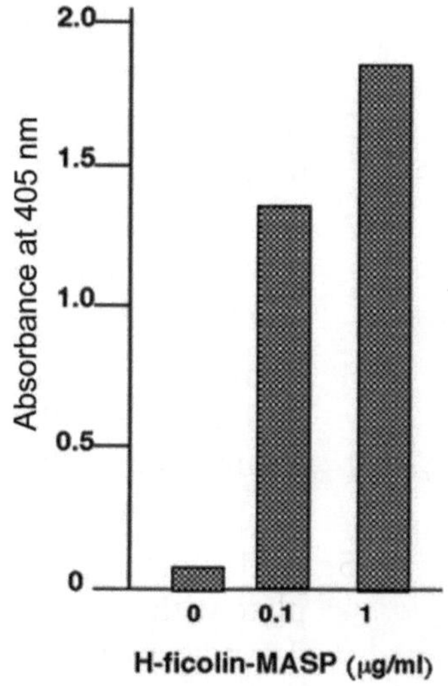

Fig. 3 C4 activation by H-ficolin-MASP bound to PSA. After H-ficolin-MASP (0, 0.1, 1 μg/mL) was incubated in the wells coated with PSA, C4 was added to the wells. After incubation, deposition of C4b onto the wells was determined

3. The plate is washed six times with PBST and developed with 150 μl of 0.1 % H_2O_2 and 0.04 % ortho-phenylenediamine in 0.1 M sodium citrate buffer (pH 5.5) for 15 min. The reaction is stopped by addition of 50 μl of 2.5 M H_2SO_4 and the color development is measured at 492 nm (*see* **Note 19**).

3.6 Assay for H-Ficolin-Mediated Complement Activation [21, 27]

1. Coat wells of a 96-well microtiter plate with PSA as described above.
2. Add BLOCK ACE to wells (300 μl/well) and incubate at 37 °C for 2 h.
3. Wash wells three times with TBST-Ca^{2+}.
4. Add H-ficolin diluted with TBST-Ca^{2+} to wells (100 μl/well) and incubate for 1 h at 37 °C (*see* **Note 20**).
5. Wash wells three times with TBST-Ca^{2+}.
6. Add human C4 (10 μg/mL) diluted in TBST-Ca^{2+} to wells (100 μl/well) and incubate for 1 h at 37 °C.
7. Wash wells three times with TBST-Ca^{2+}.
8. Add HRP-anti-C4 antibody to wells (100 μl/well) and incubate for 1 h at 37 °C.
9. Wash wells three times with TBST-Ca^{2+} and then once with TBS-Ca^{2+}.
10. Add a mixture of 0.1 M citrate buffer, 3 % H_2O_2, and ABTS (100:1:1) to wells (100 μl/well) and incubate at room temperature.
11. Measure absorbance at 415 nm (Fig. 3).

3.7 Assay for M-Ficolin-Mediated Complement Activation

1. Prepare 1 mL of GlcNAc-BSA solution by tenfold dilution of GlcNAc-BSA stock with carbonate coating buffer.
2. Add GlcNAc-BSA solution to wells (100 µl/well) of a microtiter plate.
3. Cover the plate with an adhesive plastic and incubate at 37 °C for 4 h or at 4 °C overnight for sufficient coating (*see* **Note 21**).
4. Remove the coating buffer, and wash the plate twice with 200 µl of TBS. Remove the solutions by flicking the plate over a sink. The remaining drops are removed by patting the plate on a paper towel.
5. Add blocking buffer to each well (200 µl/well). Cover the plate with an adhesive plastic and incubate for 2–3 h at 37 °C. Then keep at 4 °C before use.
6. Prepare eppendorf tubes. Add varying volumes of 0.25 µg/µl of M-ficolin and 0.25 µg/µl of MASP to each tube in order to make final amounts in the well at 0, 0.1, 0.25, 0.5, 1 µg for M-ficolin and at 0, 0.1, 0.2, 0.5, 1 µg for MASP (*see* **Note 22**). Make up to total 110 µl with TBS-Ca^{2+}-3 % BSA buffer (*see* **Note 23**). Triplicate samples are needed for statistic analysis.
7. Rotate the tubes at 4 °C overnight. On the second day, rotate the tubes for additional 10 min at 37 °C.
8. Wash the blocked GlcNAc-coated microplate four times with TBST-Ca^{2+}.
9. Add M-ficolin-MASP complexes prepared in **step 7** to each well (100 µl/well). Cover the plate with an adhesive plastic and incubate for 10 min at 37 °C (*see* **Note 24**).
10. Wash the plate four times with TBST-Ca^{2+}.
11. Add human C4 diluted with blocking buffer to each well (100 µl/well). Cover the plate with an adhesive plastic and incubate on ice for 30 min.
12. Wash the plate four times with TBST-Ca^{2+}.
13. Add HRP-anti-human C4 IgG diluted with blocking buffer at a final concentration of 7.5 µg/mL to wells (100 µl/well). Cover the plate with an adhesive plastic and incubate for 30 min at 37 °C.
14. Wash the plate four times with TBST-Ca^{2+}.
15. Prepare ready-to-use TMB solution by mixing equal amount of TMB and H_2O_2 (*see* **Note 25**).
16. Add TMB solution to each well (100 µl/well) and allow to develop at room temperature for up to 6 min.
17. Add stop buffer to each well (100 µl/well).
18. Measure absorbance at 450 nm (Fig. 4).

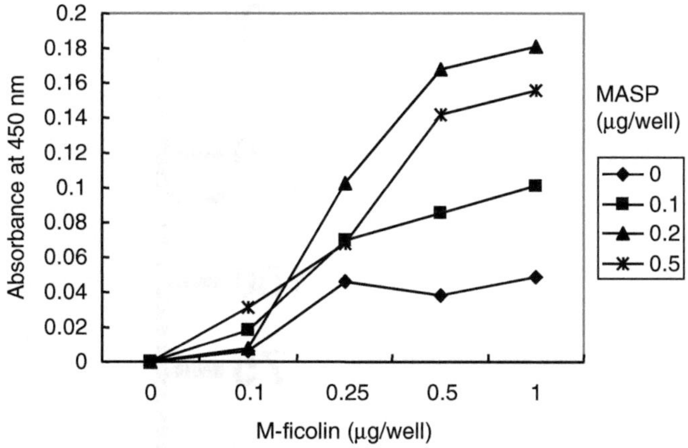

Fig. 4 C4 activation by M-ficolin-MASP complex bound to GlcNAc-BSA. After mixtures of M-ficolin (0, 0.1, 0.25, 0.5, 1 μg) and MASP (0, 0.1, 0.2, 0.5 μg) were incubated in the wells coated with GlcNAc-BSA, C4 was added to the wells. After incubation, deposition of C4b onto the wells was determined

4 Notes

1. The concentration of bacteria in the suspension is estimated by reading the optical density (absorbance) at 600 nm. An optical density of 1.0 corresponds to approximately 1.8×10^9 bacteria/mL.
2. The assay for detecting PSA is performed on a square glass slide (10 cm × 10 cm) with 0.7 % agarose gel containing 100 mM NaCl and 2 % polyethylene glycol in 10 mM Tris–HCl buffer, pH 7.4. Fractions and human serum are placed in the wells. The plate is left to stand overnight at room temperature before the precipitin line is produced between the wells. The precipitin line is examined under an inverted microscope. PSA isolated from the broth of *A. viridans* forms a clear precipitin line against H-ficolin in human serum.
3. As described in Introduction, M-ficolin is present in human serum, but has not been isolated yet. It remains unknown whether M-ficolin is complexed with MASP in serum like L-ficolin and H-ficolin. Experimentally, however, recombinant M-ficolin is able to form a complex with MASP and to activate the lectin pathway as introduced in this section.
4. Calcium ions are included in the buffers throughout the purification steps. This is because L-ficolin forms a complex with MASPs, sMAP, and MAp44 in a calcium-dependent manner in human serum. Therefore, the L-ficolin preparation purified according to this method contains these associated proteins.

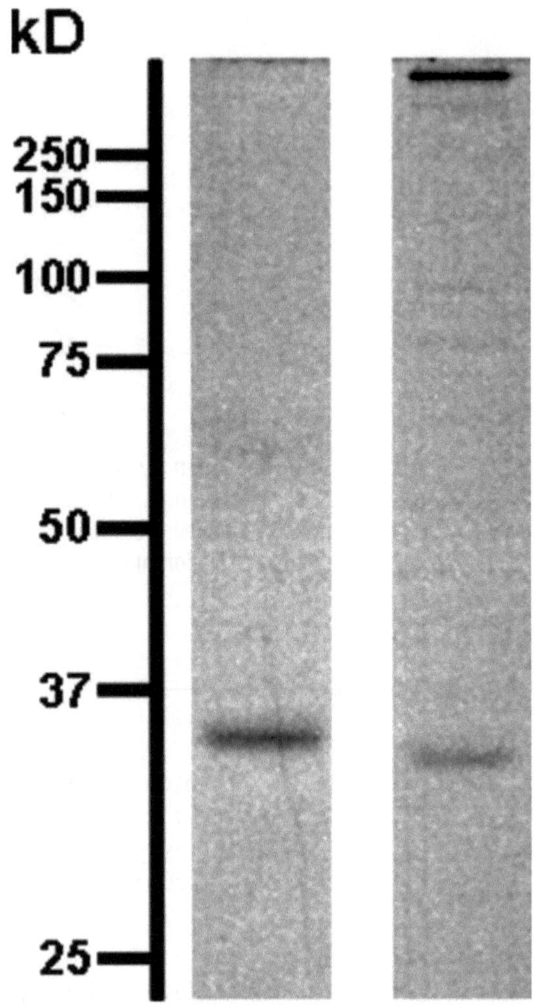

Fig. 5 SDS-PAGE profile of L-ficolin. L-Ficolin purified from human serum was subjected to SDS-PAGE (10 % gel) under reducing (*left*) and nonreducing (*right*) conditions followed by protein staining with Coomassie brilliant blue R-250

5. On the GlcNAc-agarose column, MBL is first eluted with mannose (buffer B), followed by the elution of L-ficolin with GlcNAc (buffer C). Calcium ions present in the buffers allow MBL to bind GlcNAc-agarose, since MBL is a C-type lectin and requires calcium ions for binding to its ligands. The difference in the elution profiles between these human serum lectins is because of their binding specificities. MBL binds mannose and GlcNAc, whereas L-ficolin binds GlcNAc but not mannose.

6. Purification of L-ficolin is monitored by SDS-PAGE. L-Ficolin shows an approximately 35 kDa band under reducing conditions (Fig. 5). Under nonreducing conditions, L-ficolin shows a band corresponding to a tetramer as well as a band presumably

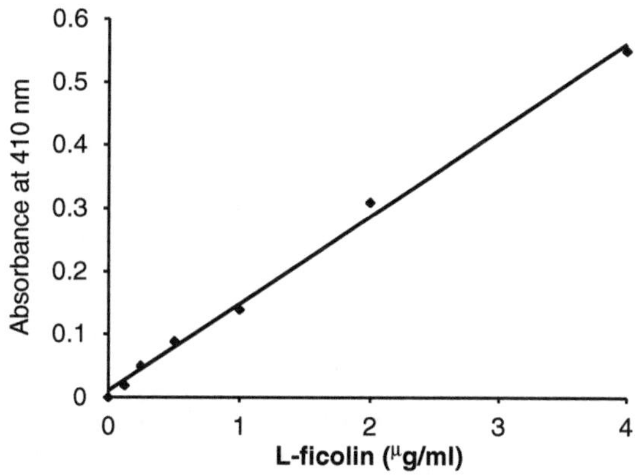

Fig. 6 Assay for L-ficolin. Absorbance as a function of a doubling dilution series of a serum containing 4,000 ng/mL of L-ficolin

corresponding to its subunit not involved in oligomerization linked by disulfide bridges. The presence of three types of MASP and their truncated proteins (sMAP and MAp44) can be detected by immunoblotting using their specific antibodies (most of the antibodies are commercially).

Instead of Mono Q, affinity chromatography using asialofetuin-Sepharose can be employed in the second step for the L-ficolin purification [28]. Asialofetuin-Sepharose is prepared by coupling of asialofetuin with cyanogen bromide-activated Sepharose. Asialofetuin is a glycoprotein-containing complex-type carbohydrates, whose nonreducing terminal lacks sialic acid. L-Ficolin binds to GlcNAc residues of asialofetuin conjugated to Sepharose and elutes with GlcNAc. The L-ficolin preparation thus obtained is slightly contaminated with IgG and IgM, which can be removed by immobilized Protein A (or Protein G) and anti-IgM.

7. Other monoclonal anti-L-ficolin antibodies may be used instead of GN1. For example, clone GN4 (at 10 μg/mL) gives similar results [29]. Alternatively, an acetylated compound such as acetylated BSA could be substituted, but that will result in lectin activity detection as opposed to protein measurement. Lectin activity correlates with total protein measurement but gives discordant values with some sera.
8. L-Ficolin is very stable in serum when stored frozen, whereas purified L-ficolin is labile even when frozen. Aliquots of a serum known to have a relatively high L-ficolin concentration (e.g., 4,000 ng/mL) are therefore used for the calibration curve at 1 in 10 dilution (Fig. 6).
9. Unknown samples diluted 1 in 20 are likely to fall within the usable range of the calibration curve. Low values should be

confirmed by repeating the assay at a 1 in 10 dilution, while very high values can be confirmed by diluting the sample 1 in 30.

10. In principle, another biotinylated second antibody could be used, but we have observed maximum sensitivity with clone GN5. Overnight incubation is chosen for convenience, but similar results are obtained with a 2 h incubation at 37 °C.
11. Light is most easily excluded by covering the ELISA plate with aluminum foil.
12. Most ELISA readers can be programmed to deduct the negative control values and then to construct a plot of Log.[A_{410}] versus Log.[protein concentration] from which the individual determinations are derived.
13. L-ficolin recognizes the acetyl group and therefore can bind to Ac-LDL in the wells [30]. As described in **Note 4**, calcium ions are required for the formation between L-ficolin and MASP. Calcium ions are included in the buffer used in this functional assay method. This allows us to assay the activation of the lectin pathway mediated by the L-ficolin-MASP complex bound to Ac-LDL. For the studies on complement activation by ficolins, buffers containing 2–10 mM Ca^{2+} are generally used. In addition to Ac-LDL, *N-acetylglucosamine-pentamer* conjugated to dipalmitoylphosphatidylethanolamine can be also used as a coating ligand for both binding and functional ELISA [31].
14. C4 has an internal thioester bond. Of the three types of MASP, MASP-2 is involved in cleaving C4. When MASP-2 in the L-ficolin-MASP complex cleaves C4, the generated C4b fragment covalently binds to proteins (Ac-LDL and/or blocking substances) on the wells through an ester or amide bond.
15. 405 nm filter can also be used to read the color development.
16. When the eluates from a 4H5-Sepharose column are collected in the test tubes of a fraction collector, neutralizing buffer (1 M Tris–HCl pH 8.2) is previously placed in each tube and an equal volume of the elute is collected, followed by mixing well immediately.
17. H-ficolin is a glycoprotein-containing mannose, GlcNAc, galactose, and fucose [17]. Lentil lectin recognizes mannose and glucose. Therefore, it is most likely that Lentil lecin-Sepharose could bind a mannose residue of H-ficolin.
18. The H-ficolin preparation from Lentil lectin-Sepharose is contaminated with immunoglobulins. They can be removed by passing through anti-IgM-Sepharose and Protein A-Sepharose. H-Ficolin thus obtained is complexed with MASPs and their truncated proteins, which can be used for the studies on complement activation. In addition to the method described here, other methods for H-ficolin purification have been reported.

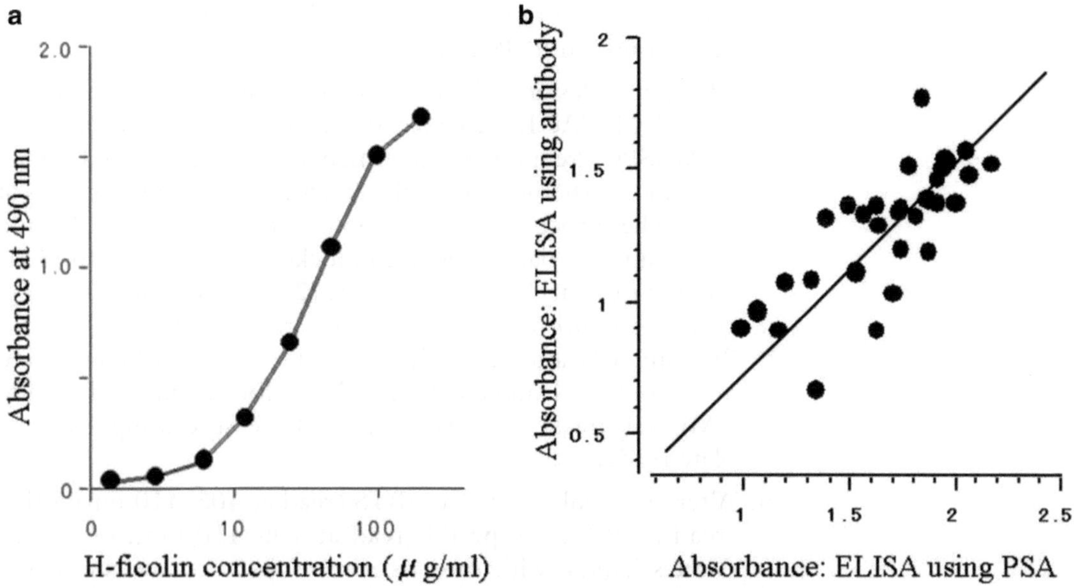

Fig. 7 Assay for H-ficolin concentration. (**a**) A standard dilution series of serum sample with known concentration of H-ficolin. (**b**) Comparison of the results of ELISA using PSA and anti-H-ficolin antibody as adsorbent against H-ficolin

These are based on the binding specificity of H-ficolin to *A. viridans* [19] and acetylated human serum albumin [32].

19. In ELISA using PSA as adsorbent, H-ficolin in dilution series of serum sample with known concentration bound to PSA in a dose-dependent manner, and this increase is clearly suppressed with 5 μg/well of PSA (Fig. 7a). H-Ficolin binding to PSA was seen in the intact serum sample, whereas binding was not seen in the inactivated serum sample exposed to 56 °C for 30 min. Furthermore, the results obtained by ELISA using PSA were practically equivalent to those obtained by ELISA using the rabbit anti-H-ficolin antibody (Fig. 7b). The concentration of H-ficolin in samples from 33 healthy blood donors is calculated as 34.5 ± 7.8 μg/mL. A sandwich ELISA has been developed using antibodies aganst H-ficolin [33].
20. Instead of PSA, acetylated-bovine serum albumin or lipopolysacchades of *H. alvei* can be used as a coating ligand for H-ficolin [20, 34].
21. This step is designed to coat GlcNAc-BSA onto the wells of the microplate. The concentration of GlcNAc-BSA should be tested by serial dilutions. We tested the concentration of GlcNAc-BSA from 0.25 μg/mL to 25 μg/mL and found that 2.5 μg/mL was best for the experiments.
22. This step is designed to form M-ficolin-MASP complexes with different ratios and to determine whether C4b deposition led by ficolin-MASP is dose-dependent or not.

23. High concentration of BSA is needed here for decreasing the background in ELISA assay.
24. This step is designed for trapping M-ficolin-MASP complex by coated GlcNAc-BSA, which subsequently leads to activation of MASPs. Preliminary experiments should be carried out to determine whether M-ficolin attaches to coated GlcNAc or not. The procedures are simply summarized as: (1) add M-ficolin in serial dilutions to blocked GlcNAc-coated plate, and incubate at 37 °C for 20 min; (2) after intensive washing, add rabbit anti-M-ficolin antibody, and incubate at 37 °C for 20 min; (3) after intensive washing, add HRP-conjugated anti-rabbit IgG, and incubate at 37 °C for 30 min; and (4) add TMB substrates for developing and measure using a microplate reader.
25. Alternative substrates are ABTS (read at 405–410 nm), OPD (read at 490 nm), pNPP (read at 405–410 nm), or others. Always handle with care, as some substrates are considered hazardous (potential carcinogens).

References

1. Matsushita M (2010) Ficolins: complement-activating lectins involved in innate immunity. J Innate Immun 2:24–32
2. Endo Y, Matsushita M, Fujita T (2011) The role of ficolins in the lectin pathway of innate immunity. Int J Biochem Cell Biol 43:705–712
3. Matsushita M, Endo Y, Taira S, Sato Y, Fujita T, Ichikawa N, Nakata M, Mizuochi T (1996) A novel human serum lectin with collagen- and fibrinogen-like domains that functions as an opsonin. J Biol Chem 271:2448–2454
4. Ma YG, Cho MY, Zhao M, Park JW, Matsushita M, Fujita T, Lee BL (2004) Human mannose-binding lectin and L-ficolin function as specific pattern recognition proteins in the lectin activation pathway of complement. J Biol Chem 279:25307–25312
5. Garlatti V, Belloy N, Martin L, Lacroix M, Matsushita M, Endo Y, Fujita T, Fontecilla-Camps JC, Arlaud GJ, Thielens NM, Gaboriaud C (2007) Structural insights into the innate immune recognition specificities of L- and H-ficolins. EMBO J 26:623–633
6. Matsushita M, Fujita T (1992) Activation of the classical complement pathway by mannose-binding protein in association with a novel C1s-like serine protease. J Exp Med 176:1497–1502
7. Sato T, Endo Y, Matsushita M, Fujita T (1994) Molecular characterization of a novel serine protease involved in activation of the complement system by mannose-binding protein. Int Immunol 6:665–669
8. Thiel S, Vorup-Jensen T, Stover CM, Schwaeble W, Laursen SB, Poulsen K, Willis AC, Eggleton P, Hansen S, Holmskov U, Reid KB, Jensenius JC (1997) A second serine protease associated with mannan-binding lectin that activates complement. Nature 386:506–510
9. Dahl MR, Thiel S, Matsushita M, Fujita T, Willis AC, Christensen T, Vorup-Jensen T, Jensenius JC (2001) MASP-3 and its association with distinct complexes of the mannan-binding lectin complement activation pathway. Immunity 15:127–135
10. Takahashi M, Endo Y, Fujita T, Matsushita M (1999) A truncated form of mannose-binding lectin-associated serine protease (MASP)-2 expressed by alternative polyadenylation is a component of the lectin complement pathway. Int Immunol 11:859–863
11. Stover CM, Thiel S, Thelen M, Lynch NJ, Vorup-Jensen T, Jensenius JC, Schwaeble WJ (1999) Two constituents of the initiation complex of the mannan-binding lectin activation pathway of complement are encoded by a single structural gene. J Immunol 162:3481–3490
12. Degn SE, Hansen AG, Steffensen R, Jacobsen C, Jensenius JC, Thiel S (2009) MAp44, a human protein associated with pattern recognition molecules of the complement system and regulating the lectin pathway of complement activation. J Immunol 183:7371–7378

13. Skjoedt MO, Hummelshoj T, Palarasah Y, Honore C, Koch C, Skjodt K, Garred P (2010) A novel mannose-binding lectin/ficolin-associated protein is highly expressed in heart and skeletal muscle tissues and inhibits complement activation. J Biol Chem 285:8234–8243
14. Matsushita M, Endo Y, Fujita T (2000) Cutting edge: complement-activating complex of ficolin and mannose-binding lectin-associated serine protease. J Immunol 164:2281–2284
15. Sugimoto R, Yae Y, Akaiwa M, Kitajima S, Shibata Y, Sato H, Hirata J, Okochi K, Izuhara K, Hamasaki N (1998) Cloning and characterization of the Hakata antigen, a member of the ficolin/opsonin p35 lectin family. J Biol Chem 273:20721–20727
16. Inaba S, Okochi K (1978) On a new precipitating antibody against normal human serum found in two patients with SLE. Igaku No Ayumi 107:690–691
17. Yae Y, Inaba S, Sato H, Okochi K, Tokunaga F, Iwanaga S (1991) Isolation and characterization of a thermolabile β-2 macroglycoprotein ("thermolabile substance" or "Hakata antigen") detected by precipitating (auto) antibody in sera of patients with systemic lupus erythematosus. Biochim Biophys Acta 1078:369–379
18. Munthe-Fog L, Hummelshøj T, Honoré C, Madsen HO, Permin H, Garred P (2009) Immunodeficiency associated with FCN3 mutation and ficolin-3 deficiency. N Engl J Med 360:2637–2644
19. Tsujimura M, Ishida C, Sagara Y, Miyazaki T, Murakami K, Shiraki H, Okochi K, Maeda Y (2001) Detection of serum thermolabile β-2 macroglycoprotein (Hakata antigen) by enzyme-linked immunosorbent assay using polysaccharide produced by *Aerococcus viridans*. Clin Diagn Lab Immunol 8:454–459
20. Swierzko A, Lukasiewicz J, Cedzynski M, Maciejewska A, Jachymek W, Niedziela T, Matsushita M, Lugowski C (2012) New functional ligands for ficolin-3 among lipopolysaccharides of Hafnia alvei. Glycobiology 22:267–280
21. Matsushita M, Kuraya M, Hamasaki N, Tsujimura M, Shiraki H, Fujita T (2002) Activation of the lectin complement pathway by H-ficolin (Hakata antigen). J Immunol 168:3502–3506
22. Honoré C, Rørvig S, Hummelshøj T, Skjoedt MO, Borregaard N, Garred P (2010) Tethering of Ficolin-1 to cell surfaces through recognition of sialic acid by the fibrinogen-like domain. J Leukoc Biol 88:145–158
23. Honoré C, Rørvig S, Munthe-Fog L, Hummelshøj T, Madsen HO, Borregaard N, Garred P (2008) The innate pattern recognition molecule Ficolin-1 is secreted by monocytes/macrophages and is circulating in human plasma. Mol Immunol 45:2782–2789
24. Liu Y, Endo Y, Iwaki D, Nakata M, Matsushita M, Wada I, Inoue K, Munakata M, Fujita T (2005) Human M-ficolin is a secretory protein that activates the lectin complement pathway. J Immunol 175:3150–3156
25. Frederiksen PD, Thiel S, Larsen CB, Jensenius JC (2005) M-ficolin, an innate immune defence molecule, binds patterns of acetyl groups and activates complement. Scand J Immunol 62:462–473
26. Matsushita M, Thiel S, Jensenius JC, Terai I, Fujita T (2000) Proteolytic activities of two types of mannose-binding lectin-associated serine protease. J Immunol 165:2637–2642
27. Tsujimura M, Miyazaki T, Kojima E, Sagara Y, Shiraki H, Okochi K, Maeda Y (2002) Serum concentration of Hakata antigen, a member of ficolins, is linked with inhibition of *Aerococcus viridans* growth. Clin Chim Acta 325:139–146
28. Matsushita M, Fujita T (2002) Immunobiology 205:490–497
29. Kilpatrick DC, Fujita T, Matsushita M (1999) P35, an opsonic lectin of the ficolin family, in human blood from neonates, normal adults, and recurrent miscarriage patients. Immunol Lett 167:109–112
30. Faro J, Chen Y, Jhaveri P, Oza P, Spear GT, Lint TF, Gewurz H (2008) L-ficolin binding and lectin pathway activation by acetylated low-density lipoprotein. Clin Exp Immunol 151:275–283
31. Inoshita H, Matsushita M, Koide S, Kusaba G, Ishii M, Onda K, Gi MJ, Nakata M, Ohsawa I, Horikoshi S, Ohi H, Tomino Y (2009) A novel measurement method for activation of the lectin complement pathway via both mannose-binding lectin (MBL) and L-ficolin. J Immunol Methods 349:9–17
32. Zacho RM, Jensen L, Terp R, Jensenius JC, Thiel S (2012) Studies of the pattern recognition molecule H-ficolin: specificity and purification. J Biol Chem 287:8071–8081
33. Munthe-Fog L, Hummelshøj T, Ma YJ, Hansen BE, Koch C, Madsen HO, Skjødt K, Garred P (2008) Characterization of a polymorphism in the coding sequence of FCN3 resulting in a Ficolin-3 (Hakata antigen) deficiency state. Mol Immunol 45:2660–2666
34. Hein E, Honoré C, Skjoedt MO, Munthe-Fog L, Hummelshøj T, Garred P (2010) Functional analysis of Ficolin-3 mediated complement activation. PLoS One 5:e15443

Chapter 13

Purification and Functional Analysis of Human Properdin

Joseph O'Flynn, Maria C. Faber Krol, Mohamed R. Daha, and Cees van Kooten

Abstract

Properdin is a member of the alternative pathway of complement. It is unique in that it is the only known positive regulator of the complement system. Properdin can stabilize and promote complement activation, but in addition is also capable of initiating the alternative pathway, making it a unique protein. This chapter focuses on the methods required for purifying human properdin and testing its functionality.

Key words Properdin, Complement, Human, Anion exchange, C3b

1 Introduction

Properdin is a member of the alternative pathway (AP) in the complement system. Discovered by Louis Pillemer in 1954, it is named after the latin word "perdere" meaning to destroy, as it is the only known positive regulator in the complement system [1]. It is a highly positively charged protein which can form various multimeric structures [2, 3]. Properdin is encoded for on the X chromosome in humans and a properdin deficient state does exist in humans which is associated with increased susceptibility to meningococcal disease [4, 5]. Furthermore, a properdin deficient mice has been generated by targeting the mouse properdin gene present on the X chromosome, allowing for the investigation of properdins capabilities in vivo [6]

A monomeric chain of properdin (53 kDa) consists of six type 1 thrombospondin repeats (TSR) [7, 8]. These monomeric subunits can form head to tail associations with each other to generate dimeric, trimeric, and tetrameric properdin structures [2, 9]. Serum-derived properdin exists in three states: dimeric, trimeric, or tetrameric in an approximate ratio of 1:2:1, respectively [10].

Mihaela Gadjeva (ed.), *The Complement System: Methods and Protocols*, Methods in Molecular Biology, vol. 1100,
DOI 10.1007/978-1-62703-724-2_13, © Springer Science+Business Media New York 2014

In contrast to most complement components which are produced by the liver, properdin is produced mainly by white blood cells including monocytes, lymphocytes, and neutrophils [11–13].

Activation of the alternative pathway can occur by two means:

The traditional view is via binding of C3b to a surface followed by attachment of Factor B to the C3b molecule. The Factor B is cleaved by Factor D resulting in the formation of alternative pathway C3 convertase, which becomes bound and stabilized by properdin, allowing the enzyme to cleave more C3 to C3b [14, 15]. Properdin has a high affinity for C3b allowing for its unique feature in stabilizing the C3 convertase prolonging the functionality of the enzyme five- to tenfold [3, 10].

More recently a novel mechanism was proposed where the initial event is the interaction and binding of properdin to a specific surface. The properdin molecule binds hydrolyzed C3 or C3b followed by attachment of Factor B. The Factor B is cleaved via Factor D producing the AP C3 convertase [16]. Both mechanisms of AP activation result in the development of a C3 convertase which can generate more C3b promoting further AP activation should it be unregulated.

The capacity of properdin to act as initiator and stabilizer in the generation of AP C3 convertase allows it to amplify and modulate complement activation in a unique manner via C3b generation. The illustration that properdin can act as initiator as well as stabilizer has led to the investigations into the various other ligands, other than C3b, which it may bind. Properdin can bind various ligands including zymosan, lipopolysaccharide (LPS), bacteria, necrotic cells, and apoptotic cells allowing it to act as an anchor for the alternative pathway.

One study illustrated the ability of properdin to bind zymosan and bacteria such as Escherichia coli, acting as a platform for C3 convertase generation [17]. Another study investigating the ability of properdin to bind LPS coated on a plate demonstrated properdins ability to bind LPS and promote AP C3 convertase production [6]. Studies by Xu et al. [18] demonstrated properdins ability to bind late apoptotic and necrotic jurkat cells in the absence of C3, this deposited properdin acts a platform for C3 convertase generation on the surface. Properdin has also been shown to interact with early apoptotic T lymphocytes leading to assembly of the AP C3 convertase on the cell surface, demonstrating properdins role in the removal of dying cells [19]. These intriguing findings of properdins ability to interact with various foreign and self antigens have led to a rejuvenation of interest in properdins role in various disease states.

In this chapter, we describe the methods required for the purification of human properdin from serum and to test its functionality in vitro.

2 Materials

2.1 Sample Preparation

1. Normal human serum (approx 550 ml).
2. Glass wool.
3. Centrifuge.

2.2 Serum Purification

1. Conductometer.
2. Polyethyleneglycol 4000.
3. Sodium chloride (NaCl).
4. Tris.
5. Ethylenediaminetetraacetic acid (EDTA).
6. DEAE buffer: 25 mM Tris, 70 mM NaCl, 2 mM EDTA pH 8.0, 6.5 mS.

2.3 Anion Exchange Purification Materials

1. Fraction collector.
2. Pump.
3. Diethylaminoethyl sepharose column (DEAE-seph).
4. BCA Protein assay.
5. Human properdin ELISA.

2.4 C3b Column Preparation and Purification Materials

1. Purified human C3.
2. Trypsin.
3. Trypsin Inhibitor Soybean.
4. Spectra/Por 6 standard RC dialysis tubing MWCO 50 kDa.
5. Sodium hydrogen carbonate ($NaHCO_3$).
6. pH meter.
7. CNBr-activated sepharose.
8. Hydrochloric acid (HCL).
9. Glassfilter connected to a vacuum system.
10. Sodium acetate (NaAc).
11. Coupling buffer: 0.1 M $NaHCO_3$, 0.5 M NaCl, pH 8.3.
12. Bead blocking buffer: 0.1 M Tris–HCl, 0.5 M NaCl pH 8.0.
13. Wash buffer 1: 0.1 M Tris–HCl, 0.5 M NaCl pH 8.0.
14. Wash buffer 2: 0.1 M NaAc, 0.5 M NaCl pH 4.0.
15. Elution buffer: 0.5 M NaCl PBS 2 mM EDTA (33.5 mS).

2.5 Functional Analysis Requirements

1. Maxisorp 96-well ELISA plate.
2. Phosphate-buffered saline sterile (PBS).
3. Albumin from bovine serum (BSA).

4. TWEEN 20.
5. Rabbit antihuman properdin antibody.
6. Goat anti-rabbit IgG horseradish peroxidase (HRP) antibody.
7. 2,2′-Azino-Bis(3-Ethylbenzthiazoline-6-Sulfonic acid) (ABTS).
8. ELISA blocking buffer: 1 % BSA/PBS.
9. ELISA diluant buffer: PBS Tween (0.05 %) 1 % BSA.

3 Method of Properdin Purification and Functional Analysis

The purification begins with normal human serum which is filtered and treated with polyethyleneglycol. The precipitated material is then passed through an anion exchange column. The fall through is then added to a C3b column for purification of human properdin.

3.1 Sample Preparation

1. Remove any fibrin or other precipitates by passing the cold human serum (550 ml) through glass wool.
2. Centrifuge the filtered material at 2,053 × *g* for 10 min.

3.2 Serum Purification

1. Add 5 % polyethyleneglycol (PEG) (27.5 g/550 ml serum) 4000 to the filtrate, ensuring the mixture is at least 2 °C.
2. Stir for 15 min on ice.
3. Allow the mixture to stand for 45 min on ice.
4. Centrifuge the mixture at 7,519 × g for 20 min in a refrigerated centrifuge 4 °C (*see* **Note 1**).
5. Dissolve the pellet in 100 ml DEAE buffer.

3.3 Anion Exchange Purification of PEG-Treated Serum

1. Rinse the DEAE-Sepharose (2.5 × 40 cm) column in DEAE buffer (*see* **Note 2**).
2. Centrifuge the sample reconstituted in DEAE buffer at 2,053 × g for 10 min.
3. Apply the supernatant to the DEAE-SEPH column connected to the pump and fraction collector, with a flow rate of 1 ml/min at 4 °C, collecting 10 ml fractions using the fraction collector (*see* **Note 3**).
4. Test every second fraction in a human properdin ELISA, detecting properdin using a specific antihuman properdin antibody.

3.4 C3b Column Preparation and Purification of Properdin

1. Purified human C3 (30 mg, pre-warmed to 37 °C) is exposed to trypsin 1 % w/w for 1 min at 37 °C to generate C3b and C3a.
2. This trypsinization reaction is inhibited by trypsin inhibitor 2 % w/w for 2 min at 37 °C.

3. The trypsinized C3 pool is dialyzed in PBS overnight at 4 °C using a 50,000 Da dialysis membrane, to remove the small molecular weight fragments such as C3a.
4. Dialyze the trypsinized C3 pool in the coupling buffer pH 8.3 overnight at 4 °C.
5. Suspend 4 g of activated Sepharose in 50 ml of 1 mM HCl for 15 min at 4 °C.
6. Filter the Sepharose in a glass filter using a vacuum system, washing with cold 1 mM HCl (approx 500 ml) followed by washing in the coupling buffer (approx 500 ml).
7. Remove the washed Sepharose gel from the glass filter and mix in a 1:1 volume ratio with the C3b pool in coupling buffer.
8. Leave the mix to rotate on a roller overnight at 4 °C.
9. Wash the Sepharose beads in a glass filter using the coupling buffer (approx 500 ml), the purified C3b is then coupled to the activated Sepharose beads.
10. Block any uncoupled groups on the beads using bead blocking buffer pH 8.0 for 2 h at room temperature.
11. Wash in a glass filter with wash buffer 1 pH 8.0 (approx 500 ml) three times.
12. Wash in a glass filter with wash buffer 2 pH 4.0 (approx 500 ml) three times.
13. Repeat **steps 11** and **12** at least three times.
14. A final wash in a glass filter using 500 ml of PBS.
15. The filtered Sepharose beads reconstituted in PBS 2 mM EDTA and poured into a column (1.5 cm × 15 cm).
16. Pool the ELISA positive properdin fractions following the DEAE purification.
17. Centrifuge the fractions at 2,000 × *g* for 10 min.
18. Apply the supernatant to the C3b column using PBS 2 mM EDTA, with a flow rate of 0.2 ml/min (*see* **Note 4**) at 4 °C.
19. Elute the properdin using elution buffer (33.5 mS) (*see* **Note 5**).
20. Test the fractions in a human properdin ELISA, detecting properdin using a specific antihuman properdin antibody (*see* Fig. 1).

3.5 Functional Analysis of Properdin

1. Coat the premade human C3b (5 μg/ml) using PBS on an ELISA plate overnight at 4 °C.
2. Block the wells using ELISA blocking buffer 1 h 37 °C.
3. Add the purified human properdin (5 μg/ml titrated in doubling dilutions) diluted in ELISA diluant buffer to the coated C3b wells for 1 h 37 °C.

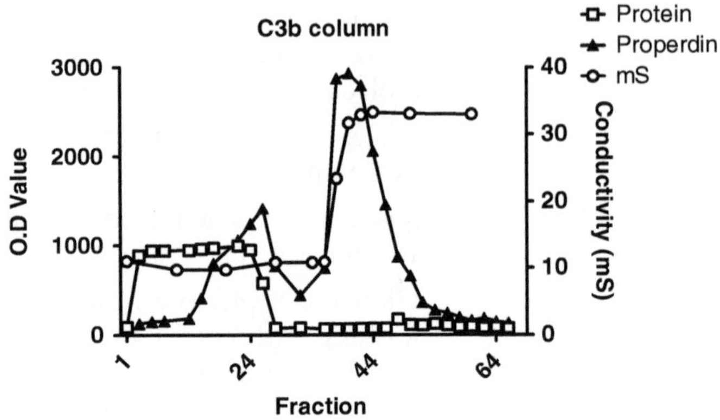

Fig. 1 Elution profile of isolated human properdin from C3b column

4. Detect the bound properdin using a specific rabbit antihuman properdin antibody diluted in ELISA diluant buffer for 1 h 37 °C.
5. Use a goat anti-rabbit HRP antibody diluted in ELISA diluant buffer for 1 h 37 °C.
6. Colorimetric reaction determined using ABTS at room temperature, with the absorbance measured at 415 nm.

4 Notes

1. Remove the supernatant following centrifugation and keep the pellet.
2. Prepare the columns, buffers, and equipment in advance. Ensure the equipment is functional and the columns are clean and leak proof. In particular, the pH and mS (conductivity) of the buffers can be temperature sensitive; the buffers should be equilibrated to the required operational temperature.
3. The properdin should be present in the fall through of the DEAE column. The fractions should be tested for properdin but can also be tested for total protein concentration using the BCA protein assay. It is useful to perform a C3 ELISA on fractions so as to rule out any contaminating C3 in properdin fractions.
4. Connect the C3b column to the pump and fraction collector. The properdin will remain bound to the C3b beads within the column.
5. The 0.5 M NaCl should be sufficient to elute the properdin from the column; however 1.0 M NaCl can also be used. The conductivity (mS), total protein concentration (BCA protein assay) and properdin levels should be ascertained for every second fraction.

Acknowledgments

This work was supported by a grant from the European Union (TranSVIR FP7-PEOPLE-ITN-2008 #238756).

References

1. Pillemer L, Blum L, Lepow IH, Ross OA, Todd EW, Wardlaw AC (1954) The properdin system and immunity. I. Demonstration and isolation of a new serum protein, properdin, and its role in immune phenomena. Science 120:279–285
2. Smith CA, Pangburn MK, Vogel CW, Muller-Eberhard HJ (1984) Molecular architecture of human properdin, a positive regulator of the alternative pathway of complement. J Biol Chem 259:4582–4588
3. Fearon DT, Austen KF (1975) Properdin: binding to C3b and stabilization of the C3b-dependent C3 convertase. J Exp Med 142: 856–863
4. Goundis D, Holt SM, Boyd Y, Reid KB (1989) Localization of the properdin structural locus to Xp11.23-Xp21.1. Genomics 5:56–60
5. Densen P, Weiler JM, Griffiss JM, Hoffmann LG (1987) Familial properdin deficiency and fatal meningococcemia. Correction of the bactericidal defect by vaccination. N Engl J Med 316:922–926
6. Kimura Y, Miwa T, Zhou L, Song WC (2008) Activator-specific requirement of properdin in the initiation and amplification of the alternative pathway complement. Blood 111: 732–740
7. Nolan KF, Schwaeble W, Kaluz S, Dierich MP, Reid KB (1991) Molecular cloning of the cDNA coding for properdin, a positive regulator of the alternative pathway of human complement. Eur J Immunol 21:771–776
8. Sun Z, Reid KB, Perkins SJ (2004) The dimeric and trimeric solution structures of the multidomain complement protein properdin by X-ray scattering, analytical ultracentrifugation and constrained modelling. J Mol Biol 343:1327–1343
9. Kemper C, Atkinson JP, Hourcade DE (2010) Properdin: emerging roles of a pattern-recognition molecule. Annu Rev Immunol 28:131–155
10. Pangburn MK (1989) Analysis of the natural polymeric forms of human properdin and their functions in complement activation. J Immunol 142:202–207
11. Schwaeble W, Huemer HP, Most J, Dierich MP, Strobel M, Claus C, Reid KB, Ziegler-Heitbrock HW (1994) Expression of properdin in human monocytes. Eur J Biochem 219:759–764
12. Schwaeble W, Dippold WG, Schafer MK, Pohla H, Jonas D, Luttig B, Weihe E, Huemer HP, Dierich MP, Reid KB (1993) Properdin, a positive regulator of complement activation, is expressed in human T cell lines and peripheral blood T cells. J Immunol 151:2521–2528
13. Wirthmueller U, Dewald B, Thelen M, Schafer MK, Stover C, Whaley K, North J, Eggleton P, Reid KB, Schwaeble WJ (1997) Properdin, a positive regulator of complement activation, is released from secondary granules of stimulated peripheral blood neutrophils. J Immunol 158: 4444–4451
14. Fearon DT (1979) Activation of the alternative complement pathway. CRC Crit Rev Immunol 1:1–32
15. Pangburn MK, Muller-Eberhard HJ (1984) The alternative pathway of complement. Springer Semin Immunopathol 7:163–192
16. Hourcade DE (2006) The role of properdin in the assembly of the alternative pathway C3 convertases of complement. J Biol Chem 281:2128–2132
17. Spitzer D, Mitchell LM, Atkinson JP, Hourcade DE (2007) Properdin can initiate complement activation by binding specific target surfaces and providing a platform for de novo convertase assembly. J Immunol 179:2600–2608
18. Xu W, Berger SP, Trouw LA, de Boer HC, Schlagwein N, Mutsaers C, Daha MR, van Kooten C (2008) Properdin binds to late apoptotic and necrotic cells independently of C3b and regulates alternative pathway complement activation. J Immunol 180: 7613–7621
19. Kemper C, Mitchell LM, Zhang L, Hourcade DE (2008) The complement protein properdin binds apoptotic T cells and promotes complement activation and phagocytosis. Proc Natl Acad Sci USA 105:9023–9028

Chapter 14

Purification and Functional Characterization of C4b-Binding Protein (C4BP)

Frida C. Mohlin and Anna M. Blom

Abstract

C4b-binding protein (C4BP) is a soluble, 570 kDa large glycoprotein, present in plasma at a concentration of approximately 200 mg/L. C4BP is the main inhibitor of the classical and lectin pathways of complement, where it controls C4b-mediated reactions. Here, we describe a method for purification of C4BP from human plasma, which is based on barium chloride precipitation, anion exchange chromatography, and gel filtration. We also describe a functional assay, in which C4BP's cofactor activity to factor I, in the degradation of C4b, can be assessed.

Key words Complement inhibitor, C4b-binding protein, Purification, Protein S, Coagulation, Apoptosis

1 Introduction

C4b-binding protein (C4BP), the main soluble inhibitor of the classical and lectin pathways, is a large glycoprotein (570 kDa) with an estimated plasma concentration of 200 mg/L [1]. C4BP exists in several isoforms, having different combinations of α- (70 kDa) and β-chains (45 kDa). The major isoform, which constitutes about 75–80 % of C4BP in plasma, is composed of seven identical α-chains and one β-chain, which are linked together in their C-terminal parts (Fig. 1a) [2]. Other less abundant forms are composed of six α-chains and one β-chain or exclusively of seven α-chains [3, 4]. The isoform pattern can be modified by factors with differential effects on the expression of the two genes coding for α- and β-chains [4].

The α- and β-chains contain eight and three complement control protein (CCP) domains, respectively. The C-terminal extensions (60 amino acid residues long) of both α- and β-chains contain two cysteine residues each and an amphipathic helical region, which is required for covalent intracellular polymerization of the molecule [5]. When analyzed by electron microscopy, C4BP

Mihaela Gadjeva (ed.), *The Complement System: Methods and Protocols*, Methods in Molecular Biology, vol. 1100,
DOI 10.1007/978-1-62703-724-2_14,

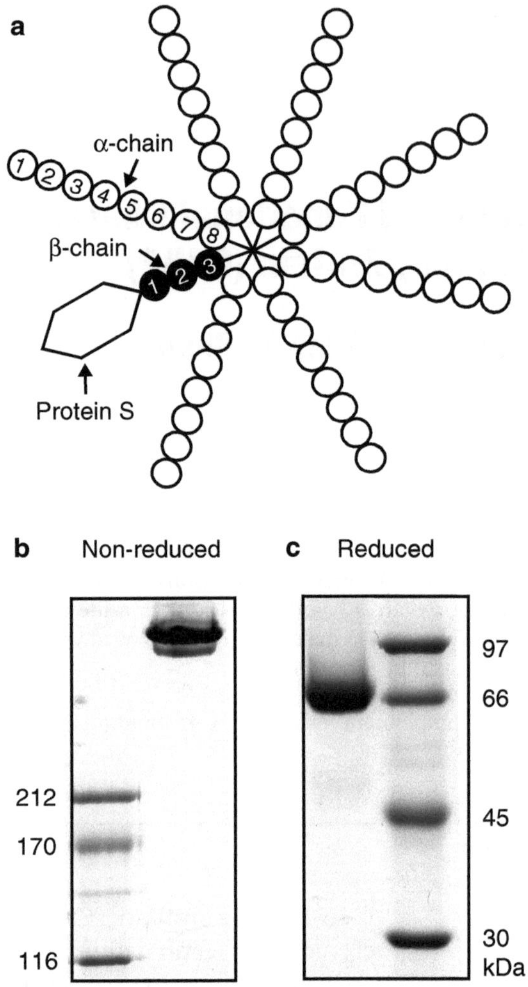

Fig. 1 Analysis of C4BP using SDS-PAGE followed by Coomassie Brilliant Blue staining. (**a**) The most common isoform of C4BP is composed of seven identical α-chains and one unique β-chain, which are covalently linked by their C-termini and form a spider-like structure. The α- and β-chains contain eight and three complement control protein (CCP) domains, respectively. The β-chain is always in complex with the vitamin K-dependent anticoagulant protein S. (**b**) C4BP migrates as a 570 kDa band when analyzed on a 5 % SDS-PAGE, under non-reducing conditions. (**c**) When analyzed on a 10 % SDS-PAGE, under reducing conditions, a 70 kDa band will appear, corresponding to both protein S and the α-chains of C4BP. The β-chain of C4BP is usually too weak to be seen on a gel

displays a spider or octopus-like shape with each of the extended tentacles being formed by one α-chain [6, 7]. The β-chain contains a high-affinity binding site for the anticoagulant, vitamin K-dependent protein S (PS) and all β-chain-containing C4BP molecules in plasma circulate in complex with PS [8, 9]. PS is a 70 kDa protein, containing a γ-carboxyglutamic acid domain (Gla-domain), which binds negatively charged phospholipids and helps to localize the C4BP-PS complex to dying cells [10, 11]. This allows opsonization of dying cells with C1q and C3b for more efficient phagocytosis but prevents overt inflammation. C4BP is an acute phase reactant and its plasma level can be elevated up to fourfold during inflammation [12]. During the acute phase, the synthesis of the α-chains, but not of the β-chain, increases and as a consequence, the plasma levels of the isoforms of C4BP lacking β-chain increase, whereas the level of β-chain-containing C4BP remains unaffected [13]. Interestingly, PS bound to C4BP is unable to participate in the anticoagulant protein C system [14]. It is crucial that the balance between free and bound PS is maintained at stable levels as lack of free PS leads to thrombosis [15, 16].

C4BP is best known as an inhibitor of the classical and lectin pathways, where it controls C4b-mediated reactions in at least three ways. First, C4BP acts as a cofactor to the serine proteinase factor I, in the proteolytic inactivation of C4b, which prevents the formation of the classical C3-convertase (C4bC2a) [2]. Second, C4BP prevents the assembly of the classical C3-convertase, by binding nascent C4b and finally it accelerates the natural decay of the complex [17]. C4BP also acts as a cofactor to factor I in the cleavage of C3b, in the fluid phase, thereby inhibiting to some extent the alternative pathway of complement as well but not to the level exerted by factor H [18, 19].

Apart from PS, C4b, and C3b, C4BP also interacts with heparin, DNA [11], low-density lipoprotein receptor-related protein (LRP) [20], and many bacterial ligands [21]. Binding of C4BP is a common strategy used by bacterial pathogens in order to attenuate activation of complement on their surface and ensuing phagocytosis.

There are several methods by which C4BP can be purified. The classical purification method, using commercially available products, is based on barium chloride precipitation to enrich C4BP-PS complex along with many Gla-domain containing coagulation proteins, followed by anion exchange chromatography and gel filtration. C4BP can also be purified using affinity chromatography with monoclonal antibodies [22] or bacterial peptides [23]. However, most of the antibodies are not commercially available and the peptides derived from streptococcal M-proteins may be difficult to synthesize.

2 Materials

2.1 Buffers and Stock Solutions

Prepare all solutions using ultrapure deionized water.

1. 1 M benzamidine (Prepare fresh in water, *see* **Note 1**).
2. 0.5 M phenylmethylsulfonyl fluoride, PMSF (Extremely toxic! Dissolve in methanol and store at RT, *see* **Note 2**).
3. 1 M $BaCl_2$.

4. 0.15 M NaCl.
5. 0.2 M EDTA, pH 7.4.
6. 0.1 M sodium phosphate buffer, pH 6.0.
7. 0.1 M sodium phosphate buffer, pH 6.0, supplemented with 0.8 M NaCl.
8. Tris-buffered saline (TBS): 50 mM Tris–HCl, 150 mM NaCl, pH 8.0.

2.2 Chromatography Resins

1. DEAE-Sephacel, weak anion exchanger (GE Healthcare): ~250 mL, packed in a 5 cm × 20 cm column.
2. Sephacryl S-400, gel filtration (GE Healthcare): ~600 mL, packed in a 3 cm × 100 cm column.

2.3 Chromatography Equipment

Depending on the availability, different types of chromatography equipment can be used, from advanced automated purification systems (e.g., ÄKTA systems from GE Healthcare) to much simpler alternatives, e.g., only a peristaltic pump. However, to facilitate the purification process we recommend the use of at least a peristaltic pump connected to an absorbance measuring unit that can follow protein elution in real time and finally a fraction collector.

2.4 Other Materials

1. 0.45 μm filter membranes (*see* **Note 3**).
2. Dialysis tubing, molecular weight cutoff: approximately 12–14 kDa.

3 Methods

The entire procedure should be carried out at 4 °C or on ice and the time of the whole procedure should be minimized.

3.1 Barium Chloride Precipitation

Barium chloride precipitates all proteins containing Gla-domains, such as those participating in the coagulation cascade. C4BP-PS complex is precipitated due to the presence of PS.

1. Use fresh or fresh frozen human citrate plasma. Add protease inhibitors: 10 mM benzamidine and 1 mM PMSF (*see* **Notes 1**, **2**, and **4**).
2. Add 80 mL of 1 M $BaCl_2$ per liter plasma, dropwise, while stirring (*see* **Note 5**).
3. Incubate for 60 min while stirring.
4. Centrifuge at 6,500 × g, for 30 min, at 4 °C.
5. Remove the supernatant and wash the pellet (which contains C4BP) twice with cold 0.15 M NaCl, i.e., add 0.15 M NaCl, resuspend the precipitate (*see* **Note 6**), centrifuge, and discard the supernatant.

6. Dissolve the pellet in ~150 mL cold 0.2 M EDTA, pH 7.4, per liter plasma, while stirring. This will take some time (*see* **Note 7**).
7. Dialyze the dissolved pellet excessively against 0.1 M sodium phosphate, pH 6.0, over night.

3.2 DEAE-Sephacel and S-400 Chromatography

All buffers used for chromatography should be cold and filtered through a 0.45 μm membrane.

1. Equilibrate the DEAE-Sephacel column with 5 column volumes (CV) of 0.1 M sodium phosphate, pH 6.0 and apply the dialysate, filtered through a 0.45 μm membrane (*see* **Note 3**), from the barium chloride precipitation.
2. Wash the column with 5 CV of 0.1 M sodium phosphate, pH 6.0.
3. Elute C4BP (flow rate: 100 mL/h) with a 1,600 mL linear gradient, from 0 to 0.8 M NaCl in 0.1 M sodium phosphate, pH 6.0. Collect 10 mL per fraction.
4. Detect in which fractions C4BP is present (*see* Subheading 3.3) and concentrate those by ultrafiltration. The final volume should be less than 5 % of the CV of the gel filtration column. The smaller the sample volume that is applied on a gel filtration column, the better resolution.
5. Equilibrate the Sephacryl S-400 gel filtration column with 2 CV of TBS and apply the concentrate from the DEAE-Sephacel column. The flow rate should constantly be 60–90 mL/h. Continue adding TBS, while collecting 8 mL fractions. Detect in which fractions C4BP is present (*see* Subheading 3.3), measure protein concentration and store in aliquots at −70 °C. Avoid repeated cycles of freezing and thawing. To ensure that the correct protein, which is functionally active, has been purified, a functional assay can be performed (*see* Subheading 3.4).

3.3 C4BP Detection

To detect in which fractions C4BP is present, different methods can be used, depending on the availability:

1. SDS-PAGE: 5 % for non-reduced and 10 % for reduced C4BP (*see* **Note 8**), followed by Coomassie Brilliant Blue staining. C4BP migrates as a 570 kDa (Fig. 1b) or 70 kDa (Fig. 1c) band under non-reducing and reducing conditions, respectively. PS is a 70 kDa protein and therefore cannot be distinguished from the α-chains of C4BP, under reducing conditions. The β-chain of C4BP is usually too weak in comparison to the α-chains to be seen on the reduced gel.

2. SDS-PAGE: 5 % for non-reduced and 10 % for reduced C4BP (*see* **Note 8**), followed by Western Blotting, using a commercially available C4BP antibody. Typically a monoclonal antibody is recommended for detection of the non-reduced protein while polyclonal antibodies usually work both under reducing and non-reducing conditions.
3. ELISA: using commercially available C4BP antibodies.

3.4 A Functional C4BP Assay

To ensure that the correct protein has been purified and that it is functionally active, a degradation assay can be performed, measuring C4BP's cofactor activity to factor I, in the degradation of C4b in fluid phase. Here, we describe the assay using ^{125}I -labeled C4b. If radioactivity cannot be used, western blotting followed by detection of degradation products of C4b with a specific antibody (such as polyclonal rabbit anti C4c from Dako), is another option.

1. Mix in TBS 100 μg/mL C4BP, 50 μg/mL C4b, 7 μg/mL factor I (*see* **Note 9**), and trace amounts of ^{125}I-labeled C4b (*see* **Note 10**), in a total volume of 40 μl. Incubate for 1.5 h at 37 °C.
2. Terminate the reaction by adding SDS-PAGE sample buffer, containing 25 mM DTT. Incubate at 95 °C for 3 min.
3. Separate the samples on a 10–15 % gradient SDS-PAGE.

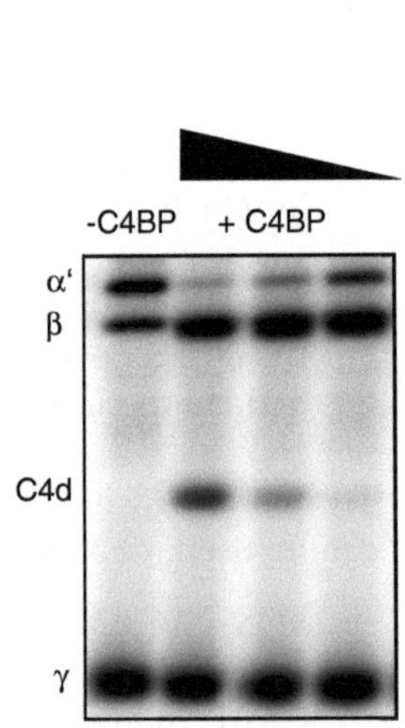

Fig. 2 A functional assay studying the cofactor activity of C4BP to factor I in the degradation of C4b in fluid phase. C4b, C4BP, factor I, and trace amounts of ^{125}I-C4b were incubated for 1.5 h at 37 °C. The reaction was terminated by adding SDS-PAGE sample buffer, containing a reducing agent and heating at 95 °C for 3 min. The proteins were separated on a 10–15 % SDS-PAGE and visualized by autoradiography. In the negative control, where no C4BP was added, the three different C4b chains can be seen: α′- (89 kDa), β- (73 kDa), and γ-chain (33 kDa). When C4BP is added, the α′-chain will be degraded and the C4d degradation fragment will appear (45 kDa). The degree of C4b degradation is dependent of C4BP concentration

4. Visualize the radioactive gels by autoradiography. C4b is composed of α′- (89 kDa), β- (73 kDa), and γ-chain (33 kDa), which all can be seen on the reduced gel and in the presence of factor I and C4BP, the α′-chain will be degraded and the C4d fragment (45 kDa) will appear (Fig. 2).

4 Notes

1. Benzamidine is inactivated by oxidation and should therefore be prepared fresh before use.
2. PMSF is extremely toxic and can be exchanged for 4-(2-aminoethyl)-benzene-sulfonyl fluoride (AEBSF, Calbiochem), which is more expensive but less toxic and more stable alternative. Since PMSF is rapidly degraded in water, the stock solution should be in methanol.
3. When filtering protein containing solutions, it is recommended to use cellulose acetate filters, which exhibit low protein binding.
4. Aprotinin (Trasylol, Bayer), 1 mM, can also be added as a protease inhibitor.
5. To avoid inadequate precipitation, it is of great importance to add the barium chloride slowly and dropwise.
6. When resuspending the precipitate in cold 0.15 M NaCl, the proteins will remain precipitated and thus the solution will not become clear.
7. If the pellet will not dissolve properly, try adding more buffer.
8. Since non-reduced C4BP is very large, 570 kDa, a 5 % SDS-PAGE has to be used and the best results are obtained when it is run very slowly. When the front of the sample dye has passed through the gel, continue on running for quite some time, to reassure that the protein has entered the gel.
9. Purified C4b and factor I are commercially available.
10. ^{125}I-label C4b with 0.5 MBq/μg of protein, using the chloramine T method [24].

References

1. Dahlbäck B (1983) Purification of human C4b-binding protein and formation of its complex with vitamin K-dependent protein S. Biochem J 209:847–856
2. Scharfstein J, Ferreira A, Gigli I et al (1978) Human C4b-binding protein, isolation and characterization. J Exp Med 148:207–222
3. Hillarp A, Hessing M, Dahlbäck B (1989) Protein S binding in relation to the subunit composition of human C4b-binding protein. FEBS Lett 259:53–56
4. Sanchez Corral P, Criado Garcia O, Rodriguez de Cordoba S (1995) Isoforms of human C4b-binding protein. I. Molecular basis for the C4BP isoform pattern and its variations in human plasma. J Immunol 155:4030–4036
5. Kask L, Hillarp A, Ramesh B et al (2002) Structural requirements for the intra-cellular

subunit polymerization of the complement inhibitor C4b-binding protein. Biochemistry 41:9349–9357
6. Dahlbäck B, Smith CA, Müller Eberhard HJ (1983) Visualization of human C4b-binding protein and its complexes with vitamin K-dependent protein S and complement protein C4b. Proc Natl Acad Sci USA 80:3461–3465
7. Happonen KE, Sjoberg AP, Morgelin M et al (2009) Complement inhibitor C4b-binding protein interacts directly with small glycoproteins of the extracellular matrix. J Immunol 182:1518–1525
8. Hillarp A, Dahlbäck B (1988) Novel subunit in C4b-binding protein required for protein S binding. J Biol Chem 263:12759–12764
9. Härdig Y, Dahlbäck B (1996) The amino-terminal module of the C4b-binding protein beta-chain contains the protein S binding site. J Biol Chem 271:20861–20867
10. Webb JH, Blom AM, Dahlbäck B (2002) Vitamin K-dependent protein S localizing complement regulator C4b-binding protein to the surface of apoptotic cells. J Immunol 169:2580–2586
11. Trouw LA, Nilsson SC, Goncalves I et al (2005) C4b-binding protein binds to necrotic cells and DNA, limiting DNA release and inhibiting complement activation. J Exp Med 201:1937–1948
12. Barnum SR, Dahlbäck B (1990) C4b-binding protein, a regulatory component of the classical pathway of complement, is an acute-phase protein and is elevated in systemic lupus erythematosus. Complement Inflamm 7:71–77
13. Garcia de Frutos P, Alim RI, Härdig Y et al (1994) Differential regulation of alpha and beta chains of C4b-binding protein during acute-phase response resulting in stable plasma levels of free anticoagulant protein S. Blood 84:815–822
14. Dahlback B (1986) Inhibition of protein Ca cofactor function of human and bovine protein S by C4b-binding protein. J Biol Chem 261:12022–12027
15. Zöller B, Garcia de Frutos P, Dahlbäck B (1995) Evaluation of the relationship between protein S and C4b-binding protein isoforms in hereditary protein S deficiency demonstrating type I and type III deficiencies to be phenotypic variants of the same genetic disease. Blood 85:3524–3531
16. Simmonds RE, Zöller B, Ireland H et al (1997) Genetic and phenotypic analysis of a large (122-member) protein S-deficient kindred provides an explanation for the familial coexistence of type I and type III plasma phenotypes. Blood 89:4364–4370
17. Gigli I, Fujita T, Nussenzweig V (1979) Modulation of the classical pathway C3 convertase by plasma protein C4b binding and C3b inactivator. Proc Natl Acad Sci USA 76:6596–6600
18. Seya T, Nakamura K, Masaki T et al (1995) Human factor H and C4b-binding protein serve as factor I cofactors both encompassing inactivation of C3b and C4b. Mol Immunol 32:355–360
19. Blom AM, Kask L, Dahlbäck B (2003) CCP1-4 of the C4b-binding protein α-chain are required for Factor I mediated cleavage of C3b. Mol Immunol 39:547–556
20. Spijkers PP, Denis CV, Blom AM et al (2008) Cellular uptake of C4b-binding protein is mediated by heparan sulfate proteoglycans and CD91/LDL receptor-related protein. Eur J Immunol 38:809–817
21. Blom AM, Hallstrom T, Riesbeck K (2009) Complement evasion strategies of pathogens-acquisition of inhibitors and beyond. Mol Immunol 46:2808–2817
22. Blom AM, Webb J, Villoutreix BO et al (1999) A cluster of positively charged amino acids in the N-terminal modules of the C4BP α-chain is crucial for C4b binding and factor I cofactor function. J Biol Chem 274:19237–19245
23. Persson J, Lindahl G (2005) Single-step purification of human C4b-binding protein (C4BP) by affinity chromatography on a peptide derived from a streptococcal surface protein. J Immunol Methods 297:83–95
24. Greenwood FC, Hunter WM, Glover JS (1963) The preparation of ^{125}I-labelled human growth hormone of high specific activity. Biochem J 89:114–123

Chapter 15

Purification and Functional Characterization of Factor I

Sara C. Nilsson and Anna M. Blom

Abstract

Factor I (FI) is a soluble, 88 kDa glycoprotein present in plasma at a concentration of approximately 35 mg/L. FI inhibits all complement pathways as it degrades activated C4b and C3b when these are bound to a cofactor such as C4b-binding protein or factor H. Here, we describe a method for purification of FI from human plasma, which is based on affinity chromatography followed by anion exchange chromatography. We also describe a functional assay, in which activity of FI can be assessed.

Key words Complement inhibitor, Factor I, Atypical hemolytic uremic syndrome

1 Introduction

Factor I (FI) is an 88 kDa serum glycoprotein that is expressed in the liver by hepatocytes [1], but also by other cells such as monocytes, fibroblasts, keratinocytes, and endothelial cells. The average serum concentration of FI is ~35 mg/L and increases during inflammation since FI is an acute phase protein.

FI is a multidomain protein synthesized as a single polypeptide chain and processed to yield the heavy (50 kDa) and the light (38 kDa) chains [2], which are then covalently linked via a disulfide bridge (Fig. 1). The protein also undergoes glycosylation and each chain contains three *N*-linked glycans. FI can be expressed recombinantly in mammalian or insect cells but only partial proteolytic processing of the single chain FI precursor occurs under such conditions and only the processed protein has catalytic activity [3, 4]. The heavy chain consists of the FI membrane attack complex domain (FIMAC), a CD5-like domain (also known as the scavenger receptor cysteine-rich domain), low-density lipoprotein receptor 1 and 2 domains (LDLr1 and 2), and a small region of unknown homology. The light chain of FI comprises the serine protease (SP) domain [5] where the catalytic triad in the active

Mihaela Gadjeva (ed.), *The Complement System: Methods and Protocols*, Methods in Molecular Biology, vol. 1100,
DOI 10.1007/978-1-62703-724-2_15,

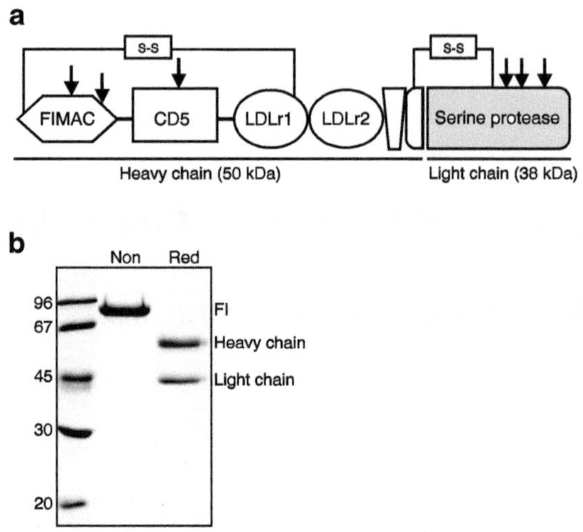

Fig. 1 (**a**) Schematic overview of FI and its domains FIMAC, CD5, LDLr1/2, and SP. The sites for N-linked glycosylations are marked with *arrows*. (**b**) FI purified from plasma analyzed on SDS-PAGE. Five micrograms FI was analyzed on a 10 % SDS-PAGE gel and stained with Coomassie. In a non-reduced state intact FI migrates as an 88 kDa protein. Under reducing conditions the heavy chain of 50 kDa and light chain of 38 kDa become apparent

site is formed by His362, Asp411, and Ser507. FI contains 40 cysteines and 36 of them are involved in intra-domain disulfide bridges, and the remaining four cysteines (C15-C237, C309-C435) connect the FIMAC and LDLr1 domains and the SP domain with the heavy chain [6]. Recently a structure of FI has been solved by X-ray crystallography [7].

FI cleaves C4b and C3b at a few specific sites only in the presence of cofactors. Degradation of C4b is supported by C4b-binding protein (C4BP), membrane cofactor protein (MCP), and complement receptor 1 (CR1). C3b can be degraded to iC3b in the presence of factor H (FH), MCP and CR1 and then further to C3d only in the presence of CR1. Purified native FI, in the absence of cofactors, cleaves peptide aminomethyl coumarin substrates [8], which can be used to assess its amidolytic activity.

Complete FI deficiency results mainly in recurrent infections with encapsulated microorganisms and sometimes in renal disease or an autoimmune disorder [9–11]. Heterozygous defects in FI lead to atypical hemolytic syndrome [3, 12–14].

The easiest way to purify FI is by using affinity chromatography with commercially available monoclonal antibody (MRC-OX21). FI is a quite robust protein and retains its activity after elution from an antibody.

2 Materials

2.1 Starting Materials

MRC-OX21 mouse monoclonal (IgG_1) directed against FI. The cell line producing MRC-OX21 was from European Collection of Cell Cultures (ECACC) No. 91060417. The antibody was expressed in two-compartment CELLine bioreactor (INTEGRA Biosciences) using fetal bovine serum with low IgG (Invitrogen). The antibody was then purified on a HiTrap Protein G column (GE Healthcare).

500 mL fresh frozen plasma.

2.2 Buffers and Reagents

Prepare all buffers using pure deionized water. The buffers applied on a column should be filtered through a 0.45 μm filter. When dialyzing plasma or purified FI use a membrane with a molecular weight cutoff of 10–14,000.

1. 0.1 M $NaHCO_3$, pH 8.0.
2. Isopropanol.
3. 1 M HCl.
4. 1 M ethanolamine–HCl, pH 8.0.
5. 0.1 M glycine pH 2.2 + 0.5 M NaCl.
6. Tris-buffered saline (TBS): 50 mM Tris–HCl, 150 mM NaCl, pH 8.0.
7. 0.5 M EDTA, pH 7.4 (stock solution).
8. TBS + 0.5 mM EDTA, pH 7.4.
9. 10 % NaN_3.
10. 0.5 M phenylmethylsulfonyl fluoride (PMSF) (stock in methanol, store at room temperature, toxic, *see* **Note 1**).
11. 1 M benzamidine (prepare fresh in water, *see* **Note 2**).
12. 3 M $MgCl_2$, pH 6.8–7.0 (*see* **Note 3**).
13. 30 mM Tris–HCl, pH 9.0.
14. 30 mM Tris–HCl, 400 mM NaCl, pH 9.0.
15. 200 mM aminocaproic acid (EACA) (stock in water, store at −20 °C) + 2 M NaCl.
16. 50 mM Na-phosphate buffer, 150 mM NaCl, 15 mM EDTA pH 7.4.
17. 50 mM Na-phosphate buffer, 150 mM NaCl, 15 mM EDTA pH 7.4, 0.02 % NaN_3.

2.3 Chromatography Resins

1. Lysine-Sepharose (GE Healthcare).
2. Affi-Gel 10 (Bio-Rad).
3. Mono Q column (GE Healthcare).

2.4 Chromatography Equipment

1. XK 26 column (GE Healthcare).

Depending on the availability, different types of chromatography equipment can be used, from advanced automated purification systems (e.g., ÄKTA systems from GE Healthcare) to much simpler alternatives, e.g., only a peristaltic pump. However, to facilitate the purification process we recommend the use of at least a peristaltic pump connected to an absorbance-measuring unit that can follow protein elution in real time and finally a fraction collector.

2.5 Buffers and Reagents for Dot Blot and ELISA

1. Washing solution: 150 mM Tris, 50 mM NaCl, 0.1 % Tween 20, pH 8.0.
2. Washing solution 10× stock: 1.5 M Tris–HCl, 0.5 M NaCl, 1 % Tween 20, pH 8.0.
3. Fish gelatin: 100 % stock (Norland HiPure liquid fish gelatin, Norlands Products).
4. Blocking solution: 3 % fish gelatin in washing solution.
5. Alkaline phosphatase (AP) buffer: 100 mM Tris–HCl, 100 mM NaCl, 10 mM $MgCl_2$, pH 9.5.
6. 75 mg/mL Nitro blue tetrazolium (NBT) (stock in dimethylformamide, Fermentas).
7. 50 mg/mL 5-bromo-4-chloro-3-indolyl phosphate, p-toluidine salt (BCIP-T) (stock in 70 % dimethylformamide, Fermentas).
8. MRCOX-21 antibody (monoclonal antibody against human FI).
9. Goat anti-human FI sera (polyclonal antibody against human FI, Quidel).
10. Rabbit anti-mouse Ig-AP.
11. Rabbit anti-goat Ig-horseradish peroxidase (HRP).
12. Goat anti-mouse Ig-HRP.
13. 1,2-phenylenediamine dihydrochloride (OPD) tablets (Dako).
14. 0.5 M H_2SO_4.
15. TBS: 50 mM Tris–HCl, 150 mM NaCl, pH 8.0.
16. HRP buffer for western blot: 10 mg diaminobenzidine (DAB), 100 mL TBS, 1 mL 0.06 M $NiCl_2$, 10 μL H_2O_2.

2.6 Buffers and Materials for Assay Testing Function of FI

1. Veronal buffer (VBS) stock (25 mM): 9.0 mM Na-barbituric acid, 15.5 mM barbituric acid, and 720 mM NaCl pH 7.35 (*see* **Note 4**).
2. GVB–Ni: 0.1 % gelatin, 2.5 mM VBS, 100 mM NaCl, and 2.5 mM $NiCl_2$ (*see* **Note 5**).
3. GVB–EDTA: 0.1 % gelatin, 2.5 mM VBS, 100 mM NaCl, and 2 mM EDTA (*see* **Note 5**).

4. DGVB^{++}: 0.1 % gelatin, 2.5 mM VBS, 140 mM glucose, 1 mM $CaCl_2$, and 0.15 mM $CaCl_2$ (*see* **Note 5**).
5. Flow cytometry medium (FCM): PBS, 1 % bovine serum albumin, 15 mM EDTA, and 30 mM NaN_3.
6. TBS: 50 mM Tris–HCl, 150 mM NaCl, pH 8.0.
7. Sheep erythrocytes (Complement Technology Ltd).
8. Purified C3, factor B (FB), and factor D (FD) (Complement Technology).
9. FI and FH can be purified from plasma or bought from Complement Technology.
10. V-bottom plate with 96 wells (Nunc).
11. Mouse anti-human C3d (Quidel).
12. Mouse anti-human iC3b (Quidel).
13. Goat anti-mouse Ig–fluorescein isothiocyanate (FITC) (Goat F(ab')2 (Dako).

2.7 Equipment Required for Assay Testing Function of FI

1. Thermomixer (e.g., Eppendorf).
2. Flow cytometer.

3 Methods

3.1 Coupling of MRC-OX21 to Affi-Gel 10

Affi-Gel 10 (Bio-Rad) is a N-hydroxysuccinimide ester of a derivatized cross-linked agarose gel bead support and couples to ligands spontaneously in aqueous solution. Ether bonds link the spacer arm to chemically cross-linked agarose gel beads while amide bonds couple the protein ligand to the terminal carboxyl of the spacer arm. The gel is resistant to urea, guanidine HCl, heat, solvents, acidic and basic conditions (pH 2–11).

1. Dialyze MRC-OX21 (*see* **Note 6** for amount) against 0.1 M $NaHCO_3$, pH 8.0. Dialyze first against 2 L buffer for 2 h and then overnight with additional 3 L. After dialysis, measure the absorbance at 280 nm.
2. Gently shake the Affi-Gel 10 vial and transfer ~50 mL to a Buchner funnel.
3. Wash rapidly, using vacuum, with 3 volumes isopropanol and then with 3 volumes of cold deionized H_2O.
4. Transfer the gel to a beaker and add the dialyzed MRC-OX21 and incubate with gentle agitation for 1.5–2 h at room temperature (*see* **Note 7**).
5. To block the remaining esters add 0.1 mL/1 mL gel of freshly made 1 M ethanolamine–HCl, pH 8.0. Incubate with gentle agitation for 1 h at room temperature.

6. Transfer the gel to a XK-26 column and continue working at 4 °C.
7. Wash the column with 5 column volumes (CV) of 0.1 M $NaHCO_3$, pH 8.0 using a flow of 2 mL/min.
8. Continue washing with 5 CV of 0.1 M glycine pH 2.2 supplemented with 0.5 M NaCl.
9. Equilibrate the column with 5 CV of TBS + 0.5 mM EDTA pH 7.4.
10. If the column is not to be used immediately, store it at 4 °C (*see* **Note 8**).

3.2 Purification of FI on the MRC-OX21 Column

The purification of FI should be performed at 4 °C.

1. The MRC-OX21 column is prepared as described above (*see* Subheading 3.1).
2. Add protease inhibitors, 5 mM EDTA, 1 mM PMSF, and 10 mM benzamidine, to 500 mL human plasma (preferably fresh frozen) (*see* **Notes 1** and **2**).
3. Dialyze the plasma against TBS + 0.5 mM EDTA pH 7.4 (2 × 10 L) at 4 °C, overnight (*see* **Note 7**).
4. Filter the dialyzed plasma through a 0.45 μm filter. If there is a visible precipitate it is advisable to centrifuge the plasma first for 20 min at 5,000 × *g* (*see* **Note 9**).
5. Equilibrate the MRC-OX21 column with 5 CV of TBS + 0.5 mM EDTA pH 7.4.
6. Load 100 mL filtered plasma on the column with a flow of 2 mL/min. Collect the flow through and check with a dot blot (*see* Subheading 3.3.1) if most of the FI is bound to the column. If not the plasma can be loaded once more on the column.
7. Wash the column with 6 CV of TBS + 0.5 mM EDTA pH 7.4 to remove unbound proteins.
8. Elute FI from the MRC-OX21 column with 5 CV of 3 M $MgCl_2$ pH 6.8–7.0. Collect fractions of 8 mL.
9. Pool the fractions that contain FI. The fractions can be run on a SDS-PAGE and/or western blot to analyze the yield and purity of the FI (*see* Subheadings 3.3.3 and 3.3.4). FI migrates as 88 kDa (Fig. 1b) or 50 kDa and 38 kDa (Fig. 1b) band under non-reducing and reducing conditions, respectively. If the FI is pure, dialyze against TBS at 4 °C, overnight. Freeze in aliquots at −80 °C. Repeat the purification four more times to us up the whole prepared plasma.
10. If FI is not pure enough it can be further purified on a Mono Q column, which is a strong anion exchanger.
11. Dialyze the FI-containing fractions against 30 mM Tris–HCl pH 9.0.

12. Equilibrate the Mono Q column with 5 CV of 30 mM Tris–HCl pH 9.0, with a flow of 1 mL/min.
13. Apply the dialyzed FI to the Mono Q column and wash with 10 CV 30 mM Tris–HCl pH 9.0.
14. Elute FI with a 50 mL gradient to 400 mM NaCl in 30 mM Tris–HCl pH 9.0. Collect fractions of 1 mL. FI elutes in the middle of the gradient. Separate the fractions on a SDS-PAGE and stain with Coomassie Brilliant Blue or silver salts.
15. Pool the fractions containing FI and dialyze against the desired buffer or freeze directly in aliquots at −80 °C. Avoid repeated freezing and thawing.

3.3 Detection of FI

3.3.1 Dot Blot

An easy and fast method to analyze if a sample contains FI is a dot blot.

1. Load 3–5 μL of each sample on an ultra bind US450 membrane (Pall Life Sciences).
2. Block nonspecific binding sites on the membrane by incubating with blocking solution for 30 min.
3. Add 1 μg/mL MRC-OX21 in blocking solution and incubate for 30–60 min at room temperature with gentle agitation.
4. Wash the membrane with washing solution for 3 × 5 min.
5. Add a secondary antibody, e.g., polyclonal rabbit anti-mouse conjugated to alkaline phosphatase (Dako), diluted 2,000× in blocking solution and incubate as before (*see* **Note 10**).
6. Wash the membrane with washing solution for 3 × 5 min.
7. Develop the blot by adding AP buffer supplemented with 330 μg/mL NBT (Fermentas) and 165 μg/mL BCIP-T (Fermentas) (*see* **Note 11**). Stop the development by rinsing the membrane with water.

3.3.2 ELISA

The concentration of FI can be measured using ELISA using purified FI or normal human serum/plasma as a standard. The volume is 50 μL per well in all steps if not stated otherwise.

1. Coat MaxiSorp plates (Nunc) with polyclonal goat anti-human FI sera (Quidel) diluted 1,000× in 50 mM sodium carbonate buffer pH 9.5, at 4 °C overnight.
2. Wash the plate four times with the washing solution (300 μL/well).
3. Block the wells with 250 μL blocking solution for 1 h at 37 °C.
4. Add the dilutions of FI of serum/plasma (a standard curve) prepared in blocking solution and only blocking solution as a negative control, incubate for 1 h at 37 °C.
5. Wash the plate four times with the washing solution (300 μL/well).

6. Add 1 μg/mL MRC-OX21 diluted in blocking solution and incubate for 1 h at 37 °C.
7. Wash the plate four times with the washing solution (300 μL/well).
8. Add polyclonal goat anti-mouse antibody conjugated to HRP diluted 2,000× in blocking solution and incubate for 1 h at 37 °C.
9. Wash the plate four times with the washing solution (300 μL/well).
10. Develop the plate by adding 2 OPD tablets dissolved in 6 mL water and 2.5 μL H_2O_2.
11. Stop the reaction with 0.5 M H_2SO_4 and measure the absorbance at 490 nm.

3.3.3 SDS-PAGE

FI can be analyzed on a 10 % SDS-PAGE gel and stained with Coomassie Brilliant Blue (Fig. 1b) or silver salts. Under non-reducing conditions FI migrates as a single band of 88 kDa and at reducing conditions it migrates as a heavy chain of 50 kDa and light chain of 38 kDa.

3.3.4 Western Blot

FI can also be analyzed using western blotting. For non-reducing conditions MRCOX-21 followed by goat anti-mouse antibodies are preferable to use and for reducing conditions goat anti-human FI followed by polyclonal rabbit anti-goat antibodies are a good choice (*see* **Note 12**).

3.4 Functional Assay for FI

The activity of FI can be determined using fluid-phase C3b and C4b degradation assay (*see* Chap. 14) or membrane bound C3b as a substrate in presence of a cofactor (e.g., C4BP, FH, MCP, or CR1) [15]. In the assay using membrane bound C3b, sheep erythrocytes are coated with C3b, which is then cleaved by FI together with FH. Two monoclonal antibodies, anti-C3d and anti-iC3b, are used to detect the cleavage products of C3b using flow cytometry (Fig. 2). Most anti-C3 antibodies recognize to various extent many forms of C3 such as C3b, iC3b and C3d and therefore it is advisable to use a ratio of the geometric means for iC3b–C3d to estimate activity of FI. Anti-C3d antibody determines how much C3b was deposited in total on the surface of the erythrocytes and anti-iC3b antibody how much iC3b is formed after cleavage with FI and FH. A high ratio of iC3b–C3d indicates degradation of FI.

1. Wash ~3 mL sheep erythrocytes (1×10^9 cells/mL) 3–5 times in 10 mL ice-cold GVB–Ni until the supernatant is transparent. Between each wash centrifuge the erythrocytes for 800 × *g* for 5 min. After the last washing resuspend the pellet (~0.5 mL) in 5.5 mL GVB–Ni.

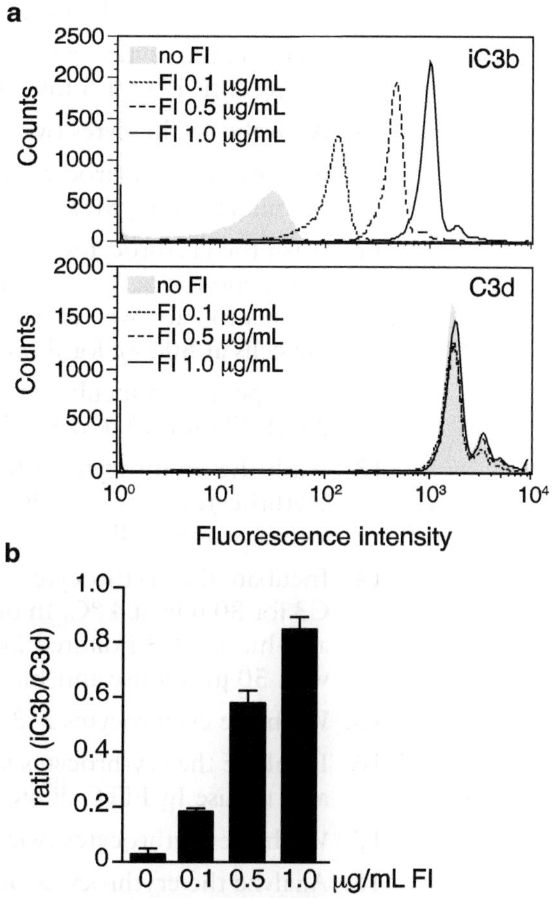

Fig. 2 C3b was deposited on the surface of sheep erythrocytes by incubation with C3, FB, and FD. (**a**) A histogram shows the amount of iC3b and C3d present on the erythrocytes after incubation with 0.1, 0.5, and 1.0 μg/mL FI together with 20 μg/mL FH. (**b**) The amount of deposited C3b and liberated iC3b was detected using specific antibodies and the results are presented as a ratio iC3b-C3d

2. Transfer 200 μL erythrocytes (from the 6 mL solution) to an eppendorf tube and add to a final concentration of 0.2 mg/mL C3, 0.02 mg/mL FB, and 0.4 μg/mL FD and incubate in a thermomixer at 800 rpm for 30 min at 30 °C.
3. Spin down the erythrocytes in a tabletop centrifuge for 3 min at 800×*g*. Wash the erythrocytes twice with 1 mL ice-cold GVB–EDTA. Resuspend the pellet with 200 μL ice-cold GVB-EDTA.
4. Incubate the erythrocytes (200 μL) with 0.02 mg/mL FB and 0.4 μg/mL FD for 5 min at 30 °C, 800 rpm.
5. Wash the erythrocytes twice with 1 mL ice-cold GVB–EDTA.
6. Incubate the erythrocytes (200 μL) with 0.2 mg/mL C3 for 20 min at 30 °C, 800 rpm.

7. Wash the cells erythrocytes with 1 mL ice-cold GVB–Ni.
8. Incubate the erythrocytes (200 μL) with 0.02 mg/mL FB and 0.4 μg/mL FD for 5 min at 30 °C, 800 rpm.
9. Wash the erythrocytes twice with 1 mL ice-cold GVB–EDTA.
10. Incubate the erythrocytes (200 μL) with 0.2 mg/mL C3 for 20 min at 30 °C, 800 rpm.
11. Wash the erythrocytes twice with 1 mL ice-cold $DGVB^{++}$ and resuspend the pellet in 5 mL $DGVB^{++}$. Transfer 100 μL erythrocytes to each well in a 96-well V-bottom plate. Spin down the cells at 800 × *g* for 3 min and discard the supernatant.
12. Resuspend and incubate the erythrocytes with 25 μL FI and 25 μL FH for 60 min at 37 °C, 800 rpm (*see* **Note 13**).
13. Wash the erythrocytes 3 times in 200 μL FCM and split the erythrocytes to two wells. Transfer 100 μL to each well and spin down the cells.
14. Incubate the erythrocytes with monoclonal antibodies against C3 for 30 min at 4 °C. In one well incubate with 50 μL mouse anti-human C3d diluted 200× in FCM and in the other well with 50 μL mouse anti-human iC3b diluted 200× in FCM.
15. Wash the erythrocytes 2–3 times with FCM.
16. Incubate the erythrocytes for 30 min at 4 °C with 50 μL goat anti-mouse Ig-FITC diluted 100× in FCM.
17. Wash the erythrocytes twice in FCM (*see* **Note 14**).
18. Analyze the erythrocytes on a flow cytometer (*see* **Note 15**).

4 Notes

1. PMSF is toxic and can be exchanged for 4-(2-aminoethyl)-benzene-sulfonyl fluoride (AEBSF, Calbiochem), which is more expensive but less toxic and more stable alternative. Since PMSF is rapidly degraded in water, the stock solution should be in methanol.
2. Benzamidine is inactivated by oxidation and should therefore be prepared fresh before use.
3. To adjust the pH add a Tris base.
4. First dissolve barbituric acid in hot H_2O (~100 mL at 150–200 °C), let it cool down, and then add to another beaker with the rest of the components dissolved. Sterile filter and store at 4 °C. Use the buffer when it is ice-cold.
5. When preparing buffer containing gelatin first boil the gelatin in 10–15 mL H_2O. When it is dissolved let it cool down and then add the rest of the chemicals to the solution.

6. It is advisable to couple 2–10 mg protein per mL gel. A column of 50 mL is a preferable size of choice, requiring 250 mg of antibody for coupling.
7. The sample added should be at least 0.5 mL ligand solution per milliliter of gel. Measure the absorbance at 280 nm of the supernatant to estimate how much of the protein that has bound to the gel. Before measuring the absorbance, the pH of the sample should be lowered by adding 1 M HCl to a final concentration of 0.01 M HCl because at neutral or basic pH the N-hydroxysuccinimide released during the coupling will absorb at 280 nm.
8. Addition of 0.02 % NaN_3 will prevent bacterial growth in the column.
9. It is optional to remove plasminogen from plasma before applying it on the MRC-OX21 column. Plasminogen is a zymogen of the active serine protease plasmin and can be activated by several different enzymes such as tissue/urokinase plasminogen activator, kallikrein, and factor XII. Plasmin may eventually degrade many plasma proteins during the purification including FI. Therefore the following step may be added in case one experiences problems with degradation.
   (a) Wash 100 mL lysine-Sepharose on a sintered glass funnel with 200 mL of 200 mM EACA + 2 M NaCl and then with 500 mL of 50 mM Na-phosphate buffer, 150 mM NaCl, 15 mM EDTA, pH 7.4.
   (b) Add 100 mL of lysine-Sepharose to the plasma (plasminogen will bind to the gel) and incubate for 1 h at 4 °C with gentle agitation (do not use magnetic stirrer). Centrifuge for 20 min at 2,830 × *g*, 4 °C to remove the gel. The supernatant contains FI, which can be further applied on a MRC-OX21 column (*see* Subheading 3.2).
   (c) Regenerate the gel with 200 mL of 200 mM EACA + 2 M NaCl, plasminogen will be eluted. Wash the gel with 500 mL of 50 mM Na-phosphate buffer, 150 mM NaCl, 15 mM EDTA, pH 7.4, and 0.02 % NaN_3 (*see* **Note 8**).
10. A polyclonal antibody against FI (e.g., goat anti-human FI, Quidel) can also be used to detect FI on a dot blot.
11. A secondary antibody conjugated to HRP also works for detection on dot blot, but then a different development buffer is needed. Mix 10 mg DAB with 100 mL TBS, when it is dissolved add 1 mL 0.06 M $NiCl_2$ and 10 μL H_2O_2. Add the solution to the membrane. Stop the development by rinsing the membrane with water.
12. The light chain of FI is usually detected with lower intensity compared to the heavy chain when using polyclonal antibodies.

13. Dilute FI and FH in TBS and make two times the concentration due to the dilution factor. The final volume should be 50 μL. Optimization of the concentrations is required but it is advisable to test concentrations in the range of 0.5–10 μg/mL FI and 5–20 μg/mL FH.
14. The final volume of the samples depends on the type of flow cytometer, which is used to analyze the samples. When analyzing many samples, it is preferable to use a 96-well plate autosampler and then a volume of 150 μL per well may be sufficient.
15. To be able to adjust the settings of the flow cytometer, analyze untreated erythrocytes before you run the actual samples.

References

1. Morris KM, Aden DP, Knowles BB et al (1982) Complement biosynthesis by the human hepatoma-derived cell line HepG2. J Clin Invest 70:906–913
2. Goldberger G, Arnaout MA, Aden D et al (1984) Biosynthesis and postsynthetic processing of human C3b/C4b inactivator (factor I) in three hepatoma cell lines. J Biol Chem 259:6492–6497
3. Nilsson SC, Karpman D, Vaziri-Sani F et al (2007) A mutation in factor I that is associated with atypical hemolytic uremic syndrome does not affect the function of factor I in complement regulation. Mol Immunol 44:1835–1844
4. Ullman CG, Chamberlain D, Ansari A et al (1998) Human complement factor I: its expression by insect cells and its biochemical and structural characterisation. Mol Immunol 35:503–512
5. Chamberlain D, Ullman CG, Perkins SJ (1998) Possible arrangement of the five domains in human complement factor I as determined by a combination of X-ray and neutron scattering and homology modeling. Biochemistry 37:13918–13929
6. Tsiftsoglou SA, Willis AC, Li P et al (2005) The catalytically active serine protease domain of human complement factor I. Biochemistry 44:6239–6249
7. Roversi P, Johnson S, Caesar JJ et al (2011) Structural basis for complement factor I control and its disease-associated sequence polymorphisms. Proc Natl Acad Sci USA 108:12839–12844
8. Tsiftsoglou SA, Sim RB (2004) Human complement factor I does not require cofactors for cleavage of synthetic substrates. J Immunol 173:367–375
9. Amadei N, Baracho GV, Nudelman V et al (2001) Inherited complete factor I deficiency associated with systemic lupus erythematosus, higher susceptibility to infection and low levels of factor H. Scand J Immunol 53:615–621
10. Nilsson SC, Trouw LA, Renault N et al (2009) Genetic, molecular and functional analyses of complement factor I deficiency. Eur J Immunol 39:310–323
11. Sadallah S, Gudat F, Laissue JA et al (1999) Glomerulonephritis in a patient with complement factor I deficiency. Am J Kidney Dis 33:1153–1157
12. Bienaime F, Dragon-Durey MA, Regnier CH et al (2010) Mutations in components of complement influence the outcome of Factor I-associated atypical hemolytic uremic syndrome. Kidney Int 77:339–349
13. Esparza-Gordillo J, Jorge EG, Garrido CA et al (2006) Insights into hemolytic uremic syndrome: segregation of three independent predisposition factors in a large, multiple affected pedigree. Mol Immunol 43:1769–1775
14. Kavanagh D, Kemp EJ, Mayland E et al (2005) Mutations in complement factor I predispose to development of atypical hemolytic uremic syndrome. J Am Soc Nephrol 16:2150–2155
15. Nilsson SC, Kalchishkova N, Trouw LA et al (2010) Mutations in complement factor I as found in atypical hemolytic uremic syndrome lead to either altered secretion or altered function of factor I. Eur J Immunol 40:172–185

Chapter 16

C1 Inhibitor: Quantification and Purification

Lilian Varga and József Dobó

Abstract

C1 inhibitor is a multipotent serpin capable of inhibiting the classical and the lectin pathways of complement, the fibrinolytic system, and contact/kinin system of coagulation. Deficiency of C1 inhibitor manifest as hereditary angioedema (HAE), an autosomal dominant hereditary disease. Measuring the C1 inhibitor level is of vital importance for the diagnosis of HAE and also for monitoring patients receiving C1 inhibitor for therapy. Determination of the antigenic C1 inhibitor level by the radial immunodiffusion (RID) technique is described in detail in this chapter. The presented purification method of plasma C1 inhibitor is primarily based on its high carbohydrate content and its affinity to the lectin jacalin.

Key words C1 inhibitor antigen, Radial immunodiffusion (RID), Mancini technique, Quantitative determination, Jacalin–agarose, Kallikrein–kinin system, Coagulation, Classical pathway of complement, Lectin pathway of complement

1 Introduction

As suggested by the name, C1 inhibitor (C1inh) has originally been identified by its inhibitory activity toward the serine proteases present in the C1 complex [1]. Actually, C1inh is "multipotent" protein, which—by suppressing many serine proteases (C1r, C1s, MASP-1, MASP-2, factor XIIa, plasma kallikrein, factor XIa, thrombin, plasmin, tissue plasminogen activator)—has an essential role in the regulation of the plasma enzyme cascades (complement, contact, coagulation, and fibrinolytic systems), and an anti-inflammatory property mediated by its non-enzymatic interactions [2, 3]. C1inh is a highly glycated, 71.1-kDa protein consisting of a single polypeptide chain. Because of its high carbohydrate content it runs on SDS-polyacrylamide gels at an apparent molecular weight (MW) of about 105 kDa. Its mean concentration in the plasma is 200 mg/L, which may double in inflammatory conditions, because C1inh is an acute phase protein. Clinically, the heterozygous deficiency of C1inh manifests as hereditary angioedema (HAE).

Mihaela Gadjeva (ed.), *The Complement System: Methods and Protocols*, Methods in Molecular Biology, vol. 1100, DOI 10.1007/978-1-62703-724-2_16, © Springer Science+Business Media New York 2014

HAE is inherited as an autosomal dominant trait. In 85 % of patients, the amount of C1inh in the blood is as low as 10–30 % of normal (HAE type I). The remaining 15 % of the patients with HAE have antigenically normal or increased amounts of C1inh in their blood, because the mutant gene produces a non-functional protein (HAE type II). HAE is characterized by attacks of generalized, subcutaneous, or submucosal edema, resolving within several days. Edema formation in the upper airways is a life-threatening condition, which can lead to suffocation owing to the narrowing of the airway lumen. The edema of the intestinal wall causes colicky pain, potentially accompanied by diarrhea, and vomiting. Edematous swelling, involving the extremities or the face, is a nuisance that also interferes with everyday activities. All these symptoms are produced by bradykinin, which accumulates in the absence of C1inh. In addition to the hereditary forms, acquired deficiency of C1inh may also occur, either alone or accompanying other disorders. Its clinical manifestations are not different from those of the hereditary forms [4]. Supplementation with purified C1inh concentrate, extracted from the plasma of healthy blood donors has been used for the acute therapy of HAE for more than three decades. Recombinant human C1inh, obtained from the milk of transgenic rabbits, has also been introduced in the recent years. Additionally, therapeutic agents inhibiting the production, or suppressing the actions of bradykinin have been developed [5].

Measuring the serum level of C1inh is necessary for establishing the diagnosis of HAE. In this disease, the concentrations of both functional C1inh and C4 are decreased; the level of antigenic C1inh is low in type I, but can be normal or even elevated in type II [6]. Determining the C1inh serum level may prove useful also in other disorders [7, 8]. Monitoring the effects of supplementation with C1inh concentrate, which is not necessarily restricted to HAE [3], may also require measuring serum C1inh levels. Chromogenic substrate based and ELISA based commercial kits are available for determining the functional C1inh. In addition to its clinical applications, the production and quantitative determination of the C1inh protein might become necessary also in research and development. This chapter describes a well-established in-house radial immunodiffusion (RID) laboratory technique for this purpose.

Because of its therapeutic significance well-established methods exist for the purification of C1inh from human plasma. The method described in this chapter is based on the procedure described by Pilatte et al. [9] with only minor modifications. An additional anion-exchange step is added to the protocol to ensure a preparation of the highest purity for various laboratory applications, for instance as a C1inh standard for quantitative determination.

2 Materials

2.1 Materials for Quantitative Determination of Human C1inh by RID

Prepare the solutions and reagents at room temperature, with water of ultrapure quality (ASTM type 1 conductivity at 25 °C is 0.056 μS/cm). Any deviation from this practice is emphasized in the description. It is recommended to use reagents of analytical grade, or of a quality at least similar to those referred to in the examples. A preservative should not be added to the reagents or buffers, in order to avoid potential, undesirable interactions during immunodiffusion. Instead, the reagents should be prepared fresh and not be stored beyond the recommended date of expiry.

2.1.1 Agarose Gel Components

1. 0.1 M EDTA (pH = 8.6, storage time: 1 month at 4 °C): Dissolve Na_2–EDTA·$2H_2O$ (MW = 372.2). Adjust the pH of the solution to 8.6 by adding 2 M NaOH.
2. Barbital buffer (pH = 8.6, storage time: 1 day at 4 °C): 0.03 M (2.95 g) sodium-barbital (sodium 5,5-diethylbarbiturate $C_8H_{11}N_2NaO_3$ MW = 206.2), and 0.03 M (1.95 g) sodium acetate ($CH_3COONa·3H_2O$, MW = 136.08), 450 mL water, and 1 mL concentrated HCl.
3. Barbital–EDTA buffer*:* mix 450 mL barbital buffer with 50 mL 0.1 M EDTA.
4. Water bath.
5. Thermometer capable of measuring temperature from 0 to 100 °C.
6. Agarose solution*:* Dissolve 1.5 (w/v)% agarose (standard electroendosmosis agarose from SERVA) in barbital–EDTA buffer, using a boiling-water bath and then, allow to cool to 56 °C (*see* **Notes 1** and **2**).
7. Pipette or a graduated cylinder suitable for measuring 15 mL volume.
8. Anti-C1inh polyclonal antiserum to human C1inh that has been used in immunochemical techniques including RID (e.g., goat anti-human C1inh, Quidel) (*see* **Note 3**).
9. 100 × 100 mm clean, dry, non-scratched glass plate, degreased with ethanol.
10. Horizontal work surface.
11. Bevel-sharpened metal tube of 2 mm diameter.
12. Pasteur pipette with rubber bulb, for removing the gel.
13. Template for marking out the wells (A template for a 6 by 6 hole grid is appropriate for a 100 × 100 mm glass plate: the wells will be at 13-mm distance from each other, and at 17 mm from the edge of the plate).

2.1.2 Immunodiffusion Components

1. C1inh standards: A set of purified C1inh standards of known concentration, or serial dilution of pooled normal human serum (NHS) with a known C1inh concentration.
2. Low and high controls: serum samples with known, low and high C1inh concentration.
3. Humidity chamber: crafted for example from a plastic box and lid (15 × 25 × 5 cm) with several layers of wet filter paper added to its bottom; this can accommodate two 100 × 100 mm plates for incubation. In order to prevent colonization by fungi, the filter paper placed to the bottom of the humidity chamber should be wetted with purified water containing 0.01 (w/v)% sodium azide (NaN_3).

2.1.3 Washing Components

1. Washing solution (storage time after opening: 1 week at +4 °C): 0.154 M NaCl (physiological saline).
2. Washtub (a 15 × 25 × 5 cm plastic box with lid).

2.1.4 Components for Drying and Dyeing

1. Protein dye solution (storage time: 1–6 months at room temperature, depending on usage): Dissolve 2 g Amido black 10B (Merck) in a mixture of 100 mL acetic acid, 500 mL methanol, and 400 mL purified water.
2. Dye-free diluent (storage time: 1–6 months at room temperature, depending on usage): a mixture of 100 mL acetic acid, 500 mL methanol, and 400 mL purified water.
3. Filter paper.
4. Dryer, or exsiccation chamber.

2.1.5 Additional Equipment for Evaluation

1. Vernier caliper providing a precision to 0.05 mm.
2. Statistical software for calculating unknown values from the standard curve.

2.2 Materials for Purification of C1inh from Human Plasma

2.2.1 Chromatographic Resins and Equipment

1. Jacalin–agarose. Stored in a buffer containing 0.02 % NaN_3 at 4°C.
2. Phenyl Sepharose 6 Fast Flow (high sub).
3. Econo-Pac, or similar 15 mm diameter, gravity-flow column.
4. Q Sepharose High Performance (*see* **Note 4**).
5. XK16/20 (16 mm diameter) empty column (*see* **Note 4**).
6. Chromatography equipment capable of forming a linear gradient (e.g., one of the ÄKTA systems from GE Healthcare).

2.2.2 Materials and Solutions for Purification

Prepare the solutions with water of ultrapure quality. Adjust the pH at room temperature, then store as indicated.

1. Approximately 200 mL of fresh frozen, citrated, human plasma (*see* **Note 5**).

2. Polyethylene glycol, average MW = 3,350 (PEG-3350).
3. Melibiose.
4. Phosphate Buffered Saline (PBS): 150 mM NaCl, 20 mM sodium-phosphate, pH = 7.4. Make fresh every week. Store at 4 °C.
5. High-salt PBS: 500 mM NaCl, 20 mM sodium-phosphate, pH = 7.4. Make fresh every week. Store at 4 °C.
6. 500 mM EDTA pH = 8.0 stock solution: weigh out 37.2 g $Na_2EDTA \cdot 2H_2O$ (MW = 372.2), add 150 mL water, and titrate with 10 M NaOH to simultaneously dissolve the powder and adjust the pH to 8.0. Make it to a final volume of 200 mL with water. Store at room temperature.
7. 100 mM p-nitrophenyl-p′-guanido-benzoate (NPGB) stock solution: dissolve 337 mg of NPGB-hydrochloride (MW = 337) in DMF in a 10-mL final volume. Store at 4 °C for the short term (weeks), or at −20 °C for years.
8. 100 mM Pefabloc SC stock solution: dissolve 240 mg of Pefabloc SC (MW = 240) in water in a 10-mL final volume. Store at −20 °C. Stable for several months if frozen (*see* **Note 6**).
9. PBS containing 10 mM EDTA, 25 μM NPGB: make 300 mL if you start with 200 mL of plasma. Prepare it by adding the stock solutions of EDTA and NPGB to PBS, and neglect the volume increase. Add NPGB while the solution is stirred vigorously to avoid precipitation. Make fresh.
10. High-salt PBS containing 10 mM EDTA, 25 μM NPGB: make 400 mL if you start with 200 mL of plasma. Prepare as above, but with high-salt PBS.
11. High-salt PBS containing 10 mM EDTA, 25 μM NPGB, 125 mM melibiose: make 50 mL if you start with 200 mL of plasma. Dissolve melibiose in the buffer prepared in the previous step. Prepare just before use.
12. 4 M $(NH_4)_2SO_4$ solution: dissolve 132 g $(NH_4)_2SO_4$ (MW = 232) in water in a 250-mL final volume.
13. 0.4 M $(NH_4)_2SO_4$ in PBS: dilute 25 mL 4 M $(NH_4)_2SO_4$ with PBS. Adjust the final volume to 250 mL.
14. Buffer A for anion exchange chromatography: 20 mM Tris–HCl, 0.1 mM EDTA, pH = 7.5.
15. Buffer B for anion exchange chromatography: 1 M NaCl, 20 mM Tris–HCl, 0.1 mM EDTA, pH = 7.5.
16. Optional, but recommended: precast gradient SDS-polyacrylamide gels and gel running solutions.

3 Methods

3.1 Quantitative Determination of Human C1inh by RID

RID (radial immunodiffusion) is a precipitation assay where the antigens, present in the sample dispensed into a well carved into the gel, diffuse in the radial direction while undergoing progressive dilution. The antibodies, suspended homogeneously in the agarose gel, and the antigens form precipitin complexes; these are arranged in a circle, the diameter of which increases with time. However, this expansion slows down after a while, and a precipitation ring appears in the equivalence zone following a sufficiently long incubation. This ring does not expand any further and persists for months, without a change. The area enclosed by the precipitation ring upon reaching its ultimate diameter is directly proportional to the antigen concentration in the sample, and is inversely proportional to the antibody concentration in the medium [10]. The method proposed herein has been developed for measuring C1inh level in serum, primarily. It is recommended for laboratories testing a moderate number of samples per occasion. Additionally, it is a less expensive and technology-intensive method, but it does not yield instant results. RID is used extensively and its accuracy matches that of other techniques, such as nephelometry, or turbidimetry [11, 12]. The readings are highly consistent with each other, although—as it has been reported for different means of protein determinations—discrepancies occur. Higher [13–15], or lower levels [16] that are detected occasionally may be attributed to the application of different standards or method of antibody preparation [17], or the buffer used [18]. During a trial performed by the International Union of Immunological Societies Subcommittee for the Standardization and Quality Assessment of Complement Measurements in 15 complement laboratories worldwide, we found differences between values measured with various types of nephelometers, or with RID. Specifically, the concentration of the C1inh in pooled serum from HAE patients was significantly lower by the RID method, compared to nephelometry and accordingly, the same applies to C4 level (Kirschfink et al., unpublished results). In our study comparing the concentration of antigenic and functional C1inh (based on C1s:C1inh complex detection with a Quidel ELISA kit) in 64 adult HAE patients, and 64 sex- and age-matched controls, we found a significant relationship (Spearman's rho = 0.610; $p < 0.0001$) (unpublished result). Others demonstrated a correlation of similar strength between these parameters of HAE patients determined by other methods (nephelometry vs. chromogenic assay) [19]. In a study conducted on HAE patients and healthy controls, Drouet et al. [20] detected a highly significant correlation (Spearman's rho = 0.91, $p < 0.0001$) comparing RID with an enzymatic functional test. An extremely close correlation has been described between the results obtained with RID and with the functional chromogenic substrate assay for C1inh in patients with malignancies [21].

3.1.1 Gel Casting

A gel slab of 1.5 mm thickness is required. The quantity of the gel should be determined taking into account the number of the wells necessary to accommodate the test samples, standards, and controls.

1. The glass plates should be marked in advance.
2. Heat the gel over a hot-water bath until transparent (*see* **Note 7**). A single 100 × 100 mm gel slab requires 15 mL of gel, and can accommodate 36 wells.
3. Let the gel cool to 56 °C, add the antibody (e.g., 120 μL of goat anti-human C1inh, Quidel A300), mix gently, and,
4. Pour the gel onto the glass plate placed on a horizontal table (*see* **Note 8**).
5. Keep the slab at room temperature for 30 min to allow congealing (*see* **Note 9**).

3.1.2 Dispensing the Samples

1. Dilute the samples, standards, and controls in the barbital-EDTA buffer. It is expedient to test human sera at 2× dilution (*see* **Note 10**). Undiluted (1×) NHS, as well as its 2×, 4×, and 8× (etc.) dilutions are suitable as standards.
2. Punch the wells into the slab at the correct sites using the template and then, dispense 5 μL of each sample into the appropriate wells (*see* **Notes 11** and **12**). Samples should be dispensed slowly, taking care to avoid foaming and spilling.
3. Record the wells position correspondingly to all test samples, standards, controls, and the marking of the glass plate (see Fig. 2) on a data sheet (Fig. 1).
4. Incubate the slabs at room temperature for 24 h in a horizontal humidity chamber.

3.1.3 Washing

1. Incubate the slabs in 500 mL (154 mM NaCl) washing fluid.
2. Remove washing fluid after 60 min and pour fresh washing fluid onto the slabs (*see* **Note 13**).
3. Repeat **steps 1** and **2**.

3.1.4 Drying

1. The slabs should be flushed with purified water.
2. Covered with filter paper and then,
3. Dried.
4. After drying, the gel is fixed as a very thin film like layer on the glass plate (*see* **Notes 14** and **15**).

3.1.5 Dyeing

1. Following the removal of the filter paper, the dried slab should be incubated in a dyeing vessel filled with the dyeing solution, and incubated for 20 min.
2. Upon removal from the dye, the slab is drained and then, transferred into the dye-free (differentiating) solution.

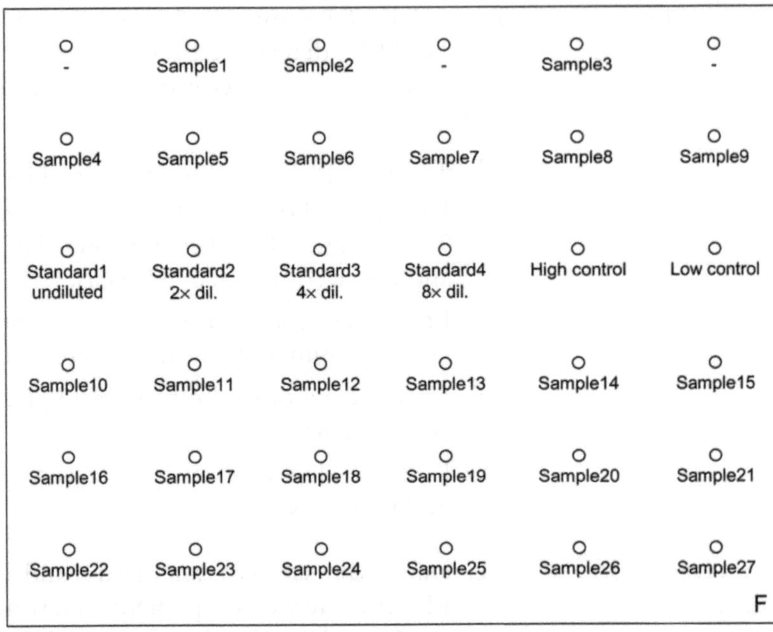

Fig. 1 A sample scheme depicting the layout of the numbered test samples, standards, and controls dispensed onto the RID plate shown in the photo displayed as Fig. 2. The scheme exhibits the actual degrees of dilution along with the identification of the glass plate (marked "F" in the right lower corner)

3. This step is then repeated with fresh dye-free solution, until the slab becomes transparent in the non-stained regions outside the precipitation rings.
4. The slabs are flushed with purified water and dried (*see* **Note 16**).

3.1.6 Reading the Results

1. Measure the diameter of the precipitation rings (example seen in Fig. 2) with a Vernier caliper.
2. Based on the linear relationship between the squares of diameters and protein concentrations, use a statistical software to determine the antigen concentrations in the samples with the help of the standard curve plotted from the diameters of standards with known C1inh content (Fig. 3). If you lack standards with known concentrations, the C1inh content of the samples may be expressed as a percentage of NHS (*see* **Notes 17–19**).

3.2 Purification of C1inh from Human Plasma

The procedure described here is based on the protocol originally generated by Pilatte et al. [9]. C1inh is a markedly hydrophilic protein with very high carbohydrate content. It binds to the lectin jacalin, which is also used to purify IgA from serum, or plasma. An initial PEG fractionation step is used to remove the interfering IgA, which is followed by jacalin–agarose affinity chromatography. The third step is hydrophobic interaction chromatography. Under the conditions applied C1inh does not bind to the Phenyl Sepharose

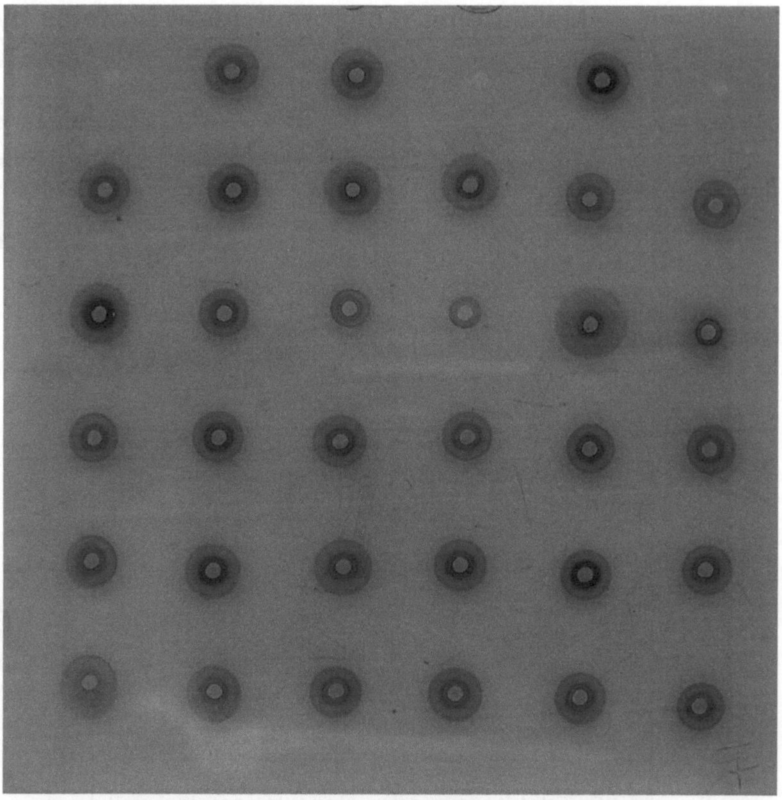

Fig. 2 Photograph of a finished gel used to measure C1-inhibitor concentration by RID. The test samples, standards, and controls are listed by location on the scheme shown in Fig. 1. See the diameters read from the gel and the calculated results on Fig. 3

resin, and essentially it is the only protein in the flow-through. A final "polishing" anion exchange step is used to remove any residual contaminating proteins and compounds in order to obtain a stable preparation [22, 23]. The procedure takes about 3 days: on the first day prepare the solutions and pack the columns, on day 2 and 3 perform the purification procedure. It is recommended to check the purity of the samples by SDS-PAGE analysis (Fig. 4a). C1inh runs at an apparent MW of 95–110 kDa depending on the gel-type used, but its actual MW is only 71.1 kDa [24].

1. Thaw a unit (~200 mL) of fresh frozen human plasma at 37 °C in a water bath. It will take about 20 min. The subsequent steps are carried out in the cold room at 2–8 °C. Amounts indicated from now on are based on a 200-mL starting volume.
2. Add protease inhibitor stocks of EDTA, NPGB, and Pefabloc SC (*see* **Note 6**) to achieve final concentrations of 10 mM, 100 μM, and 1 mM, respectively. The volume will slightly increase to ~206 mL. Add NPGB while the solution is stirred to avoid precipitation.

Measurement of complement proteins by RID

Dilution	1	2	4	8	16	32	64	128	256
standards diameter (mm*100)	755	603	506	403					
samples diameter (mm*100)		658	655		654				
	636	615	687	710	614	596			
	755	603	506	403	901	358			
	603	605	642	603	758	608			
	630	665	680	624	623	602			
	689	658	617	654	622	585			

Protein tested:	C1-Inhibitor
Sample dilution:	2
Reference reagent	
concentration:	200
unit:	mg/L

Results:

C1-inhibitor concentrations of samples : (mg/L)					
	271	268		266	
246	223	305	334	222	203
392	210	115	33	604	3
210	212	253	210	396	215
239	279	297	233	232	209
308	271	225	266	230	191

C1-inhibitor concentrations of samples: (%)					
	135	134		133	
123	111	153	167	111	101
196	105	58	17	302	1.5
105	106	126	105	198	108
120	140	148	116	116	104
154	135	113	133	115	96

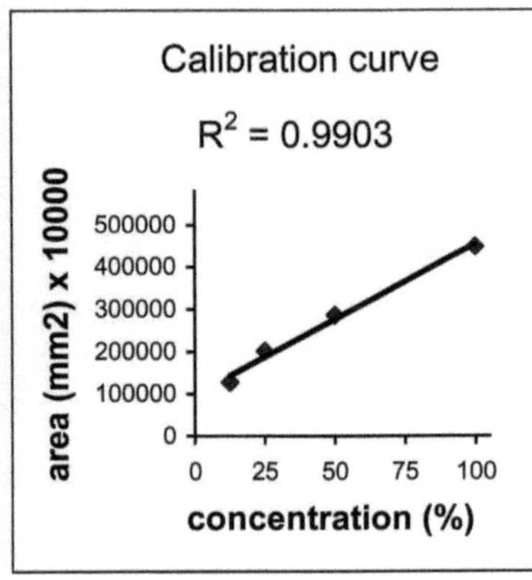

Fig. 3 Calculation of C1inh concentration in the test samples loaded onto the gel shown in Fig. 2 using Microsoft Office Excel 2003 (mancini.xls, *see* the Supplement). It should be noted, however, that any statistical software is appropriate for calculating the concentrations from the linear relationship between the squares of the precipitation rings and C1inh content. The results are expressed either as percentages of the standard, or as absolute values—when a standard of known C1inh content is used. In our example, the absolute C1inh concentration in the sample was 0.2 g/L. Calculation of C1inh concentrations by a statistical software: Undiluted (containing 200 mg/L C1inh), 2×, 4×, and 8× dilutions pooled NHS were used as standard (diameters are in the *turquoise field*). Diameters of samples and controls are input accordingly to wells arranged on the slab. Relative (given as a percent of standard) C1inh concentrates are shown in the *red field*, absolute C1inh concentrates are shown in the *green field* (Color figure online)

3. Add 44 g of solid PEG-3350 to the plasma (~206 mL) gradually while it is continuously stirred on a magnetic stirrer. Continue stirring for 45 min.
4. Remove the precipitate by centrifugation for 30 min, at 10,000 × *g*, 4 °C.

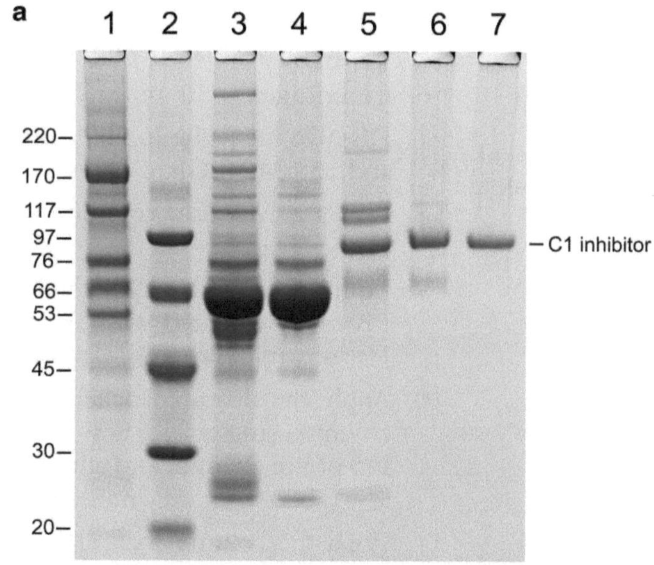

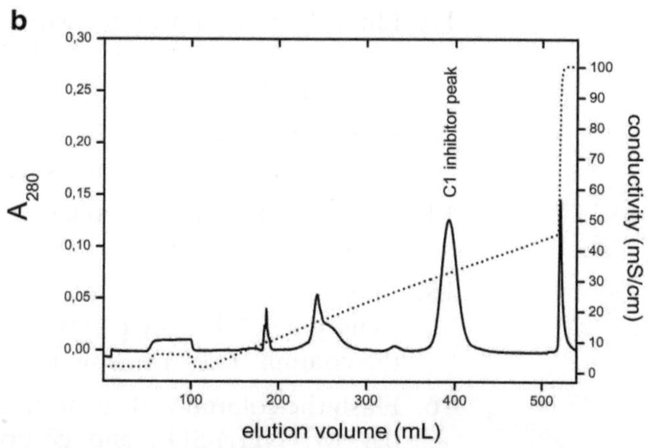

Fig. 4 Purification of C1inh from human plasma. (**a**) SDS-PAGE analysis of samples taken at different stages of the purification. *Lane 1*: High MW marker (GE Healthcare). *Lane 2*: Low MW marker (GE Healthcare). The molecular weights are indicated on the side for both markers. *Lane 3*: Human plasma sample (~10 μg of total protein). *Lane 4*: The dissolved second PEG precipitate (~7 μg of total protein). *Lane 5*: The proteins eluted from jacalin–agarose (~2 μg total protein). *Lane 6*: the flow-through of the Phenyl Sepharose column after dialysis (~1 μg C1inh). *Lane 7*: The final product after the anion-exchange step (~1 μg C1inh). A NuPAGE 4–12 % Bis–Tris gel was run under reducing conditions using NuPAGE MES running buffer (from Invitrogen). (**b**) Anion-exchange chromatography on a Q Sepharose High Performance column. After application of the sample a linear gradient of 0–400 mM NaCl was applied in 20 mM Tris–HCl, 0.1 mM EDTA, pH7.5 buffer. C1inh is found in a peak eluting at about 30 mS/cm (~300 mM NaCl). The *solid line* is the absorbance at 280 nm, the *dotted line* is the conductivity

5. Add 52 g of solid PEG-3350 gradually to the supernatant (~220 mL) while stirring. Continue stirring for 45 min.
6. Centrifuge for 30 min at 10,000 × *g*, 4 °C. Keep the pellet.
7. Dissolve the pellet in 200 mL PBS containing 10 mM EDTA and 25 μM NPGB.
8. Pack a gravity flow column (15 mm diameter) with 10 mL of jacalin–agarose.
9. Equilibrate the 10-mL jacalin–agarose column with 50 mL of PBS supplemented with 10 mM EDTA, and 25 μM NPGB. Use gravity flow.
10. Apply the dissolved pellet (~200 mL) to the jacalin–agarose column using gravity flow by pipetting 10-mL aliquots on the top of the column, and allow to drip through. The flow rate is low (about 1–2 mL/min), so be patient.
11. Wash the column with 300 mL of high-salt PBS containing 10 mM EDTA, and 25 μM NPGB.
12. Elute the bound proteins with 50 mL high-salt PBS containing 10 mM EDTA, 25 μM NPGB, and 125 mM melibiose (*see* **Note 20**).
13. Add 1/9 volume (5.5 mL–50 mL) of 4 M $(NH_4)_2SO_4$ to adjust the final concentration of $(NH_4)_2SO_4$ to approx. 0.4 M.
14. Pack a 5-mL Phenyl Sepharose column and equilibrate with 30 mL of PBS containing 0.4 M $(NH_4)_2SO_4$.
15. Apply the sample (~55 mL) to the Phenyl Sepharose column using gravity flow by pipetting 10-mL aliquots on the top of the column. Keep the flow-through.
16. Flush the column with an additional 40 mL of PBS containing 0.4 M $(NH_4)_2SO_4$, and combine it with the initial flow-through (*see* **Note 21**).
17. Dialyze the combined flow-through (~95 mL) from the Phenyl Sepharose column against 4 L of 20 mM Tris–HCl, 0.1 mM EDTA, pH = 7.5 (*see* **Note 22**).
18. Pack a 20-mL Q Sepharose High Performance XK16/20 (16 mm diameter) column (*see* **Note 4**). The last chromatographic step can be performed at room temperature.
19. Apply the dialyzed sample to the 20-mL Q Sepharose High Performance column equilibrated in the same buffer (20 mM Tris–HCl, 0.1 mM EDTA, pH = 7.5).
20. Elute C1inh using a 20-column-volume (400 mL) 0–400 mM NaCl gradient in 20 mM Tris–HCl, 0.1 mM EDTA, pH = 7.5. Collect 10 mL (= 0.5 column volume) fractions throughout the gradient. The main peak eluting at around 300 mM NaCl (~30 mS/cm) contains pure C1inh (Fig. 4b). Wash the column with 1 M NaCl in the same buffer (*see* **Note 23**).

21. Combine the fractions (30–50 mL total) containing pure C1inh and determine the concentration using the extinction coefficient $\varepsilon = 0.382$ mL/mg/cm [25]. The procedure will yield 10–15 mg of pure C1inh from 200 mL of plasma.
22. It is recommended to check the purity of the final product, and also that of the intermediate samples by SDS-PAGE analysis under reducing conditions (Fig. 4a) (*see* **Note 24**).
23. Concentrate C1inh, if required, using appropriate spin-concentrators, and store in aliquots at −20 °C or below.

4 Notes

1. After adjusting to the final volume over a hot-water bath, the gel should be filled into glass tubes, in aliquots corresponding to the volume of one gel slab (e.g., 15 mL for 100 × 100 mm gels), and stored tightly covered (to prevent exsiccation) at +4 °C for not more than 3 months.
2. When the use of a preservative is deemed necessary, 0.015 (w/v)% NaN_3 may be added to the gel. Use caution when handling this material, because its powder is highly toxic and can be absorbed through the skin. Moreover, as NaN_3 powder has explosive properties, it should be kept in a safety cabinet adapted for the storage of potentially explosive substances.
3. Before purchasing the antibody, always check whether the manufacturer recommends using the reagent for RID, as well as whether it is free from cross-reactions with other proteins present in the test sample. When introducing a new antibody, it is recommended to determine the concentration ideally suited for your needs by performing microscale titration within the recommended concentration range (such as goat anti-human C1-inhibitor from Quidel).
4. If you are inexperienced with column packing: different sizes of pre-packed columns are available, e.g., HiScreen Q Sepharose High Performance (4.7 mL), or HiLoad 16/10 Q Sepharose HP (20 mL), both from GE Healthcare. Even the smaller column has sufficient capacity to perform the last purification step described here; however, the volume of the applied gradient should be adjusted to the column size.
5. Both citrated, and EDTA plasma should work fine.
6. Pefabloc can be substituted (at the same concentration) with the much cheaper, but less water-soluble and more toxic phenyl-methyl-sulfonyl fluoride (PMSF), which is soluble in absolute ethanol, or DMF at 100 mM. Store the PMSF stock at −20 °C.
7. The gel can be heated in a microwave oven much faster than over a hot-water bath. However, caution is required, because the hot gel may boil out of the tube and cause burns.

8. The 1.5-mm thick plates of sanded edges should be handled by touching only their edges, so as not to leave fingerprints on the surface. It is recommended to wear gloves during gel casting. Do not use a waterproof marker pen, because the dye will dissolve the ink. The glass plates should be marked using a diamond scriber. Use pre-heated glassware (pipettes, graduated cylinders) for dispensing the gel. It is essential to adhere to the 53–56 °C temperature range while mixing the antibody into the gel. At lower temperatures, the gel would begin to set and interfere with the homogenous distribution of the antibody in it, whereas at higher temperatures, the antibody would undergo denaturation. Foaming should be avoided while mixing the antibody into the gel. Bubbles forming while pouring the gel may be punctured promptly, with the tip of a pipette. The pouring of the gel should be started in the middle of the plate, as by doing so, the liquid stops spreading at the edge of the plate without overflowing. Working on a horizontal surface is essential while casting the gel, as well as during the dispensing and the diffusion of the sample. The slightest deviation from horizontal distorts the precipitation ring. Therefore, you should check the horizontality of the work surface with a spirit level laid across the tabletop beforehand.
9. Once poured, the slab should be left to set over 30 min, to become suitable for punching. Alternatively, the cast may be placed into a humidity chamber at +4 °C for 10 min.
10. When testing samples with extremely low antigen concentration (such as sera from patients with type I HAE), using undiluted samples a more accurate measurement of C1inh content is possible.
11. Place an appropriate hole-grid template under the plate to assist cutting the wells at regular intervals, approx. 13 mm apart. It is important to keep a distance of at least 17 mm from the edge of the plate, as the gel slab is thinner along its edges.
12. Using a vacuum gel-puncher accelerates the process of cutting the wells. Remember to hold the puncher perpendicularly to the gel surface.
13. The removal of surplus protein is made efficient by not only replacing, but also streaming the washing fluid. A flow washer device may be used where available. As the gel can easily detach from the glass plate, the washing fluid should flow very slowly. Furthermore, do not use a washtub substantially larger than the RID plate. The washing fluid can be drained with a vacuum suction pump. Prevent the plates from sliding over each other during washing.
14. Before drying, apply the pre-wetted filter paper to the gel carefully, starting from the edge to prevent the trapping of air bubbles under the paper.

15. The gel can be dried at room temperature; however, this takes a long time (12 h). When using a dryer, avoid blowing away the covering filter paper. The latter should be removed only after the gel has dried completely, otherwise this procedure can damage the gel, which may remain wrinkled and this can interfere with interpretation.
16. Although the dye solution may be reused, once it is exhausted, the precipitation rings will stain faintly, as well as the background regions of the gel will not become transparent, but remain blotchy and granular despite soaking in differentiating solution. The dye can be removed from the differentiating solution by straining through filter paper using active carbon. This will extend its service life for the removal of excess dye.
17. The test should be repeated, if: (a) the diameters of the standard solutions are not sorted in ascending order from the lowest to the highest concentration; (b) the r^2-value is less than 0.95 for a linear standard curve.
18. The detection threshold is 3 mg/L C1inh, which is about 70 times lower than the mean concentration in NHS (200 mg/mL), and corresponds to 15 μg of total C1inh.
19. Coefficients of variation: intra-assay CV %=3.5, inter-assay CV %=4.5.
20. Regenerate the jacalin–agarose column by washing with 10 column volumes of PBS. Store in PBS containing 0.02 % NaN_3 at 4 °C.
21. Regenerate the Phenyl Sepharose column by washing with 10 column volumes of PBS. Store in 20 % ethanol at room temperature.
22. The material after the Phenyl Sepharose column is pure enough for many applications; however, an exhaustive dialysis is required to remove compounds like NPGB. Therefore we highly recommend to perform a last anion-exchange chromatographic step.
23. Store Q Sepharose High Performance in 20 % ethanol at room temperature.
24. We used precast NuPAGE 4–12 % Bis–Tris gels and NuPAGE MES running buffer (from Invitrogen) for the analysis, but other precast, or self-prepared gels should work fine.

Acknowledgements

The authors gratefully acknowledge the advice and technical help of Ms. Márta Kókai and Ms. Zsuzsa Szendrei. J. Dobó was supported by the János Bolyai Research Fellowship and OTKA grants NK77978 and NK100834.

References

1. Ratnoff OD, Lepow IH (1957) Some properties of an esterase derived from preparations of the first component of complement. J Exp Med 106:327–343
2. Zeerleder S (2011) C1-inhibitor: more than a serine protease inhibitor. Semin Thromb Hemost 37:362–374
3. Davis AE 3rd, Lu F, Mejia P (2010) C1 inhibitor, a multi-functional serine protease inhibitor. Thromb Haemost 104:886–893
4. Carugati A, Pappalardo E, Zingale LC, Cicardi M (2001) C1-inhibitor deficiency and angioedema. Mol Immunol 38:161–173
5. Tourangeau LM, Zuraw BL (2011) The new era of C1-esterase inhibitor deficiency therapy. Curr Allergy Asthma Rep 11:345–351
6. Agostoni A, Aygören-Pürsün E, Binkley KE et al (2004) Hereditary and acquired angioedema: problems and progress: proceedings of the third C1 esterase inhibitor deficiency workshop and beyond. J Allergy Clin Immunol 114(3 Suppl):S51–S131
7. Bene L, Füst G, Fekete B, Kovács A, Horváth L, Prohászka Z, Miklós K, Pálos G, Daha M, Farkas H, Varga L (2003) High normal serum levels of C3 and C1 inhibitor, two acute-phase proteins belonging to the complement system, occur more frequently in patients with Crohn's disease than ulcerative colitis. Dig Dis Sci 48:1186–1192
8. Széplaki G, Varga L, Laki J, Dósa E, Rugonfalvi-Kiss S, Madsen HO, Prohászka Z, Kocsis A, Gál P, Szabó A, Acsády G, Karádi I, Selmeci L, Garred P, Füst G, Entz L (2007) Low c1-inhibitor levels predict early restenosis after eversion carotid endarterectomy. Arterioscler Thromb Vasc Biol 27:2756–2762
9. Pilatte Y, Hammer CH, Frank MM, Fries LF (1989) A new simplified procedure for C1 inhibitor purification. A novel use for jacalin-agarose. J Immunol Methods 120:37–43
10. Mancini G, Carbonara AO, Heremans JF (1965) Immunochemical quantitation of antigens by single radial immunodiffusion. Immunochemistry 2:235–254
11. Blanchard GC, Gardner R (1980) Two nephelometric methods compared with a radial immunodiffusion method for the measurement of IgG, IgA and IgM. Clin Biochem 13:84–91
12. Davis DG, Schaefer DM, Hinchcliff KW, Wellman ML, Willet VE, Fletcher JM (2005) Measurement of serum IgG in foals by radial immunodiffusion and automated turbidimetric immunoassay. J Vet Intern Med 19:93–96
13. McCarthy RC, Fetterhoff TJ, Luckey DW (1987) Three immunoassay methods evaluated for quantifying prealbumin (transthyretin) in serum. Clin Chem 33:1430–1433
14. Bachorik PS, Cloey TA (1989) Rate immunonephelometry and radial immunodiffusion compared for apolipoproteins AI and B assay. Clin Chem 35:2236–2241
15. Cloppet H, Francina A, Coquelin H, Boucaud-Maître Y, Hutinel P, Creyssel R (1982) Laser nephelometry and radial immunodiffusion compared for immunoglobulin quantification in pathological sera. Clin Chem 28:180–182
16. Keyser JW, Fifield R, Watkins GL (1981) Standardization of immunochemical determinations of serum albumin. Clin Chem 27:736–738
17. Buffone GJ, Lewis SA (1977) Effect of analytical factors on immunochemical reference limits for complement component C3 in serum of a reference pediatric population. Clin Chem 23:994–999
18. Persson K, Kindmark CO, Pensky J, Naff G (1977) Quantitative measurement of properdin in normal human serum by electroimmunoassay and single radial immunodiffusion. Clin Exp Immunol 29:84–88
19. Cedzyński M, Madaliński K, Gregorek H, Swierzko AS, Nowicka E, Obtułowicz K, Dzierzanowska-Fangrat K, Wojda U, Rabczenko D, Kawakami M (2008) Possible disease-modifying factors: the mannan-binding lectin pathway and infections in hereditary angioedema of children and adults. Arch Immunol Ther Exp 56:69–75
20. Drouet C, Alibeu C, Ponard D, Arlaud GJ, Colomb MG (1988) A sensitive method to assay blood complement C1-inhibitor activity. Clin Chim Acta 31:121–130
21. Starcević D, Jelić-Ivanović Z, Kalimanovska V (1991) Plasma C1 inhibitor in malignant diseases: functional activity versus concentration. Ann Clin Biochem 28(Pt 6):595–598
22. Donaldson VH, Falconieri MW (1993) A modification of an affinity procedure for purification of human C1 inhibitor that provides a homogeneous stable preparation. J Immunol Methods 157:101–104
23. Beinrohr L, Murray-Rust TA, Dyksterhuis L, Závodszky P, Gál P, Pike RN, Wijeyewickrema LC (2012) Serpins and the complement system. Methods Enzymol 499:55–75
24. Perkins SJ, Smith KF, Amatayakul S, Ashford D, Rademacher TW, Dwek RA, Lachmann PJ, Harrison RA (1990) Two-domain structure of

the native and reactive centre cleaved forms of C1 inhibitor of human complement by neutron scattering. J Mol Biol 214:751–763
25. Dobó J, Major B, Kékesi KA, Szabó I, Megyeri M, Hajela K, Juhász G, Závodszky P, Gál P (2011) Cleavage of kininogen and subsequent bradykinin release by the complement component: mannose-binding lectin-associated serine protease (MASP)-1. PLoS One 6:e20036

Chapter 17

Purification, Quantification, and Functional Analysis of Complement Factor H

Bing-Bin Yu, Beryl E. Moffatt, Marina Fedorova, Claire G.S. Villiers, James N. Arnold, Eugenie Du, Astrid Swinkels, Man Chung Li, Ali Ryan, and Robert B. Sim

Abstract

Complement Factor H (FH) is an abundant, non-enzymic plasma/serum glycoprotein, which has a major role in regulating activation of the complement system. It can be purified from human plasma/serum by affinity chromatography, using a monoclonal anti-FH antibody as ligand. Other affinity chromatography ligands, including cardiolipin and trinitrophenyl-bovine serum albumin (TNP-BSA), can be used to purify human FH and also FH from a wide range of vertebrates, including mammals, birds, bony fish. Human FH protein concentration can be quantified by sandwich ELISA. The activity of FH is generally measured by assays which detect the cleavage, by complement factor I, of the complement protein C3b to form iC3b. Cleavage occurs only in the presence of a cofactor, and FH is one of a small number of cofactors for this reaction.

Key words Complement, Factor H, Factor I, Affinity chromatography, ELISA, SDS-PAGE, Proteolysis, Gel filtration, Protein G

1 Introduction

Complement Factor H is an abundant plasma and serum protein which is an importnat regulator of the activity of the complement system. It was first identified by Nilsson and Muller-Eberhard in 1965 [1], and was at that time called β1H globulin. It is a single chain glycoprotein of molecular weight about 150 kDa, which includes about 10% by weight glycan [2, 3]. It is made up of a chain of twenty small homologous domains, called CCP (complement control protein) domains, each about 60 amino acids long and containing two internal disulfide bridges. The domain type is also called a Sushi or SCR (short complement repeat) domain. The 20 domains are arranged like a string of beads, so FH is a long, flexible thread-like protein [4]. The FH gene, on human chromosome 1q32,

Mihaela Gadjeva (ed.), *The Complement System: Methods and Protocols*, Methods in Molecular Biology, vol. 1100, DOI 10.1007/978-1-62703-724-2_17, © Springer Science+Business Media New York 2014

is in a region called the RCA (regulation of complement activation) gene cluster, which contains the genes for several other complement regulatory proteins and receptors, including CR1 (CD35), CR2 (CD21), DAF (CD55), MCP (CD47), C4b-binding protein (C4bp), and five factor H-related proteins (FHRs 1–5) [5, 6]. All of these proteins are made up of CCP domains, and are homologous to FH. Several of them, especially the FHRs, may be reactive with polyclonal antisera against FH. The factor H gene has two protein products: FH, and a shorter, alternative splicing product FHL-1, (49 kDa) which consists of the first seven CCPs of FH, followed by a unique four amino acid sequence SFTL [3].

The function of FH is considered to be mainly in control of the complement alternative pathway. When C3b is formed during complement activation, it can interact with Factors B and D (FB and FD) to form the protease C3bBb (C3 convertase) which activates more C3 to form C3b. This is an amplification of C3 activation, which would eventually consume all of the C3 available. To prevent this, C3b can bind to FH instead of to FB, and the C3b in the C3bFH complex is cleaved by Factor I to form iC3b, which does not form a protease like C3bBb, and so the amplification of C3 turnover is damped down [7–9]. In this reaction FH is said to act as a cofactor for FI. The related proteins FHL-1, CR1, MCP, C4bp also have cofactor activity. The convertase C3bBb is unstable and decays (by dissociation of Bb from C3b) within minutes. FH is said to have "decay-acceleration activity," as it can displace Bb from C3b. FHL-1, CR1, DAF, C4bp also have decay-acceleration activity.

FH also binds to surfaces (e.g., wound sites, microbes) to control excessive complement activation. Many bacteria and other microorganisms have evolved surface ligands for FH, and this is assumed to protect them from complement attack [10–12]. Binding of FH to surface ligands is generally via recognition of charge clusters on the ligand: an example is the binding to the glycosaminoglycan, heparin, or to anionic phospholipid [13, 14]. The complement protein C1q also binds to charge clusters, and it is now apparent that FH and C1q compete for binding to some charge features. Since binding of C1q to charge motifs on surfaces activates the complement classical pathway, the competition for binding by FH means that FH also regulates classical pathway activation by a wide range of potential activators [14, 15].

Partial deficiencies in FH are associated with the disease atypical hemolytic uremic syndrome (aHUS) [16]. Polymorphic variation in Factor H, particularly a Tyr/His interchange at amino acid 384 of the mature protein (position 402 of the unprocessed polypeptide) is strongly associated with susceptibility to adult macular degeneration (AMD) [13, 17, 18, 19].

It is relatively easy to purify FH from human serum/plasma by affinity chromatography. For human factor H, the most convenient method is to use the anti-(human Factor H) monoclonal antibody MRCOX23 as the ligand. However, factor H from human and from other vertebrate species can be purified using a (cheap) natural ligand, anionic phospholipid (cardiolipin), or synthetic ligand (trinitrophenyl groups). FH is very stable in human plasma or serum, so outdated plasma, and plasma which has not been stored in the best conditions (e.g., multiple freeze–thaw cycles) can be used for purification. Once purified, the protein is very robust and stable, and will survive denaturation/renaturation and multiple freezing and thawing.

2 Materials

Prepare all solutions using ultrapure water and analytical grade reagents.

2.1 For Cardiolipin Chromatography

1. Cardiolipin column buffer: 10 mM potassium phosphate, 0.5 mm EDTA, pH 7.0, and the same buffer, made 0.5 M with NaCl.
2. Protein G column buffers: 10 mM HEPES, 140 mM NaCl, 0.5 mm EDTA, pH 7.0, and 0.2 M glycine, adjusted to pH 2.2 by addition of HCl.
3. Gel filtration buffer: 10 mM HEPES, 140 mM NaCl, 0.5 mm EDTA, pH 7.0.
4. Cardiolipin in ethanol solution.
5. Immobilized cardiolipin: Glass beads (acid-washed) are washed in ethanol and degassed under vacuum. Cardiolipin, 100 mg in 25 ml ethanol, is mixed with 25 g glass beads in a large glass crystallizing dish or large petri dish and left in a fume hood air current to allow the ethanol to evaporate. The beads, now coated with cardiolipin are suspended in 100 ml water, degassed and packed into a chromatography column (1.5–2 cm diam). The column is then equilibrated by passing through it 100 ml of buffer (10 mM potassium phosphate, 0.5 mm EDTA, pH 7.0). To elute proteins from the column, the same buffer, made 0.5 M with NaCl, is used (10 mM potassium phosphate, 0.5 M NaCl, 0.5 mm EDTA, pH 7.0).
6. Plasma or serum. Plasma can be anti-coagulated with EDTA, citrate or hirudin, but heparinized plasma should not be used. Plasma or serum, 5–20 ml, is dialyzed at 4 °C against 1 l of buffer (10 mM potassium phosphate, 0.5 mm EDTA, pH 7.0) for a minimum of 6 h. This causes precipitation of some proteins. Protein precipitates are removed by centrifugation for

10 min at 4 °C and 10,000 × *g*, and discarded. The plasma/serum (supernatant) should then be applied to the column immediately, as further precipitation may occur on storage.

7. Protein G: a high binding capacity immobilized protein G column is used. For washing and re-equilibration of this column (*see* **Note 2**).
8. Gel filtration/size exclusion chromatography. This is most easily done with an AKTA/FPLC system and a Superose 6 column, 1 cm diam, 30 cm length, equilibrated in 10 mM HEPES, 140 mM NaCl, 0.5 mm EDTA, pH 7.0. Other suitable gel filtration media are Sepharose 6B, Sephacryl S300, or any medium which provides separation in the range about 400–40 kDa.

2.2 For TNP-BSA Chromatography

1. TNP-BSA column buffer: Dulbecco's Phosphate-buffered saline (PBS) made by dissolving tablets in water, 1 tablet per 100 ml (*see* Subheading 2.2.3 below). 1/3 PBS is PBS diluted with two volumes of water.
2. TNP-BSA column elution buffer: PBS-0.5 mM EDTA-1 M NaCl, pH 7.4 is used.
3. Dulbecco's PBS is 2.7 mM KCl, 1.5 mM KH2PO4, 136.9 mm NaCl, 8.1 mM Na2HPO4, pH 7.4.
4. Protein G column buffers: 10 mM HEPES, 140 mM NaCl, 0.5 mm EDTA, pH 7.0, and 0.2 M glycine, adjusted to pH 2.2 by addition of HCl.
5. Gel filtration buffer: 10 mM HEPES, 140 mM NaCl, 0.5 mm EDTA, pH 7.0.
6. TNP-BSA: TNP-BSA can be made as described as follows, or can be purchased. TNP-BSA is prepared by mixing 10 ml of 1 % (w/v) BSA in PBS-0.5 mM EDTA, pH 7.4, with 2 ml of 5% (w/v) picrylsulfonic acid solution for 4 h at room temperature and pH 7.0–7.5 (maintained by monitoring pH of reaction and addition of 0.1 M NaOH), followed by dialysis against PBS-0.5 mM EDTA at 4 °C.
7. Immobilized TNP-BSA: TNP-BSA-Sepharose is prepared by mixing 100 mg TNP-BSA with 6 g cyanogen bromide-activated Sepharose 4B resin for 2 h at room temperature according to the manufacturer's instructions. Excess binding sites on the product are blocked by mixing with 100 mM ethanolamine–HCl, 150 mM NaCl, pH 8.5 at room temperature for 2 h under rotation. The TNP-BSA-Sepharose is packed into a chromatography column (1.5–2 cm diam) and equilibrated with 100 ml of 1/3 PBS-EDTA.
8. Plasma/serum: Plasma can be anti-coagulated with EDTA, citrate or hirudin, but heparinized plasma should not be used. Plasma or serum (up to 50 ml) is taken and centrifuged at

4 °C, 10,000 × *g*, 10 min to remove aggregates. The plasma/serum is then diluted with two volumes of water to reduce ionic strength. The diluted plasma/serum should then be applied to the column immediately, as protein precipitation may occur on storage.

9. Protein G: a high binding capacity immobilized protein G column (1 ml) is used. For washing and re-equilibration of this column (*see* **Note 2**).
10. Gel filtration/size exclusion chromatography. This is most easily done with an AKTA/FPLC system and a Superose 6 column, 1 cm diam, 30 cm length, equilibrated in 10 mM HEPES, 140 mM NaCl, 0.5 mm EDTA, pH 7.0. Other suitable gel filtration media are Sepharose 6B, Sephacryl S300, or any medium which provides separation in the range about 400–40 kDa.

2.3 For MRC-OX23 Chromatography

1. Sepharose-lysine column buffer: 100 mM sodium phosphate, 150 mM NaCI, 15 mM EDTA, pH 7.4, and the same buffer, made 0.5 M with 6-aminocaproic acid, pH 7.4.
2. Non-immune IgG and MRCOX23 column buffer: 25 mM Tris–HC1, 140 mM NaC1, 0.5 mM EDTA, pH 7.4.
3. Protein G column buffers: 10 mM HEPES, 140 mM NaCl, 0.5 mm EDTA, pH 7.0, and 0.2 M glycine, adjusted to pH 2.2 by addition of HCl.
4. Gel-filtration buffer: 10 mM HEPES, 140 mM NaCl, 0.5 mM EDTA, pH 7.0.
5. Chaotrope: 3 M $MgCl_2$ solution, adjusted to pH 6.8 by addition of Tris base. The pH of this solvent is adjusted to below 7 to prevent formation and precipitation of magnesium hydroxide.
6. Plasma/serum: Plasma can be anti-coagulated with EDTA, citrate or hirudin, but heparinized plasma should not be used. Plasma or serum (up to 200 ml) is taken and centrifuged at 4 °C, 10,000 × *g*, 10 min to remove aggregates.
7. Sepharose-lysine [24, 29] (*see* **Note 5**).
8. Immobilized non-immune IgG: Rabbit or human non-immune IgG can be coupled to CNBr-activated Sepharose at high density (we use about 20 mg of IgG per ml of Sepharose) as described in ref. [24]. Alternatively, the affinity materials can be purchased directly. These commercial media have a lower substitution than the 20 mg/ml mentioned above.
9. MRCOX23: The MRCOX23 hybridoma cell line is available from the European Collection of Animal Cell Cultures (ECACC) via the Health Protection Agency, UK (http://www.hpacultures.org.uk/products/celllines/hybridoma/search.jsp).

10. The purified antibody is also available commercially (e.g., AbD Serotec). We use affinity columns containing 20–50 mg of MRCOX23, coupled at about 2 mg/ml of Sepharose, to isolate batches of 10–40 mg of FH. The procedure for coupling MRCOX23 to CNBR-activated Sepharose is as follows [24]: The purified MRC OX23 (20–50 mg in 50–100 ml) is dialyzed against 2 l of 50 mM potassium phosphate, 150 mM KCl, pH 7.2–7.5, and mixed on a slow rotary stirrer (2 h, room temperature) with 10–25 ml packed volume (corresponding to about 3.5–8 g dry weight) of CNBr-activated Sepharose 4B (GE Healthcare). It is particularly important that the pH for coupling of the antibody to the resin is not greater than pH 7.5, as higher pH leads to loss of the antigen-binding capacity of the immobilized antibody. The resin is then washed with 150 ml of 2 M NaCl and mixed with 100 ml of 100 mM ethanolamine hydrochloride, 150 mM NaCl, pH 8.5, to block reactive sites. The coupling efficiency is generally 95–98 %, and about 2 mg of antibody should be bound per milliliter (packed volume) of Sepharose. The MRCOX23-Sepharose will be usable for several hundred cycles of affinity chromatography and should be stable for up to 5 years if kept refrigerated. We store it in physiological buffer with 5 mM EDTA to prevent microbial growth.

2.4 For Factor H ELISA

An ELISA can be carried out with a polyclonal or monoclonal antibody to capture FH from plasma/serum, then a polyclonal or monoclonal antibody (from a different species compared with the capture antibody) for detection, followed by a secondary antibody enzyme conjugate (*see* **Note 10**).

1. Coating buffer: 0.1 M $Na2CO_3$ (pH 9.4–9.6).
2. Washing and diluting buffer: PBS-0.1% w/v Tween20.
3. Factor H standard: if FH concentrations are to be measured in units of μg/ml, a well-characterized FH standard is required. FH can be purified as described here. Its concentration can be measured by reading OD 280, and applying an extinction coefficient calculation. However there is still uncertainty in making this calculation. The OD280 of a 1 mg/ml solution of FH was originally calculated as 1.41 [2] but this was an underestimate. A calculated extinction coefficient (E280, 1 mg/ml) is 1.81 (Protparam, Expasy database), while a new experimentally determined value is 1.96 [20].

2.5 For Factor H Functional Assay

1. Assay Buffer: 10 mM HEPES, 65 mM NaCl, pH 7.4, or similar.
2. Purified C3b or $C3(H_2O)$ at 0.5–1 mg/ml.
3. Factor I, diluted to ~ 20–50 μg/ml, prepared as described in this volume Chapter 15, or commercially available.

4. Factor H, sufficiently purified to be free of C4bp.
5. SDS-PAGE gel sample buffer: 0.2 M Tris, 2%w/v SDS, 8 M urea, pH 8.2.

3 Methods

3.1 Purification Using Immobilized Cardiolipin [22, 28] (See Note 1)

Cardiolipin is dissolved in ethanol and dried on to glass beads that are packed into a chromatography column. Plasma or serum is taken and diluted with water to reduce ionic stength, then poured through the column. Several proteins bind to the column (FH, variable amounts of IgG, IgM, IgA, beta2 glycoprotein 1, small quantity of C1q). These are eluted with high salt. IgG is removed by passage through a protein G column. FH is isolated to 95–99% purity by gel filtration on a Superose 6 column.

1. Pack glass beads (25 g, with 100 mg bound cardiolipin), (*see* Subheading 2.1.5) into a chromatography column (1.5–2 cm diam).
2. Equilibrate the column with 10 mM potassium phosphate, 0.5 mm EDTA, pH 7.0.
3. 5–20 ml of plasma or serum are dialyzed at 4°C against 10 mM potassium phosphate, 0.5 mm EDTA, pH 7.0 (*see* above, Subheading 2.1) and applied to the column of cardiolipin-glass at a flow-rate of 1–2 ml/min.
4. Wash the column extensively with the same buffer until the OD280 of the eluate falls to <0.04 AU.
5. Bound proteins are eluted as a single OD280 peak using the same buffer made 0.5 M NaCl at a flow rate of 1–2 ml/min. Fractions of the eluate are collected until its OD280 decreases to under 0.04 AU. SDS-PAGE analysis of a typical eluate is shown in Fig. 1. The eluate contains FH, IgG, IgM, traces of C1q and beta2 glycoprotein 1.
6. Remove IgG from the eluate by passage on a HiTrap protein G column (1 ml). The eluate from the cardiolipin column, in the high salt buffer can be passed directly through the protein G column at 1–2 ml/min and room temperature. IgG from most mammalian species will bind to protein G, even at high salt. For washing and re-equilibration of this column (*see* **Note 4**).
7. The run-through from the protein G column is then taken and concentrated to about 5 ml or less, to reduce the volume in preparation for gel filtration. Concentration is achieved conveniently using centrifugal filter units, with mol. wt. cutoff up to 100 kDa.
8. The sample is then subjected to gel filtration on a Superose 6 column (1 cm diam × approx 30 cm) equilibrated in 10 mM

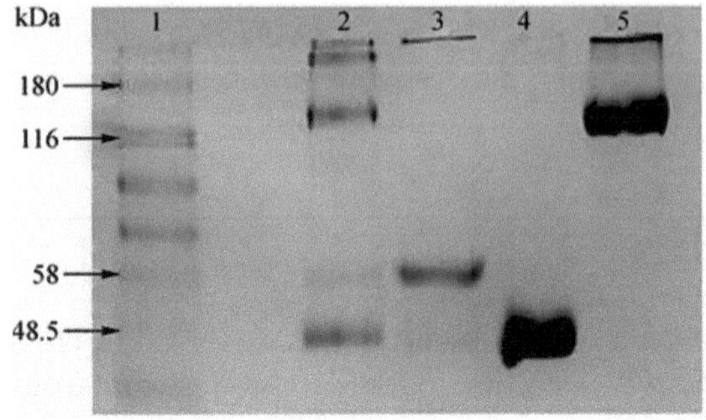

Fig. 1 Proteins which bind to Cardiolipin. Non-reduced samples. *Lane 1*, molecular weight standards; *lane 2*, proteins eluted from immobilized cardiolipin; *lane 3*, human C1q standard; *lane 4*, human beta 2 glycoprotein 1 standard; *lane 5*, human FH standard. The strong band at ~58 kDa on track 3 is the C1q A-B dimer: the faint band at about 48kDa is the C1q C-C dimer. This figure is taken from ref. [15], with permission. Factor H migrates anomalously in SDS-PAGE, generally migrating with an apparent molecular weight, versus globular protein standards, of 120,000–145,000 (unreduced) and 160,000–170,000 (reduced)

HEPES, 140 mM NaCl, 0.5 mm EDTA, pH 7.0, at room temperature with a flow rate of 0.5–1 ml/min. One ml can be loaded for each run. Large proteins, i.e., IgM and C1q, emerge close to the void volume, while FH elutes next as a symmetrical peak. Beta2 glycoprotein 1 emerges as a third peak. The FH peak is pooled, analyzed for purity by SDS-PAGE, and stored frozen at −20 °C.

3.2 Purification Using Immobilized Trinitrophenyl-Bovine Serum Albumin (TNP-BSA) [26, 27] (See Note 3)

TNP-BSA is made using BSA and picrylsulfonic acid, then immobilized on CNBr-activated Sepharose. The TNP-BSA-Sepharose is packed into a chromatography column. Plasma or serum is poured through the column. Several proteins bind (FH, variable amounts of IgG, IgM, IgA, small quantity of C1q). The binding is of very high affinity and although most of the bound protein can be eluted with high salt, complete elution requires chaotrope (3 M $MgCl_2$) or denaturant (6 M guanidine–HCl). The eluted proteins are dialysed to remove high salt or denaturant, then FH is isolated, as for the cardiolipin method, to 95–99 % purity by passage through a protein G column, then gel filtration on a Superose 6 column.

1. Plasma or serum (e.g., 20 ml) is taken and centrifuged at 4 °C, 10,000 × *g*, 10 min to remove aggregates.
2. The plasma/serum is then diluted with two volumes of water to reduce ionic strength.
3. The plasma/serum should then be applied to the column immediately, as protein precipitation may occur on storage. The diluted serum or plasma is passed at a rate of 1–2 ml/min at room temperature through a column (15 cm × 1.6 mm diam)

containing 5 ml packed volume of TNP-BSA-Sepharose equilibrated with 1/3 PBS-EDTA.

4. The column is washed with the same buffer until the OD280 of the effluent falls below 0.04 AU.
5. Bound proteins are then eluted as a single OD280 peak using PBS-0.5 mM EDTA-1 M NaCl, pH 7.4 at a flow rate of 1–2 ml/min.
6. Fractions of the eluate are collected until its OD280 decreases to under 0.04 AU.
7. SDS-PAGE analysis of a typical eluate is shown in Fig. 2. The eluate contains FH, IgG, IgM, traces of C1q.
8. IgG is removed from the eluate by passage on a HiTrap protein G column (1 ml) as described above for cardiolipin chromatography. The eluate in the high salt buffer can be passed directly through this column at 1–2 ml/min and room temperature.
9. The eluate is then taken and concentrated to about 5 ml or less, to reduce the volume in preparation for gel filtration.
10. Concentration can be achieved conveniently using centrifugal filter units, with mol. wt. cutoff up to 100 kDa.
11. The sample is then subjected to gel filtration on a Superose 6 column (1 cm diam x approx 30 cm) equilibrated in 10 mM HEPES, 140 mM NaCl, 0.5 mm EDTA, pH 7.0, at room temperature with a flow rate of 0.5–1 ml/min. One ml can be loaded for each run. Large proteins, i.e., IgM and C1q, emerge close to the void volume, while FH elutes later as a symmetrical peak. The FH peak is pooled, analyzed for purity by SDS-PAGE, and stored frozen at −20 °C.

3.3 Purification Using Immobilized MRCOX23 Monoclonal Anti-(Human FH) Antibody [23, 24] (See Note 4)

Plasma is taken and passed through a column of Sepharose-lysine. This removes plasminogen/plasmin which binds weakly to antibody columns and (plasmin) can degrade FH. The plasma is then passed through a column of Sepharose-nonimmune IgG (human or rabbit). This removes proteins which bind to IgG (e.g., C1q, some IgG, IgM (rheumatoid factor-like activity)). The plasma is then passed through a column of MRCOX23-Sepharose, which binds FH and FHL-1. Bound proteins are eluted with 3 M MgCl2, and dialysed into a physiological buffer. The eluate usually contains 95–99 % pure FH, but sometimes there is contamination with IgG or IgM (antibodies which randomly recognize MRCOX23). FHL-1 is barely detectable in outdated plasma, but if fresh plasma is used, FHL-1 may be visible by SDS-PAGE in the product. If these contaminants are present, the protein G and gel filtration steps, as described for the cardiolipin method, can be applied.

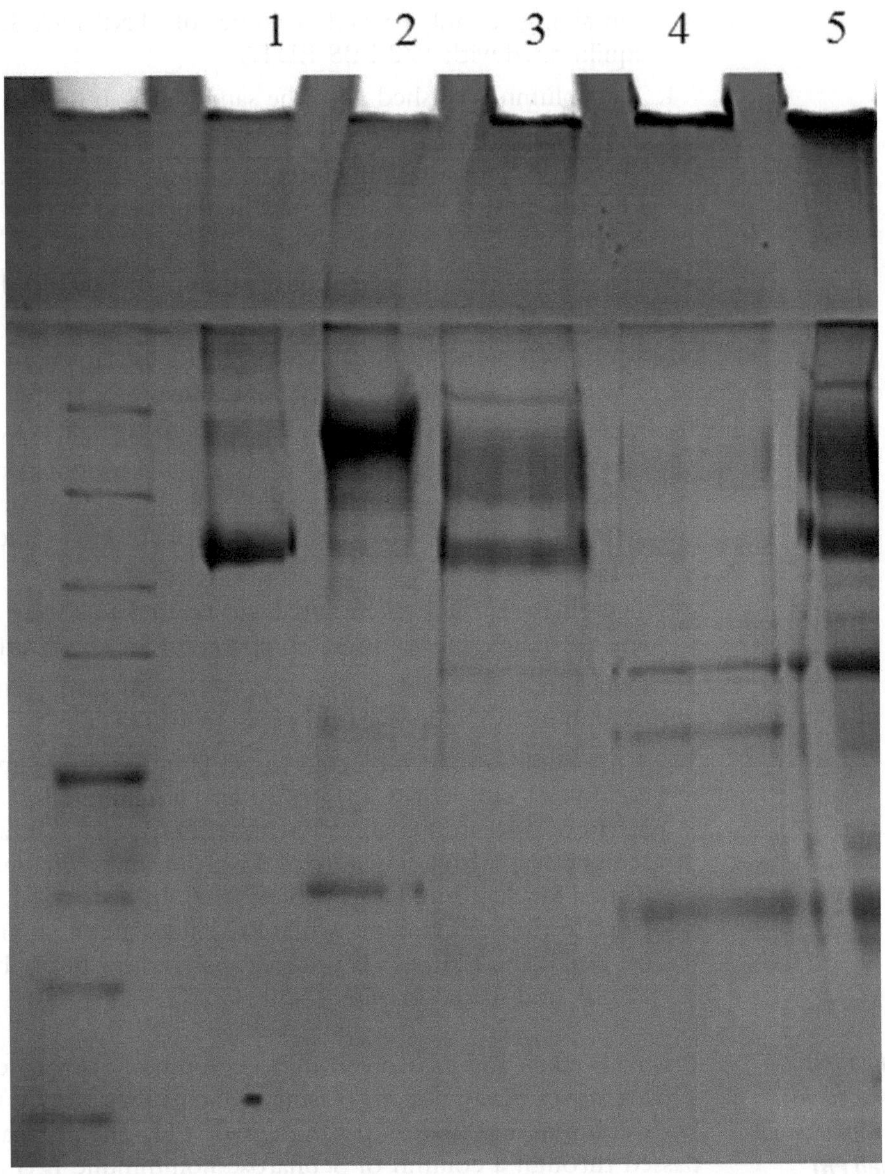

Fig. 2 Affinity chromatography on TNP-BSA-Sepharose. SDS-PAGE analysis, Coomassie Blue staining, unreduced samples. *Lane 1*, human FH standard; *2*, human IgG standard; *3*, eluate from affinity column run with horse serum; *4*, affinity resin after elution; *5*, affinity resin before elution. The staining in the wells [3–5] is mainly IgM

All procedures are carried out at 4 °C unless stated otherwise.

1. Up to 300 ml of pooled outdated human plasma (with citrate anticoagulant) or serum, made 5 mM with EDTA, is made 0.5 mM with the protease inhibitor Pefabloc-SC (4-(2-aminoethyl) benzenesulfonylfluoride) and passed through a lysine-Sepharose column (about 25 ml volume) equilibrated in 100 mM sodium phosphate, 150 mM NaCI, 15 mM EDTA, pH 7.4, to remove plasminogen/plasmin. For washing and regeneration of this column (*see* **Note 5**).

2. The eluted plasma, now diluted to a volume of about 350 ml, is again made 0.5 mM with Pefabloc-SC and dialyzed twice for 6 h against 2 l of MRCOX23 column buffer and with 0.5 mM Pefabloc-SC.
3. The guard column (non-immune IgG-Sepharose) and affinity column (MRC OX23-Sepharose, each about 18.5 × 2.0 cm diameter) are connected in series, equilibrated in the running buffer, and the plasma/serum run through at a rate of about 25 ml/h.
4. The guard column is then disconnected and the affinity column washed with 500 ml of the running buffer.
5. Factor H is eluted with 100 ml of the chaotrope, 3 M $MgCl_2$, adjusted to pH 6.8–7.0 by addition of Tris base. Factor H emerges as a single sharp peak with a trailing edge.
6. The MRC OX23 column is re-equilibrated in the running buffer and the guard column is regenerated by washing with 200 ml of 3 M $MgCl_2$, followed by re-equilibration in the running buffer.
7. Factor H eluted from the MRCOX23 column is generally >98 % pure. The material is then dialyzed against 2 l of water, to remove the $MgCl_2$, then against 2 l of 10 mM HEPES, 140 mM NaCl, 0.5 mM EDTA, pH 7.0, and the concentration adjusted, as desired, by ultrafiltration or using centrifugal filter units. Factor H is quite soluble and can readily be concentrated to 5 mg/ml or more (*see* **Notes 6–9** and **11**).

3.4 Measurement of FH in Body Fluids by ELISA [35]

The concentration of human FH in body fluids can be measured by capture or sandwich ELISA as follows. Some values for human FH concentrations in a limited number of body fluid samples are shown in Table 1. The large study described in ref. [20] finds the range of FH values in >1,500 healthy plasmas to be 63.5–847.6 μg/ml, mean 232.7 (*see* **Note 10**).

1. Microtiter plates are coated with monoclonal anti-human FH MRCOX23 (100 μl/well) at a concentration of 25 μg/ml in coating buffer.
2. Plates are left for 1 h at room temperature.
3. Plates are washed four times with PBS.
4. Plates are blocked with PBS-0.1% Tween20 (PBS-T) for 2 h at room temperature.
5. Samples of plasma or serum are assayed in doubling dilutions from 1/100 to 1/25,600 in PBS-T. Serially diluted samples (100 μl) are added to each coated well and incubated for 1 h at room temperature.
6. FH of a known concentration (diluted 1/2 to 1/512 in PBS-T, with a starting concentration of 10 μg/ml) is included as a standard and treated exactly as the plasma samples.

Table 1
Examples of Factor H concentrations in human body fluids

Body Fluid	No of samples	FH concentration (μg/ml)	
		Range and mean	
Serum	6	93–373	187.7
Synovial fluid, RA	5	28–108	62.5
Cerebrospinal fluid	5	0.32–0.63	0.45
Milk	5	0.08–0.53	0.23
Lung lavage	6	0.02–0.07	0.06
Saliva	5	0.007–0.059	0.026
Urine	5	0.0005–0.053	0.002

Healthy donors, except RA = rheumatoid arthritis

7. The wells are washed four times in PBS-T.
8. 100 μl of rabbit anti-human FH at an appropriate dilution (to be established by titration or according to suppliers instructions) in PBS-T are added to each well and incubated for 1 h at 20°C.
9. The wells are washed again with PBS-T.
10. 100 μl of goat anti-rabbit IgG alkaline phosphatase conjugate at an appropriate dilution (to be established by titration or according to suppliers instructions) in PBS-T, is added to each well.
11. The plate is incubated as before, washed again in PBS-T, and developed with buffered substrate tablets containing p-nitrophenyl phosphate.
12. The plate is read at 405 nm in a microtiter plate reader after optimum color development has occurred.

3.5 Functional Assay of FH

FH has several activities which can be measured. These include:

(1) Decay-acceleration activity, which is the capacity to inactivate the C3 convertase, C3bBb by displacing Bb from C3b. The basis for assaying this activity is presented in refs. [8] and (2) Factor I-cofactor activity, which is the capacity to form a complex with C3b, and C3b in the complex is then cleaved by Factor I to form iC3b. The basis for assaying this activity is also presented in refs. [7] and [8], and varying conditions for the assay are in refs. [25, 32, 33]. A procedure for this assay is given below. (3) Classical pathway downregulation, which can be measured by the capacity to compete with C1 or C1q for binding to targets such as cardiolipin. The basis for an assay of this type is given in refs. [14, 34]. The assay of cofactor activity (2) is the assay most frequently used for FH. This assay relies on fluid-phase incubation of C3b, factor I,

and factor H followed by analysis, by SDS-PAGE, to observe the extent of breakdown, by factor I, of the α' chain of C3b (110 kDa) to 68- and 43-kDa fragments. Often it is more convenient to use a form of C3 in which the thiolester is cleaved ($C3(H_2O)$, C3(NH3)) instead of C3b for the assay. $C3(H_2O)$ has an α chain of 118 kDa, which is cleaved to 76 kDa plus 43 kDa. This type of assay is suitable for measuring either factor I activity or the activity of cofactors, including CR1, FH, FHL-1, MCP, and C4bp.

The cleavage of $C3(H_2O)$ or C3b by FI in the presence of FH proceeds most rapidly at acid pH (~pH5) and low salt (e.g., equivalent to ~10 mM NaCl [25, 32, 33]). However, for most purposes it is preferable to perform the assay nearer to physiological conditions: pH 7.4 and half-physiological salt strength is a reasonable compromise. Since the rate of reaction is very sensitive to pH and salt strength, proteins should all be equilibrated in the same buffer before use. FH in serum/plasma cannot be assayed by this method, as C4bp in serum/plasma contributes to the activity.

1. Assemble reaction by mixing the following reagents in the order listed: 5 μg C3b or $C3(H_2O)$, Factor I, 0.1 μg, Factor H, 0.1–1 μg, and buffer to a final volume of 20 μl. Control reactions with no FH or FI should be included.
2. Incubate samples at 37 °C for different times (0, 5, 10, 20, 40, 80, 160, 320 min) and stop reaction at the appropriate time by addition of 20 μl of SDS-PAGE gel sample buffer.
3. Samples are reduced by addition of 5 μl of 0.1 M dithiothreitol in SDS-PAGE sample buffer, incubated at 95 °C for 2 min, and analyzed by SDS-PAGE followed by Coomassie Blue staining.

An example of part of such an assay (with $C3(H_2O)$) is shown in Fig. 3. During the reaction, the C3 (H_2O) alpha chain (118 kDa) is cleaved to form two fragments, 43 kDa (via an intermediate 46 kDa) and 76 kDa. The rate of cleavage is proportional to the FH activity. Rate of cleavage can be calculated by scanning the gel (densitometry) and calculating the rate of loss of alpha chain, or rate of appearance of 43 kDa chain.

No cleavage of $C3(H_2O)$ should occur in the controls without FH or without FI. If cleavage does occur in these controls, it indicates cross-contamination of the proteins.

After the first assay, the time-course can be adjusted according to the observed speed of the reaction.

4 Notes

1. The cardiolipin method is suitable only for relatively small scale purification from 20 ml plasma or less. It has been applied to the purification of FH from human, mouse, rat, horse, sheep, cattle, chicken, turkey (unpublished), and carp [14]. Protein G may not

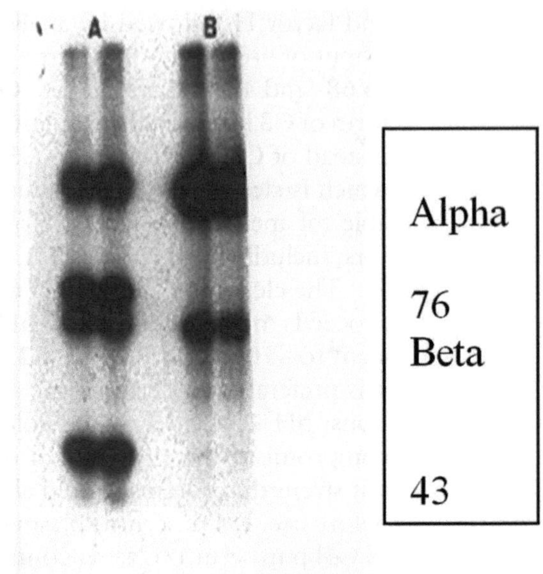

Fig. 3 Assay of Factor H activity. C3(H_2O) is shown in duplicate *tracks B*, and consists of an alpha chain and beta chain. After incubation with Factors H and I, the alpha chain is cleaved (in this case, partially) to two fragments of 76 and 43 kDa (*Tracks A*)

successfully remove IgG from all species. The glass beads can be cleaned and regenerated by washing in ethanol. We originally used porous glass beads (Waters, Corning). These have high surface area but are expensive.

2. Washing and equilibration of the Hi-trap protein G column. This column can be run manually, using, for example, a 10 ml syringe, or can be linked to an AKTA or FPLC instrument. The column is equilibrated by washing with 10 ml 10 mM HEPES, 140 mM NaCl, 0.5 mm EDTA, pH 7.0. After use, bound IgG is eluted with 10 ml of 0.2 M glycine–HCl, pH 2.2, followed by re-equilibration in the HEPES buffer.
3. The TNP method has so far only been tested by us on a relatively small scale (up to 50 ml plasma) to purify human, rat, horse (unpublished) and goat [27] FH. FH from the following additional species has been shown to bind to TNP-BSA-Sepharose, but the subsequent purification steps have not been done: ostrich, chicken, pig, dog, sperm whale, mouse, sheep, rabbit.
4. MRCOX23 when immobilized at pH 7.2–7.4 on Sepharose will bind 1 FH molecule per MRCOX23, so that, e.g., 20 mg of MRCOX23 will bind about 20 mg of FH. A 10 ml affinity column, with 20 mg of immobilized MRCOX23, is suitable for purifying FH from about 100 ml human plasma. This method is suitable only for human FH and for FH from primates in which the MRCOX23 epitope is conserved (rhesus monkey,

cynomolgus monkey, and African green monkey FH have the MRCOX23 epitope) [23].

5. Sepharose-lysine can be purchased or made as in [24, 29]. Washing and equilibration of the Sepharose-lysine column. This column is run at high salt strength to avoid nonspecific binding. The column is equilibrated with 50 ml of 100 mM sodium phosphate, 150 mM NaCI, 15 mM EDTA, pH 7.4, After running plasma/serum through it, the column is washed with 200 ml of the same buffer, then bound plasminogen/plasmin is eluted with 200 ml of 100 mM sodium phosphate, 150 mM NaCI, 0.5 M 6-aminocaproic acid, 15 mM EDTA, pH 7.4, and finally re-equilibrated with 50 ml 100 mM sodium phosphate, 150 mM NaCI, 15 mM EDTA, pH 7.4.

6. Note that $MgCl_2$ is incompatible with SDS-PAGE, so it must be removed before analysis. Care must be taken not to mix $MgCl_2$ with phosphate buffers, or expose it to alkaline buffers, to prevent precipitation of magnesium phosphates or hydroxide.

7. Contamination of the purified factor H with human IgG/IgM is observed infrequently. This arises from immunoglobulins in a few blood donors which recognize the MRCOX23 antibody. FHL-1 may also be visible in the final FH preparation. If either is present they can be separated from FH by protein G chromatography and gel filtration, as described for the cardiolipin and TNP purification methods.

8. Elution of bound protein with 3 M $MgCl_2$ is more efficient, and preserves the binding capacity of the columns for much longer than do the acid or alkaline elution techniques often used with antibody columns.

9. Factor H undergoes gradual cleavage of the single 155-kDa polypeptide chain into a form with two disulfide-linked chains (approximately 38 and 120 kDa, visible on reducing SDS-PAGE) on storage in plasma, probably by the action of plasmin or thrombin [2]. The cleavage is within the sixth CCP domain. This form has slightly modified activity [30]. If cleaved FH is observed after purification, the use of Pefabloc SC during storage of the plasma/serum is suggested.

10. We use a mouse monoclonal antibody for capture (MRCOX23) and an in-house rabbit polyclonal for detection. Polyclonal antibodies against human FH are quite widely available (e.g., sheep (The Binding Site); goat (Comptech or Sigma-Aldrich)). Several monoclonal antibodies are commercially available (e.g., AdB Serotec). Biocompare http://www.biocompare.com lists ELISA kits to measure FH from several different species, including rat, mouse, guinea pig, rabbit, and human. Hycult Biotech also lists an ELISA kit for human FH. Other antibody based assays for human FH are available, e.g., a single radial immunodiffusion kit

(The Binding Site) and an assay, suitable for multiple sample clinical laboratory use, based on nephelometry using reagents from The Binding Site [20].

11. FH binds some other ligands in addition to complement proteins C3b and Factor I. Factor H is a high avidity zinc ion-binding protein. In plasma, it is second only to alpha-2 macroglobulin as a Zn^{++} binder. The physiological significance of this is not known. In practical terms, FH can be concentrated easily by precipitation by Zn^{++} ions, or purified from minor contaminants. FH in a nonchelating buffer at physiological salt strength and pH 7.0–8.0, is made 1 mM with $ZnCI_2$. FH precipitation occurs over a period of 24 h at 4 °C. The precipitate is harvested by centrifugation at $10,000 \times g$ for 10 min, and redissolves readily in a physiological buffer containing 5 mM EDTA, at pH 7.0–8.0 [21, 31]. FH is also known as adrenomedullin binding protein 1 (AMBP-1) and there are many published papers in which FH is referred to (only) as AMBP-1.

References

1. Nilsson UR, Mueller-Eberhard HJ (1965) Isolation of beta If-globulin from human serum and its characterization as the fifth component of complement. J Exp Med 122:277–298
2. Sim RB, DiScipio RG (1982) Purification and structural studies on the complement-system control protein beta 1H (Factor H). Biochem J 205:285–293
3. Ripoche J, Day AJ, Harris TJ, Sim RB (1988) The complete amino acid sequence of human complement factor H. Biochem J 249:93–602
4. Aslam M, Perkins SJ (2001) Folded-back solution structure of monomeric factor H of human complement by synchrotron X-ray and neutron scattering, analytical ultracentrifugation and constrained molecular modelling. J Mol Biol 309:1117–1138
5. Hourcade D, Holers VM, Atkinson JP (1989) The regulators of complement activation (RCA) gene cluster. Adv Immunol 45:381–416
6. Jozsi M, Zipfel PF (2008) Factor H family proteins and human diseases. Trends Immunol 29:380–387
7. Whaley K, Ruddy S (1976) Modulation of C3b hemolytic activity by a plasma protein distinct from C3b inactivator. Science 193:1011–1013
8. Weiler JM, Daha MR, Austen KF, Fearon DT (1976) Control of the amplification convertase of complement by the plasma protein beta1H. Proc Natl Acad Sci U S A 73:3268–3272
9. Carreno MP, Labarre D, Maillet F, Jozefowicz M, Kazatchkine MD (1989) Regulation of the human alternative complement pathway: formation of a ternary complex between factor H, surface-bound C3b and chemical groups on nonactivating surfaces. Eur J Immunol 19: 2145–2150
10. Carroll MV, Lack N, Sim E, Krarup A, Sim RB (2009) Multiple routes of complement activation by Mycobacterium bovis BCG. Mol Immunol 46:3367–3378
11. Diaz A, Ferreira A, Sim RB (1997) Complement evasion by Echinococcus granulosus: sequestration of host factor H in the hydatid cyst wall. J Immunol 158:3779–3786
12. Schneider MC, Prosser BE, Caesar JJ, Kugelberg E, Li S, Zhang Q, Quoraishi S, Lovett JE, Deane JE, Sim RB, Roversi P, Johnson S, Tang CM, Lea SM (2009) Neisseria meningitidis recruits factor H using protein mimicry of host carbohydrates. Nature 458: 890–893
13. Clark SJ, Higman VA, Mulloy B, Perkins SJ, Lea SM, Sim RB, Day AJ (2006) His-384 allotypic variant of factor H associated with age-related macular degeneration has different heparin binding properties from the non-disease-associated form. J Biol Chem 281: 24713–24720
14. Tan LA, Yu B, Sim FC, Kishore U, Sim RB (2010) Complement activation by phospholipids: the interplay of factor H and C1q. Protein Cell 1:1033–1049
15. Kishore U, Sim RB (2012) Factor H as a regulator of the classical pathway activation. Immunobiology 217:162–168
16. Atkinson JP, Goodship TH (2007) Complement factor H and the hemolytic uremic syndrome. J Exp Med 204:1245–1248

17. Klein RJ, Zeiss C, Chew EY, Tsai JY, Sackler RS, Haynes C, Henning AK, SanGiovanni JP, Mane SM, Mayne ST, Bracken MB, Ferris FL, Ott J, Barnstable C, Hoh J (2005) Complement factor H polymorphism in age-related macular degeneration. Science 308:385–389
18. Day AJ, Willis AC, Ripoche J, Sim RB (1988) Sequence polymorphism of human complement factor H. Immunogenetics 27:211–214
19. Clark SJ, Perveen R, Hakobyan S, Morgan BP, Sim RB, Bishop PN, Day AJ (2010) Impaired binding of the age-related macular degeneration-associated complement factor H 402H allotype to Bruch's membrane in human retina. J Biol Chem 285:30192–30202
20. Sofat R, Mangione PP, Gallimore JR, Hakobyan S, Hughes TR, Shah T, Goodship T, D'Aiuto F, Langenberg C, Wareham N, Morgan BP, Pepys MB, Hingorani AD (2013) Distribution and determinants of circulating complement factor H concentration determined by a high-throughput immunonephelometric assay. J Immunol Methods 390 (1–2):63–73
21. Sim RB, Malhotra V, Ripoche J, Day AJ, Micklem KJ, Sim E (1986) Complement receptors and related complement control proteins. Biochem Soc Symp 51:83–96
22. Kertesz Z, Yu BB, Steinkasserer A, Haupt H, Benham A, Sim RB (1995) Characterization of binding of human beta 2-glycoprotein I to cardiolipin. Biochem J 310(Pt 1):315–321
23. Sim E, Palmer MS, Puklavec M, Sim RB (1983) Monoclonal antibodies against the complement control protein factor H (beta 1 H). Biosci Rep 3:1119–1131
24. Sim RB, Day AJ, Moffatt BE, Fontaine M (1993) Complement factor I and cofactors in control of complement system convertase enzymes. Methods Enzymol 223:13–35
25. Sim E, Sim RB (1983) Enzymic assay of C3b receptor on intact cells and solubilized cells. Biochem J 210:567–576
26. Arnold JN, Wormald MR, Suter DM, Radcliffe CM, Harvey DJ, Dwek RA, Rudd PM, Sim RB (2005) Human serum IgM glycosylation: identification of glycoforms that can bind to mannan-binding lectin. J Biol Chem 280: 29080–29087
27. Moreno-Indias I, Dodds AW, Arguello A, Castro N, Sim RB (2012) The complement system of the goat: haemolytic assays and isolation of major proteins. BMC Vet Res 26(8):91
28. Moffat BE, Willis AC, Sim RB, Smith S (2001) Complement regulatory protein Factor H in shark and carp. FASEB J 15(4):A686
29. Deutsch DG, Mertz ET (1970) Plasminogen: purification from human plasma by affinity chromatography. Science 170:1095–1096
30. Alsenz J, Schulz TF, Lambris JD, Sim RB, Dierich MP (1985) Structural and functional analysis of the complement component factor H with the use of different enzymes and monoclonal antibodies to factor H. Biochem J 232: 841–850
31. Nan R, Farabella I, Schumacher FF, Miller A, Gor J, Martin AC, Jones DT, Lengyel I, Perkins SJ (2011) Zinc binding to the Tyr402 and His402 allotypes of complement factor H: possible implications for age-related macular degeneration. J Mol Biol 408:714–735
32. Sim E, Wood AB, Hsiung L-M, Sim RB (1981) Pattern of degradation of human complement fragment C3b. FEBS Lett 132: 55–60
33. Sim E, Sim RB (1983) Enzymic assay of C3b receptor on intact cells and solubilized cells Biochem J 210:567–576
34. Tan LA, Yang AC, Kishore U, Sim RB (2011) Interactions of complement proteins C1q and factor H with lipid A and Escherichia coli: further evidence that factor H regulates the classical complement pathway. Protein Cell 2:320–332
35. Schneider MC, Exley RM, Chan H, Feavers I, Kang YH, Sim RB, Tang CM (2006) Functional significance of factor H binding to Neisseria meningitidis. J Immunol 176: 7566–7575

Chapter 18

Factor H-Related Proteins

Mihály Józsi and Seppo Meri

Abstract

Factor H-related proteins (CFHRs) are plasma glycoproteins related in structure and antigenicity to each other and to the complement inhibitory protein factor H. Such proteins are found in most mammals but their number and domain composition vary. This chapter summarizes our current knowledge on the human factor H-related proteins. In contrast to factor H, they have no strong complement inhibitory activity, although for some of them regulatory or complement modulatory activity has been reported. A common feature of CFHRs is that they bind to the C3b component of complement. Novel links between CFHRs and various diseases (C3 glomerulopathies, atypical hemolytic uremic syndrome and age-related macular degeneration) have been revealed in recent years, but we are still far from understanding their biological function.

Key words Complement, Factor H protein family, Short consensus repeat, Glomerulonephritis, Atypical hemolytic uremic syndrome, Age-related macular degeneration

1 Introduction

The human factor H protein family includes the alternative pathway regulator factor H, its splice variant factor H-like protein 1 (CFHL1), and five factor H-related proteins (CFHRs) [1]. The genes of these proteins have appeared through several gene duplication events. These genes are located in a tandem arrangement in chromosome 1 (1q32) in the so-called regulators of complement activation (RCA) gene cluster (Fig. 1). While factor H and factor H-like protein 1 are regulators of the alternative pathway, the CFHR proteins mostly lack this kind of activity. However, some of them have some complement regulatory activity and/or modulate that of factor H.

The gene cluster including the *CFH* gene and the five *CFHR* genes is prone to genomic rearrangements due to sequence duplications and homologous sequences. The *CFHR1* and *CFHR3* genes are particularly often affected [2, 3]. The combined *CFHR1/ CFHR3* deletion is relatively common and is linked to anti-factor H autoantibody-mediated atypical hemolytic uremic syndrome

Mihaela Gadjeva (ed.), *The Complement System: Methods and Protocols*, Methods in Molecular Biology, vol. 1100, DOI 10.1007/978-1-62703-724-2_18, © Springer Science+Business Media New York 2014

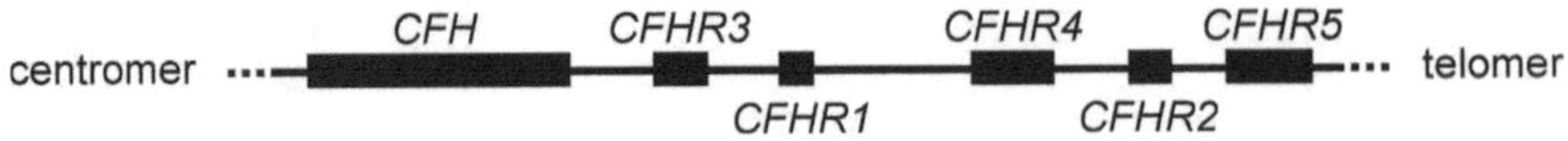

Fig. 1 Schematic overview of the factor H gene cluster. The five *CFHR* genes are found in a centromer-to-telomer tandem arrangement on the long arm of chromosome 1. There is a high sequence similarity between the *CFH* and *CFHR* genes due to several genomic duplications. *CFHR3* in particular is similar to *CFHR4*, and *CFHR1* is similar to *CFHR2*. Because of the sequence homologies, genomic rearrangements are frequent in this chromosomal region, most often causing deletions of *CFHR3/CFHR1* and *CFHR1/CFHR4* via nonallelic homologous recombination

(aHUS) [4]. They are also involved in hybrid gene formation with *CFH* in aHUS [5, 6].

The links of factor H and CFHRs to aHUS, age-related macular degeneration (AMD) and certain types of glomerulonephritis have raised considerable interest in these proteins [7]. However, little is known about their function to date. In this chapter, we provide a brief overview of the factor H-related proteins and cover recent developments in identifying novel ligands and functions among these closely related proteins.

2 Common/General Features of Human Factor H-Related Proteins

The CFHR proteins are composed of four to nine short consensus repeat (SCR) domains (also known as Sushi domains or complement control protein, CCP domains). They show various degree of sequence identity with SCRs of factor H (Fig. 2). Among themselves, CFHR1 is closely related to CFHR2 and CFHR3 is closely related to CFHR4. This is because of the genomic duplications that gave rise to these proteins.

The CFHR proteins lack SCRs related to the factor H domains that mediate complement inhibiting cofactor and decay accelerating activities (SCRs 1–4). Therefore, the CFHR proteins have been largely ignored as being smaller variants of factor H without complement regulatory role.

It is striking that all five *CFHR* genes have retained exons that encode for SCRs homologous to SCRs 19–20 of factor H. This is likely the basis for the reported interactions of CFHR1, CFHR3, CFHR4, and CFHR5 with C3b (Table 1). Association with lipoprotein particles has been observed for CFHR1, CFHR2, CFHR4, and CFHR5, but the relevance of this has remained unclear.

3 Factor H-Related Protein 1

CFHR1 is composed of five SCRs that are homologous to SCRs 6–7 and SCRs 18–20 of factor H. The sequence identity of SCRs 1–2 to SCRs 6–7 of factor H is rather low, but these CFHR1 domains are closely related to SCRs 1–2 of CFHR2 and CFHR5

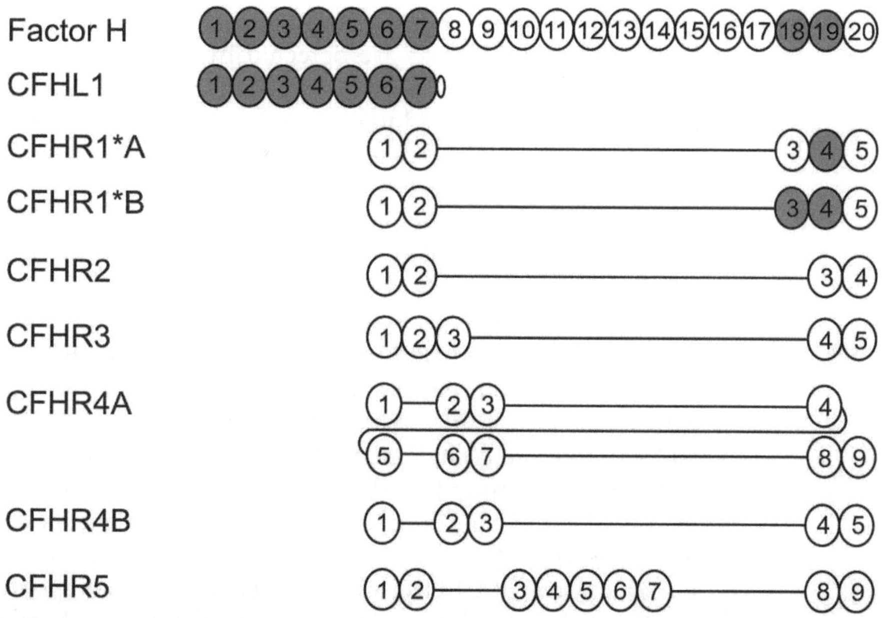

Fig. 2 The human factor H protein family. The schematic figure shows the members of the human factor H protein family with their SCR domains aligned based on amino acid sequence similarity to SCRs in factor H. SCRs 1-7 of CFHL1 is identical with those of factor H (shown by *shading*) and has a four amino acid long unique C-terminal end. The two CFHR1 isoforms differ in their sequence from each other in SCR3. SCR3 of CFHR1*B and SCR4 of both CFHR1 isoforms are identical with SCR18 and SCR19 of factor H, respectively (shown by *shading*). Note that SCRs 1-2 of CFHR1, CFHR2, and CFHR5 are closely related to each other and only distantly related to domains in factor H

Table 1
Known major ligands and related proposed functions of the CFHR proteins

Protein	Ligand	Proposed function	References
CFHR1	C3b	?	[15]
	C5	Inhibition of the alternative pathway C5 convertase	[15]
CFHR3	C3b	Enhancement of the cofactor activity of factor H, cofactor activity	[16, 32, 33]
CFHR4	C3b	Enhancement of the cofactor activity of factor H, enhancement of opsonization	[32, 33, 37]
	CRP	Enhancement of opsonization	[38, 39]
CFHR5	C3b	Cofactor activity, decay accelerating activity	[41, 42]
	CRP	?	[42]

(*see* **Note 1**). The plasma concentration of CFHR1 has been estimated as 50–100 μg/ml [8–10]. It is thus the most abundant of the CFHR proteins. A fraction of CFHR1 is associated with plasma lipoproteins [11].

Various isoforms of CFHR1 have been described. Two CFHR1 bands (37 and 43 kDa) are detected by Western blot in plasma. They represent differentially glycosylated isoforms termed CFHR1α and CFHR1β [9]. In addition, two isoforms are known based on sequence differences. These have recently been analyzed in more detail [8, 12]. The CFHR1*A (acidic) isoform differs in three amino acids in SCR3 from SCR18 of factor H, whereas SCR3 of the CFHR1*B (basic) isoform is identical with SCR18 of factor H (Fig. 2). SCR4 of both isoforms is identical with SCR19 of factor H, and SCR5 differs in two amino acids from SCR20 of factor H. Because the CFHR1*B isoform was found to be associated with aHUS, it has been speculated that it may more efficiently compete with factor H, causing reduced factor H binding to C3b and cells and thus reduced complement regulatory activity [12]. On the other hand, a recent study found that the *CFHR1*A* allele is associated with AMD [13]. The functional effects of these sequence differences in the CFHR1 alleles remain unclear. They may affect different functional activities of CFHR1 or that of factor H via competition.

A further intriguing disparity is that the lack of CFHR1 (most often due to the combined deletion of the *CFHR3* and *CFHR1* genes) is protective against AMD but predisposes to aHUS. In aHUS, this is mainly due to the association of *CFHR1* deletion with the presence of anti-factor H autoantibodies [4, 14].

The three C-terminal domains of CFHR1 are very similar to those of factor H. Consequently, similar C3b and cell glycosaminoglycan binding properties for CFHR1 and factor H and a competition between the two proteins are very likely [7, 15, 16]. CFHR1 has indeed been reported to bind to endothelial cells via its C-terminal domains [15, 17]. Reports, however, are contradicting regarding the interaction of CFHR1 with C3b. The two amino acid differences between SCR5 of CFHR1 and SCR20 of factor H may lead to somewhat different binding affinities. Two studies reported reduced binding to C3b by CFHR1 and by factor H having a CFHR1-like C-terminus due to gene conversion [15, 18]. Deletion of a large chromosomal region results in a hybrid CFH::CFHR1 protein where the two C-terminal SCRs of factor H are replaced with the SCRs 4–5 of CFHR1 [5]. The S1191L/V1197A factor H mutant is associated with aHUS. Three other studies found no significant impairment in C3b binding by these mutations (i.e., by a CFHR1-like factor H SCR19–20) [19–21], but the double-mutant showed functional impairment in protection against complement-mediated lysis [18, 21]. Moreover, in hemolysis assays no significant competition with factor H at physiologic CFHR1 concentrations has been found [17].

Whereas CFHR1 lacks complement regulatory activity at the level of C3b and the C3 convertase [9], it has been described as an inhibitor of C5 convertases and of the terminal pathway [15].

On the other hand, recent reports indicated that CFHR1 bound to the surface of *Borrelia spp.* did not confer sufficient protection from complement [22, 23]. CFHR1 also binds to other pathogens such as *Candida albicans* [24], *Aspergillus fumigatus* [25], and *Leptospira interrogans* [26], but no functional activity of it has been demonstrated yet. In addition, competition between CFHR1 and factor H for microbial ligands has been reported [27, 28]. Therefore, further studies are necessary to clarify the potential role of CFHR1 in complement regulation under physiological conditions and in the complement evasion of microbes.

Recently, it has been found that CFHR1, similar to factor H, binds to complement receptor type 3 (CR3) on human neutrophilic granulocytes and facilitates the adhesive, phagocytic, and antifungal responses of these innate immune cells [24].

Altogether, these data indicate partly similar, partly different functions of CFHR1 compared with factor H.

4 Factor H-Related Protein 2

CFHR2 is composed of four SCRs homologous to SCRs 6–7 and SCRs 19–20 of factor H. The serum concentration of CFHR2 is relatively low (<50 μg/ml, not determined exactly yet). Two isoforms, the nonglycosylated CFHR2 (24 kDa) and the glycosylated CFHR2α (29 kDa) have been described [29]. CFHR2 is associated with lipoproteins [11]. Functional analysis of this protein has not yet been published, only its binding to *Borrelia* spp. has been observed [22, 23, 30]. The latter activity, however, conferred no protection to these bacteria from complement-mediated lysis, indicating no potent inhibitory role of CFHR2 in the complement system.

5 Factor H-Related Protein 3

CFHR3 is composed of five SCRs related to SCRs 6–8 and 19–20 of factor H. CFHR3 is detected in western blot as several bands in plasma, probably representing different glycosylation forms [31]. The plasma concentration was reported to be 50–80 μg/ml [16]. This appears quite high and needs to be confirmed.

CFHR3 binds to C3b and C3d through its SCRs 4–5 [32, 33]. Competition between CFHR3 and factor H for binding to surface-bound C3b has been described [16]. There are two contrasting reports on the functional activity of CFHR3. One described no cofactor activity [32], whereas another one showed significant cofactor activity for CFHR3 [16]. Additionally, CFHR3 has been shown to enhance the cofactor activity of factor H [32]. CFHR3 binds heparin and to the M protein of group A streptococci [32, 34]. This is due to the SCR2 domain related to SCR7 of factor H. The functional relevance of these interactions is unclear. Altogether, the functional role of CFHR3 in vivo is yet unknown.

6 Factor H-Related Protein 4

Two isoforms of CFHR4 have been described. Both contain domains related to SCRs 6, 8, 9, 19, and 20 of factor H (Fig. 2). CFHR4A is composed of 9 SCRs and is detected as an 86 kDa glycoprotein in human plasma [35]. The CFHR4B isoform is composed of 5 SCRs and can be detected as a ~42–45-kDa plasma glycoprotein [36]. The five domains of CFHR4B essentially correspond to SCRs 1 and 6–9 of CFHR4A. SCRs 1–4 and 5–8 represent internally duplicated domains in CFHR4A. The plasma concentration of CFHR4 has been recently measured using a commercially available anti-CFHR4 monoclonal antibody and a CFHR4 rabbit antiserum, both of which recognize the two CFHR4 isoforms. The mean CFHR4 plasma concentration is ~25 μg/ml [37]. CFHR4 is associated with plasma lipoproteins, mainly with chylomicrons, LDL and VLDL. The relevance of this lipoprotein association is, however, unknown [36].

Both CFHR4 isoforms bind to necrotic cells and to native pentameric C-reactive protein [38]. C-reactive protein binding has been shown to be mediated via SCR1 of CFHR4A and CFHR4B and lead to activation of C4-dependent complement pathways [39]. Thus, CFHR4 may enhance opsonization by this interaction.

CFHR4B was shown to bind C3b via SCRs 4–5 [32, 33]. CFHR4 may bind to surfaces such as opsonized microbes via deposited C3b [32]. The interaction of CFHR4 with surface-bound C3b is, however, rather weak [37]. CFHR4 has no potent complement inhibitory activity although it can enhance the cofactor activity of factor H in vitro when added in excess, in non-physiological high concentrations [32, 37]. Recently, CFHR4-bound C3b has been found to form an active alternative pathway C3 convertase (CFHR4-C3bBb) that is less efficiently regulated by factor H than the C3bBb convertase. Via C3b binding and allowing assembly of the C3 convertase, CFHR4 was able to activate the alternative pathway [37].

Binding of CFHR4 to *Candida albicans* [24] and *Fusobacterium necrophorum* [40] has been reported, but its function on microbes has not yet been analyzed.

These data suggest that CFHR4 rather enhances complement activation and opsonization than inhibits it. This functionally markedly different activity from that of the complement inhibitor factor H may in part be also explained by competition between CFHR4 and factor H for binding to C3b.

7 Factor H-Related Protein 5

CFHR5 is composed of 9 SCRs with homology to SCRs 6–7, 10–14 and 19–20 of factor H [41]. This 65-kDa glycoprotein has a plasma concentration of 3–6 μg/ml [42].

Biochemical characterization of CFHR5 has shown that the protein binds to heparin and C-reactive protein, and it is associated with HDL in plasma [42]. Similarly to factor H and other CFHRs, CFHR5 binds to C3b. CFHR5 displays a weak cofactor activity for C3b cleavage and inhibits the alternative pathway C3 convertase in the fluid phase through a yet unidentified mechanism [42]. Although it does not appear as a very potent complement regulator, CFHR5 binds to C3 activation products and has been shown to be colocalized with complement deposits in the glomeruli of diseased kidneys [43].

There is a growing body of evidence that CFHR5 abnormalities are connected with glomerular disease. Sequence variations in CFHR5 have been associated with the kidney diseases aHUS [44, 45] and dense deposit disease [46]. A recently reported case of heterozygous CFHR5 deficiency due to a single nucleotide insertion that results in a premature stop codon in a patient with acute poststreptococcal glomerulonephritis further supports a role for CFHR5 in protecting against glomerular injury [47]. Interestingly, CFHR5 levels were found to be reduced in this patient as well as in patients with C3 glomerulonephritis [47].

A recently described kidney disease, CFHR5 nephropathy, is associated with the presence of an abnormal CFHR5 in which SCRs 1 and 2 of the protein are duplicated [48]. The mutation shows autosomal dominant inheritance with more than 90 % penetrance. All described patients are of Cypriot ancestry and apparently have a common ancestor [48, 49]. Clinically, the patients have microscopic or macroscopic hematuria, and a fraction of the patients (mostly men) develop proteinuria, deteriorating renal function, and end-stage renal disease [48–50]. The histological characteristics of CFHR5 nephropathy show immunostaining for complement products C3, C5, and C9 without the deposition of immunoglobulins or C1q. This suggests complement alternative pathway dysregulation as a pathogenetic factor in the disease. It is, however, unclear at present how the mutant CFHR5 causes disease or whether any other abnormalities are involved.

Regarding association of *CFHR5* sequence variants with AMD, one study reported significant association with increased risk of AMD [51], whereas another reported no association [52].

In addition, binding of CFHR5 to the OspE proteins (CRASP3-5) of *Borrelia burgdorferi* has been reported. Similar to the binding of CFHR1 and CFHR2, no functional effect of CFHR5 on complement evasion of the bacteria could be demonstrated [22, 23].

The extraordinary example of CFHR5 nephropathy warrants further studies to determine the role of CFHR5 in complement regulation in the kidney and to identify additional ligands and functions of the protein.

8 CFHR Copy Numbers and Diseases

In addition to the *CFHR* sequence variations discussed above, gene conversions and partial or whole gene deletions have been observed in the factor H-related gene cluster. Due to the high sequence similarity among these genes, genetic studies are difficult as PCR amplifications may not be specific enough (e.g., for the terminal exons of CFHR1 and CFH). The lack of certain CFHR proteins in plasma, particularly that of CFHR1 and CFHR3, has been observed by western blot analyses, indicating a relatively frequent deletion of these genes. Multiplex ligation-dependent probe amplification (MLPA) assays have been developed to detect the lack of various exons in the *CFH* and *CFHR* genes. This facilitated the recognition of disease-associated copy number variations and hybrid genes in this genomic region [2–6].

Deletions of one or more of the *CFHR* genes have been described in healthy individuals and in patients with distinct diseases. Especially the homozygous deletion of *CFHR1* has been associated with the presence of anti-factor H autoantibodies [4, 12, 14, 53]. This suggests that CFHR1 could have a role in maintaining immunological tolerance to factor H.

Antibodies to factor H in association with the *CFHR3/CFHR1* deletion have been found in aHUS patients [3, 4]. The *CFHR3/CFHR1* deletion is also associated with an increased risk of systemic lupus erythematosus [54]. In contrast, the deletion has been found to be less frequent in patients with AMD [2] and IgA nephropathy [55]. The *CFHR3/CFHR1* deletion is contained in a common *CFH* haplotype associated with reduced risk of AMD [2, 56]. It is important to note that the *CFHR3/CFHR1* deletion is relatively common in the population and its frequency differs between various ethnic groups (2.2–17.3 %) [57].

Additional deletions are less frequently observed, such as combined *CFHR1/CFHR4* deletions [12, 58, 59], *CFHR3*, *CFHR1* and *CFHR2* deletion [56, 59]. As a reciprocal event, extra copies of *CFHR1* and *CFHR4* have also been observed [56, 58].

9 Functional Analysis of the Factor H-Related Proteins

The close relatedness of the factor H-related proteins to each other and to factor H poses several problems. To our knowledge, except for CFHR5, there are no well-characterized, monospecific antibodies available yet that recognize only one of these proteins. This hampers the quantification of these proteins in body fluids and their detection in tissues, and makes their purification from plasma also difficult. Most studies therefore used recombinant proteins to investigate the ligand binding characteristics and function of these proteins, as summarized above.

The most striking feature of the CFHR proteins is the homology of their two most C-terminal SCR-domains with each other and with those of factor H. Since SCR 19–20 domains of factor H are the main C3d/C3b and host surface recognition sites, the CFHRs may have a modulating effect on these functions. How and why this occur remains to be determined.

10 Conclusion

The CFHR proteins represent a group of interesting molecules that share structural homology in their C-termini. Their association with C3b/C3d, possible binding to lipoproteins and pentraxins and involvement in various complement-related diseases suggest important functional activities. More effort should thus be devoted to studies on their functions and roles in various inflammatory disorders.

11 Note

1. Two recent reports showed that SCRs 1–2 of CFHR1, CFHR2 and CFHR5 contain a dimerization motif, which allows formation of homo- and heterodimers among these proteins [60, 61]. The oligomer formation enhances the avidity of these proteins for C3b and its fragments, and results in enhanced competition with factor H. This process, termed complement deregulation, causes increased complement activation by interfering with the complement inhibitor factor H. Disease-associated mutant CFHR1, containing internally duplicated SCRs 1–4 [61], and mutant CFHR5 with duplicated SCRs 1–2 [60], form higher order oligomers that more efficiently deregulate complement than the native proteins.

Acknowledgements

M.J. is supported by the "Lendület" Program of the Hungarian Academy of Sciences (grant LP2012-43/2012). S.M. is supported by the Sigrid Jusélius Foundation, Helsinki University Central Hospital Funds and the Immunobiology Research Program, University of Helsinki.

References

1. Zipfel PF, Skerka C, Hellwage J et al (2002) Factor H family proteins: on complement, microbes and human diseases. Biochem Soc Trans 30:971–978
2. Hughes AE, Orr N, Esfandiary H et al (2006) A common CFH haplotype, with deletion of CFHR1 and CFHR3, is associated with lower risk of age-related macular degeneration. Nat Genet 38:1173–1177
3. Zipfel PF, Edey M, Heinen S et al (2007) Deletion of complement factor H-related genes CFHR1 and CFHR3 is associated with atypical hemolytic uremic syndrome. PLoS Genet 3:e41
4. Józsi M, Licht C, Strobel S et al (2008) Factor H autoantibodies in atypical hemolytic uremic syndrome correlate with CFHR1/CFHR3 deficiency. Blood 111:1512–1514
5. Venables JP, Strain L, Routledge D et al (2006) Atypical haemolytic uraemic syndrome associated with a hybrid complement gene. PLoS Med 3:e431
6. Francis NJ, McNicholas B, Awan A et al (2012) A novel hybrid CFH/CFHR3 gene generated by a microhomology-mediated deletion in familial atypical hemolytic uremic syndrome. Blood 119:591–601
7. Józsi M, Zipfel PF (2008) Factor H family proteins and human diseases. Trends Immunol 29:380–387
8. Estaller C, Koistinen V, Schwaeble W et al (1991) Cloning of the 1.4-kb mRNA species of human complement factor H reveals a novel member of the short consensus repeat family related to the carboxy terminal of the classical 150-kDa molecule. J Immunol 146:3190–3196
9. Timmann C, Leippe M, Horstmann RD (1991) Two major serum components antigenically related to complement factor H are different glycosylation forms of a single protein with no factor H-like complement regulatory functions. J Immunol 146:1265–1270
10. Skerka C, Horstmann RD, Zipfel PF (1991) Molecular cloning of a human serum protein structurally related to complement factor H. J Biol Chem 266:12015–12020
11. Park CT, Wright SD (1996) Plasma lipopolysaccharide-binding protein is found associated with a particle containing apolipoprotein A-I, phospholipid, and factor H-related proteins. J Biol Chem 271:18054–18060
12. Abarrategui-Garrido C, Martínez-Barricarte R, López-Trascasa M et al (2009) Characterization of complement factor H-related (CFHR) proteins in plasma reveals novel genetic variations of CFHR1 associated with atypical hemolytic uremic syndrome. Blood 114:4261–4271
13. Martínez-Barricarte R, Recalde S, Fernández-Robredo P et al (2012) Relevance of complement factor H-related 1 (CFHR1) genotypes in age-related macular degeneration. Invest Ophthalmol Vis Sci 53:1087–1094
14. Dragon-Durey MA, Blanc C, Marliot F et al (2009) The high frequency of complement factor H related CFHR1 gene deletion is restricted to specific subgroups of patients with atypical haemolytic uraemic syndrome. J Med Genet 46:447–450
15. Heinen S, Hartmann A, Lauer N et al (2009) Factor H-related protein 1 (CFHR-1) inhibits complement C5 convertase activity and terminal complex formation. Blood 114:2439–2447
16. Fritsche LG, Lauer N, Hartmann A et al (2010) An imbalance of human complement regulatory proteins CFHR1, CFHR3 and factor H influences risk for age-related macular degeneration (AMD). Hum Mol Genet 19:4694–4704
17. Strobel S, Abarrategui-Garrido C, Fariza-Requejo E et al (2011) Factor H-related protein 1 neutralizes anti-factor H autoantibodies in autoimmune hemolytic uremic syndrome. Kidney Int 80:397–404
18. Heinen S, Sanchez-Corral P, Jackson MS et al (2006) De novo gene conversion in the RCA gene cluster (1q32) causes mutations in complement factor H associated with atypical hemolytic uremic syndrome. Hum Mutat 27:292–293
19. Ferreira VP, Herbert AP, Cortés C et al (2009) The binding of factor H to a complex of physiological polyanions and C3b on cells is impaired in atypical hemolytic uremic syndrome. J Immunol 182:7009–7018
20. Morgan HP, Schmidt CQ, Guariento M et al (2011) Structural basis for engagement by complement factor H of C3b on a self surface. Nat Struct Mol Biol 18:463–470
21. Herbert AP, Kavanagh D, Johansson C et al (2012) Structural and functional characterization of the product of disease-related factor H gene conversion. Biochemistry 51:1874–1884
22. Siegel C, Hallström T, Skerka C et al (2010) Complement factor H-related proteins CFHR2 and CFHR5 represent novel ligands for the infection-associated CRASP proteins of *Borrelia burgdorferi*. PLoS One 5:e13519
23. Hammerschmidt C, Hallström T, Skerka C et al (2012) Contribution of the infection-associated complement regulator-acquiring surface protein 4 (ErpC) to complement resistance of *Borrelia burgdorferi*. Clin Dev Immunol 2012:349657
24. Losse J, Zipfel PF, Józsi M (2010) Factor H and factor H-related protein 1 bind to human neutrophils via complement receptor 3, mediate attachment to *Candida albicans*, and enhance neutrophil antimicrobial activity. J Immunol 184:912–921

25. Behnsen J, Hartmann A, Schmaler J et al (2008) The opportunistic human pathogenic fungus Aspergillus fumigatus evades the host complement system. Infect Immun 76:820–827
26. Castiblanco-Valencia MM, Fraga TR, Silva LB et al (2012) Leptospiral immunoglobulin-like proteins interact with human complement regulators factor H, FHL-1, FHR-1, and C4BP. J Infect Dis 205:995–1004
27. Haupt K, Kraiczy P, Wallich R et al (2007) Binding of human factor H-related protein 1 to serum-resistant *Borrelia burgdorferi* is mediated by borrelial complement regulator-acquiring surface proteins. J Infect Dis 196:124–133
28. Reuter M, Caswell CC, Lukomski S et val (2010) Binding of the human complement regulators CFHR1 and factor H by streptococcal collagen-like protein 1 (Scl1) via their conserved C termini allows control of the complement cascade at multiple levels. J Biol Chem 285:38473–38485
29. Skerka C, Timmann C, Horstmann RD et al (1992) Two additional human serum proteins structurally related to complement factor H. Evidence for a family of factor H-related genes. J Immunol 148:3313–3318
30. Dieterich R, Hammerschmidt C, Richter D et al (2010) Inadequate binding of immune regulator factor H is associated with sensitivity of *Borrelia lusitaniae* to human complement. Infect Immun 78:4467–4476
31. Skerka C, Kühn S, Günther K et al (1993) A novel short consensus repeat-containing molecule is related to human complement factor H. J Biol Chem 268:2904–2908
32. Hellwage J, Jokiranta TS, Koistinen V et al (1999) Functional properties of complement factor H-related proteins FHR-3 and FHR-4: binding to the C3d region of C3b and differential regulation by heparin. FEBS Lett 462:345–352
33. Hellwage J, Jokiranta TS, Friese MA et al (2002) Complement C3b/C3d and cell surface polyanions are recognized by overlapping binding sites on the most carboxyl-terminal domain of complement factor H. J Immunol 169:6935–6944
34. Kotarsky H, Hellwage J, Johnsson E et al (1998) Identification of a domain in human factor H and factor H-like protein-1 required for the interaction with streptococcal M proteins. J Immunol 160:3349–3354
35. Józsi M, Richter H, Löschmann I et al (2005) FHR-4A: a new factor H-related protein is encoded by the human FHR-4 gene. Eur J Hum Genet 13:321–329
36. Skerka C, Hellwage J, Weber W et al (1997) The human factor H-related protein 4 (FHR-4). A novel short consensus repeat-containing protein is associated with human triglyceride-rich lipoproteins. J Biol Chem 272:5627–5634
37. Hebecker M, Józsi M (2012) Factor H-related protein 4 activates complement by serving as a platform for the assembly of an alternative pathway C3 convertase via its interaction with C3b. J Biol Chem 287:19528–19536
38. Mihlan M, Hebecker M, Dahse HM et al (2009) Human complement factor H-related protein 4 binds and recruits native pentameric C-reactive protein to necrotic cells. Mol Immunol 46:335–344
39. Hebecker M, Okemefuna AI, Perkins SJ et al (2010) Molecular basis of C-reactive protein binding and modulation of complement activation by factor H-related protein 4. Mol Immunol 47:1347–1355
40. Friberg N, Carlson P, Kentala E et al (2008) Factor H binding as a complement evasion mechanism for an anaerobic pathogen, Fusobacterium necrophorum. J Immunol 181: 8624–8632
41. McRae JL, Cowan PJ, Power DA et al (2001) Human factor H-related protein 5 (FHR-5). A new complement-associated protein. J Biol Chem 276:6747–6754
42. McRae JL, Duthy TG, Griggs KM et al (2005) Human factor H-related protein 5 has cofactor activity, inhibits C3 convertase activity, binds heparin and C-reactive protein, and associates with lipoprotein. J Immunol 174: 6250–6256
43. Murphy B, Georgiou T, Machet D et al (2002) Factor H-related protein-5: a novel component of human glomerular immune deposits. Am J Kidney Dis 39:24–27
44. Monteferrante G, Brioschi S, Caprioli J et al (2007) Genetic analysis of the complement factor H related 5 gene in haemolytic uraemic syndrome. Mol Immunol 44:1704–1708
45. Maga TK, Nishimura CJ, Weaver AE et al (2010) Mutations in alternative pathway complement proteins in American patients with atypical hemolytic uremic syndrome. Hum Mutat 31:E1445–E1460
46. Abrera-Abeleda MA, Nishimura C, Smith JL et al (2006) Variations in the complement regulatory genes factor H (CFH) and factor H related 5 (CFHR5) are associated with membranoproliferative glomerulonephritis type II (dense deposit disease). J Med Genet 43:582–589
47. Vernon KA, Goicoechea de Jorge E, Hall AE et al (2012) Acute presentation and persistent glomerulonephritis following streptococcal infection in a patient with heterozygous complement factor H-related protein 5 deficiency. Am J Kidney Dis 60:121–125
48. Gale DP, Goicoechea de Jorge E, Cook HT et al (2010) Identification of a mutation in complement factor H-related protein 5 in patients of Cypriot origin with glomerulonephritis. Lancet 376:794–801

49. Athanasiou Y, Voskarides K, Gale DP et al (2011) Familial C3 glomerulopathy associated with CFHR5 mutations: clinical characteristics of 91 patients in 16 pedigrees. Clin J Am Soc Nephrol 6:1436–1446
50. Gale DP, Pickering MC (2011) Regulating complement in the kidney: insights from CFHR5 nephropathy. Dis Model Mech 4: 721–726
51. Zhang H, Morrison MA, Dewan A et al (2008) The NEI/NCBI dbGAP database: genotypes and haplotypes that may specifically predispose to risk of neovascular age-related macular degeneration. BMC Med Genet 9:51
52. Narendra U, Pauer GJ, Hagstrom SA (2009) Genetic analysis of complement factor H related 5, CFHR5, in patients with age-related macular degeneration. Mol Vis 15:731–736
53. Moore I, Strain L, Pappworth I et al (2010) Association of factor H autoantibodies with deletions of CFHR1, CFHR3, CFHR4, and with mutations in CFH, CFI, CD46, and C3 in patients with atypical hemolytic uremic syndrome. Blood 115:379–387
54. Zhao J, Wu H, Khosravi M et al (2011) Association of genetic variants in complement factor H and factor H-related genes with systemic lupus erythematosus susceptibility. PLoS Genet 7:e1002079
55. Gharavi AG, Kiryluk K, Choi M et al (2011) Genome-wide association study identifies susceptibility loci for IgA nephropathy. Nat Genet 43:321–327
56. Schmid-Kubista KE, Tosakulwong N, Wu Y et al (2009) Contribution of copy number variation in the regulation of complement activation locus to development of age-related macular degeneration. Invest Ophthalmol Vis Sci 50:5070–5079
57. Hageman GS, Hancox LS, Taiber AJ et al (2006) Extended haplotypes in the complement factor H (CFH) and CFH-related (CFHR) family of genes protect against age-related macular degeneration: characterization, ethnic distribution and evolutionary implications. Ann Med 38:592–604
58. Sudmant PH, Kitzman JO, Antonacci F et al (2010) Diversity of human copy number variation and multicopy genes. Science 330:641–646
59. Kubista KE, Tosakulwong N, Wu Y et al (2011) Copy number variation in the complement factor H-related genes and age-related macular degeneration. Mol Vis 17:2080–2092
60. Goicoechea de Jorge E, Caesar JJE, Malik TH et al (2013) Dimerization of complement factor H-related proteins modulates complement activation in vivo. Proc Natl Acad Sci USA 110:4685–4690
61. Tortajada A, Yébenes H, Abarrategui-Garrido C et al (2013) C3 glomerulopathy-associated CFHR1 mutation alters FHR oligomerization and complement regulation. J Clin Invest 123:2434–2446

Chapter 19

Functional Evaluation of Factor H genetic and Acquired Abnormalities: Application for Atypical Hemolytic Uremic Syndrome (aHUS)

Lubka T. Roumenina, Roxane Roquigny, Caroline Blanc, Nelly Poulain, Stéphanie Ngo, Marie-Agnès Dragon-Durey, and Véronique Frémeaux-Bacchi

Abstract

The atypical hemolytic uremic syndrome (aHUS) is a paradigm of a disease, caused by overactivation of the alternative complement pathway secondary to a not well-understood trigger event. About 60 % of the patients present genetic or acquired abnormalities in the proteins of the alternative complement pathway. In 40 % of the cases the affected protein is the complement regulator Factor H (FH)—30 % due to mutations and 10 % because of anti-FH autoantibodies. Here we describe the detailed protocol for a rapid test to analyse the functional defect associated with genetic or acquired FH-related abnormalities. It can be applied for the characterization of the underlying complement defect in aHUS, based on spontaneous lysis of non-sensitized sheep erythrocytes in contact with patients' plasma or serum.

Key words Complement, aHUS, C3, Endothelium, FH, Disease risk, Therapy

1 Introduction

The atypical hemolytic uremic syndrome (aHUS) is a paradigm of a disease, caused by overactivation of the alternative complement pathway secondary to a non-specific trigger event. Inefficient regulation due to deficiency and loss-of-function mutations in Factor H (FH) [1, 2], Factor I (FI) [3–5] or MCP (CD46) [6, 7] or hyperactivity due to gain-of-function mutations in C3 [8, 9] and Factor B [10, 11] or presence of anti-FH auto-antibodies [12, 13] lead to increased levels of anaphylatoxins C3a and C5a and endothelial cells and platelets-bound cell-bound C3b [14]. This complement overactivation is associated with endothelial cells damage in the kidney microvasculature, leading to thrombotic microangiopathy. Hallmarks of aHUS are (1) the mechanical

Mihaela Gadjeva (ed.), *The Complement System: Methods and Protocols*, Methods in Molecular Biology, vol. 1100, DOI 10.1007/978-1-62703-724-2_19, © Springer Science+Business Media New York 2014

hemolytic anemia, induced by rupture of erythrocytes passing by the occluded glomerular microvessels, (2) the reduced platelets count (thrombocytopenia) due to consumption for the thrombosis in the kidney and, as a result, (3) the acute renal failure [15]. The aHUS is an ultra rare (less 0.5/million new cases/year), acute and life-threatening disease progressing rapidly to end-stage renal failure after the first flare in about half of the cases. Until recently the plasmatherapy was the treatment of choice in order to remove the harmful complement activation fragments and to introduce functional regulators. Unfortunately, this strategy was frequently unsuccessful and unable to prevent the loss of renal function. The disease often re-occurred after renal transplantation, leaving the patients under hemodialysis for life. Recently a complement inhibitor monoclonal antibody has become available for treatment of aHUS, blocking C5—the source of the potent anaphylatoxin C5a and the initiator of the membrane attack complex C5b-9 [16, 17]. Rapid aHUS diagnostic and identification of the underlying complement abnormality are of importance for the patients' management.

Quantitative deficiencies of complement proteins are relatively easy to be detected using sandwich ELISA or radial immunodiffusion. More difficult to trace are the functional abnormalities, since they are associated with normal protein level [14]. A hot spot for loss-of-function mutations in FH is the C-terminal part of the protein and in particular the last two domains SCR19 and 20 [18]. These mutations result in decreased binding to C3b and glucosaminoglycans on the cell surface, impairing local complement control [19]. One approach for functional evaluation for FH is the use of a hemolytic assay, employing sheep erythrocytes, which do not activate human complement [11]. Sheep erythrocytes (in contrast to the rabbit ones) are rich in sialic acid and are capable of binding FH from the plasma to protect themselves against human complement attack [20]. Sanchez-Corral et al. demonstrated that aHUS serum and plasma samples carrying FH mutations induce lysis of the sheep erythrocytes via the alternative complement pathway [11]. The test is easy and could rapidly give indications on FH-related abnormalities (mutation and auto-antibodies), which affect about 40 % of the aHUS patients.

2 Materials

All buffers should be prepared using deionized or double distilled water and analytical grade reagents. Concentrated solutions may be prepared and stored at 4 °C for 2–3 weeks and diluted to 1× before use. Follow the regulations for work with human material.

2.1 Buffers

1. VBS EGTA-Mg: 2.5 mM barbital, 1.5 mM sodium barbital, 144 mM NaCl, 7 mM $MgCl_2$, 10 mM EGTA, pH 7.2–7.4.
2. VBS EDTA: 2.5 mM barbital, 1.5 mM sodium barbital, 144 mM NaCl, 10 mM EDTA, pH 7.2–7.4
3. 0.15 M NaCl: measure 8.766 g NaCl and dissolve in 1 l of water (MW NaCl = 58.44).
4. Stock solution of Veronal buffer saline (VBS) 5×, which will serve as a base for VBS containing buffers in the experiment, and which can be stored at 4 °C for 2–3 weeks.
5. Weigh 85 g NaCl + 3.75 g sodium diethylbarbital and dissolve on ice in 1 l of water. Separately measure 5.75 g barbital and dissolve on a hot plate (350 °C) in 500 ml of water. Mix the two solutions, adjust the pH between 7.2 and 7.4 when the solution is cold and adjust the final volume to 2 l.
6. 1 M MgCl2. Dissolve 5 g MgCl2 · 6H2O in 25 ml of water. Keep for a month at 4 °C.
7. 200 mM Ethylene glycol-bis(2-aminoethylether)-N,N,N′,N′-tetraacetic acid (EGTA): weigh 7.6 g EGTA and dissolve with heating and stirring to 100 ml of water, adjusting the pH to 7.5. Keep for a month at 4 °C.
8. 200 mM Ethylenediaminetetraacetic acid disodium salt dihydrate (EDTA): Weigh 7.4 g EDTA and dissolve with heating and stirring to 100 ml of water, adjusting the pH to 7.5. Keep for a month at 4 °C.
9. 1× VBS, EGTA-Mg: Mix 100 ml VBS 5× + 3.5 ml 1 M MgCl2 + 25 ml 200 mM EGTA. Adjust volume to 0.5 l. Prepare on the day of the experiment and discard after the end of the tests.
10. To prepare VBS EDTA 1×, 0.5 l—Mix 100 ml VBS 5× + 25 ml 200 mM EDTA. Prepare on the day of the experiment and discard after the end of the tests.

2.2 Sheep Erythrocytes

Use sheep blood as a source of sheep erythrocytes. Wash the needed amount of sheep erythrocytes (start with 100 μl of cell suspension and adjust according to the experiment) two times with EGTA-Mg. Prepare a desired volume a cell suspension of 10^8 cells/ml in VBS EGTA-Mg (take into account at least 10 % excess) (*see* **Note 1**).

2.3 Patients' and Control Samples

EDTA-plasma or serum (*see* **Note 2**) can be obtained by venopuncture, centrifuged, aliquoted, and stored at −80 °C until use.

3 Method

1. Prepare dilutions of patient and control plasma or serum in 5 ml tubes, mixing on ice according to Table 1.

   Conditions (samples and blank)

   Prepare dilutions in the manner described in Table 1 for each patient's and each healthy donor's plasma, the positive control and the standard pool plasma to be tested. The positive control consists of inhibition of FH by a selected blocking antibody (*see* **Note 3**). Add the blocking antibody to pooled plasma or serum at 250 μg/ml final concentration and dilute this sample rapidly on ice as the other samples.

   Controls for the experiment

   Tube A: 100 μl VBS EGTA-Mg 1×—for T0 (baseline hemolysis), after addition of 145 mM NaCl.

   Tube B: 100 μl VBS EDTA, for blank control of the T0 after addition of 145 mM NaCl.

   Tube C: 100 μl VBS EGTA-Mg 1×—for T100 (maximal hemolysis), after addition of water.

2. Add 100 μl of sheep erythrocytes at 1×10^8 cells/ml resuspended in VBS EGTA-Mg to each tube.

Table 1
Chart for samples preparation

Condition	1	2	3	4	5	T0	T100
Samples							
VBS EGTA-Mg 1×, μl	50	60	70	80	90	100	–
Plasma, μl	50	40	30	20	10	0	–
10^8 Cells/ml, μl	100	100	100	100	100	100	100
Controls							
VBS EDTA, μl	50	60	70	80	90	100	–
Plasma, μl	50	40	30	20	10	0	–
10^8 Cells/ml, μl	100	100	100	100	100	100	100
30 min in a water bath with gentle shaking							
NaCl 145 mM, ml	1.6	1.6	1.6	1.6	1.6		1.6
Water, ml						1.8	
Centrifuge and read the A_{414} in the supernatant							

3. Incubate the tubes in a water bath at 37 °C with gentle shaking for 30 min.
4. Add 1.6 ml of cold 145 mM NaCl to each tube except tube C to stop the reaction. In tube C add 1.8 ml water to obtain the maximal hemolysis, induced by osmotic shock.
5. Centrifuge the samples at 1,800 × g.
6. Read the optical density of the supernatant at 414 nm (A414) by a spectrophotometer and calculate the level of hemolysis according to **Note 4**. For the evaluation of the results (*see* **Notes 5–11**).

4 Notes

1. The concentration of the cell suspension can be verified by spectrophotometry. Mix 2.9 ml water + 100 μl homogenized cell suspension. The absorption at 414 nm should be 0.286 if the cells are at 10^8 cells/ml. If the A_{414} is below this value, the sample is too diluted. In this case more cells have to be added. If the value exceeds 0.286, the sample has to be diluted. The final volume of the suspension can be calculated by the equation:

$$\text{Final volume} = \left(\text{sample } A_{414} / 0.286\right) \times \text{Initial volume}$$

Re-do the same measurement after dilution and be sure not to dilute too much the sample.

2. The protocol is given for plasma, but is identical for serum. All samples should be thawed immediately before use, centrifuged at 4 °C and kept on ice. Avoid use of freeze–thawed samples. Avoid use of hemolysed or turbid samples. In each experiment an aliquot of pooled normal plasma or serum must be used. This should be a pool of 100 healthy donors' plasma or serum.
3. The positive control of the test is a blocking anti-FH monoclonal antibody. It could be directed against the C-terminal part of the protein, for example C18 [21], L20, Mab 167 or against the N-terminal part of the protein, as Ox24 [21] (*see* Fig. 1b). An example for a non-inhibitory anti-FH antibody is Ox23, Fig. 1b. All antibodies are commercially available, for example from Thermo Scientific or from Abnova for Mab 167.
4. Calculation of the level of hemolysis: The lysis corresponding to each dilution can be calculated by subtracting the A_{414} of the corresponding blank (VBS-EDTA samples) from each sample (VBS EGTA-Mg), and dividing by the A_{414} of the control of total lysis (Tube C). The % of lysis will be obtained after multiplication by 100. The spontaneous lysis in absence of

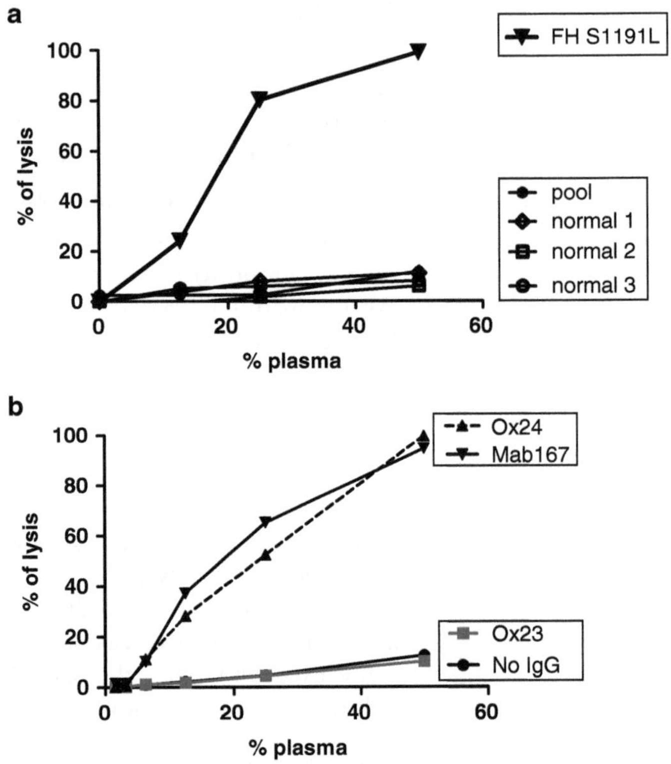

Fig. 1 Spontaneous hemolysis of sheep erythrocytes, induced by increasing concentrations of aHUS patient's plasma (**a**) or normal plasma, supplemented with blocking anti-Factor H antibodies (**b**). The patient is a carrier of Factor H C-terminal mutation S1191L. Plasma from normal donors did not induce lysis. Anti-FH antibody which does not block the functional activity (Ox23) did not induce any lysis. Cells were incubated with the plasma for 30 min at 37 °C and released hemoglobin was measured by spectrophotometry

plasma is evaluated by the A_{414} of tubes A and B for the two buffers respectively.

$$\%\text{ of lysis} = \left(A_{414}\text{EGTA} - \text{Mg} - A_{414}\text{EDTA} - \text{T0 EDTA} - \text{T0 EGTA}\right) / \left(A_{414}\text{water} - \text{T0 EGTA}\right) \times 100$$

The results can be represented in a graph, plotting the % of hemolysis versus the % of plasma in the samples, Fig. 1a representing the positive control (Ox24 and Mab 167 monoclonal antibodies treated plasma) and Fig. 1b representing an aHUS patient sample.

The results can be also compared for one particular dilution of the plasma, as presented at Fig. 2. A sample can be considered as positive if it exceeds the average lysis obtained from the standard plasma or serum pool and at least ten individual normal donors + 2× standard deviation.

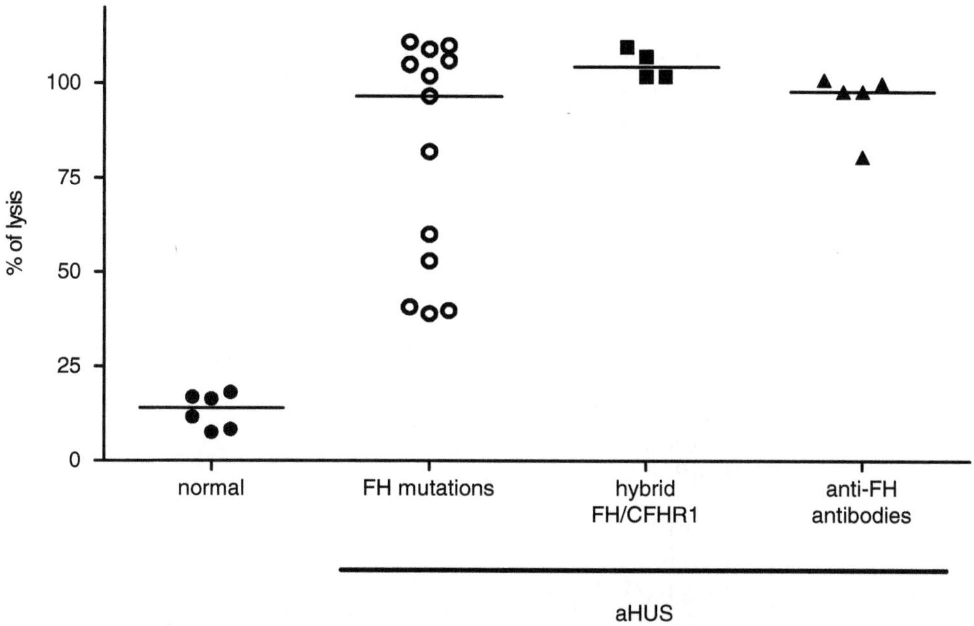

Fig. 2 Spontaneous hemolysis of sheep erythrocytes, induced by incubation with 50 % of aHUS patients' plasma. Patients with Factor H mutations (N- and C-terminal), FH/CFHR1 hybrid gene as well as anti-factor H auto-antibodies were tested. Cells were incubated with the plasma for 30 min at 37 °C and released hemoglobin was measured by spectrophotometry

5. The test is positive in case of FH mutations [22–24] and anti-FH Abs [21], as is evident from the literature and from our experience, presented at Figs. 1 and 2. Usually the anti-FH antibodies, the C-terminal mutations, and the FH/CFHR1 hybrid protein give stronger lysis [25], compared to the mutations in the rest of the protein. A list of examples of the FH mutations inducing lysis in this test is given in Table 2. Rarely the presence of some mutant FH in the plasma or serum does not induce increased lysis with this test [26]. Therefore negative results do not completely exclude a FH-related defect.
6. In presence of a plasma or serum with FH mutations or anti-FH antibodies, the lysis can be prevented by addition of purified FH [11, 21, 24].
7. C3 consumption in the plasma or serum sample interferes with the results. Reduced C3 and/or FB levels in the patient sample (below the normal range) could result in an inefficient lysis, despite of the presence of a FH-related defect. Therefore the results of this test should be always interpreted in correlation with the C3 and FB levels.
8. If the sample was transported or remained at room temperature or a long time, complement may be consumed in vitro in

Table 2
Examples of aHUS associated FH genetic and acquired abnormalities, inducing spontaneous lysis of sheep erythrocytes

Abnormality	References
Mutations	
A161S	Our laboratory, Fig. 2
C870R	Sanchez-Corral et al. 2004 [11]
W1183L	Heinen et al. 2006 [22]
W1183R	Stahl et al. 2008 [24]
V1186E	Kird et al. 2012 [25]
L1189R	
V1197A	
E1198K	
E1198stop	
R1210C	
S1191W	
L1189F	
S1191L/V1197A	
Antibodies	
Anti-FH antibodies, autoimmune aHUS	Our laboratory, Figs. 1 and 2
Monoclonal antibodies	Strobel et al. [21]
Ox24 Mab	
L20 Mab	
167Mab	
C18 Mab	

the tube. The antigenic level of C3 and FB will remain normal but the proteins will be not functional. False negative result may be obtained in this case. In general, serum samples are more sensitive to such artificial complement consumption, compared to plasma-EDTA.

9. Some samples appear positive without any presence of anti-FH antibodies or subsequent detection of a mutation in FH by a direct sequencing. For some of these patients, large rearrangements in the gene locus where FH gene is located were detected by Multiplex ligation-dependent probe amplification (MLPA) (Fig. 2). Therefore a strong positive result and no defect detected by sequencing is an indication for an in dept analysis for the presence of hybrid FH/CFHR1 genes. In this case FH exchanges its C-terminal exones with CFHR1, leading to a production of a protein carrying the same sequence as the native FH, except two amino-acid residues in the cell surface recognition domain SCR20 (S1191L and V1197A). These substitutions, especially S1191L, are known to perturb the cell surface protection [22, 27], Fig. 1 rendering the hybrid FH/

CFHR1 protein unable to protect sheep erythrocytes from lysis [25], Fig. 2. Other genetic rearrangements between the FH related genes give rise to hybrid molecules such as hybrid FH/CFHR3 gene, which induced only limited lysis [28].

10. There is still limited data in the literature for the test specificity and whether it could be used to detect other complement abnormalities. In our experience the mutant C3 containing samples are negative in this test. Rarely for some positive samples remain unexplained by a presence of a FH-related defect. Therefore, other aHUS associated unknown factors could influence this test. In our experience, the test is never positive for healthy donors.
11. For diagnostic purposes for a routine screening the experimental approach could be simplified, taking only two dilutions of the plasma or serum samples—50 and 20 %. In case of a positive result, a validation with an extended dose response may be performed. Cascade dilution of the plasma could be performed to speed up the test, as was done for the experiments in Fig. 1a, b.

Acknowledgments

This work was supported by grants from Agence Nationale de la Recherche (ANR Genopath 2009–2012 09geno031011 and ANR Biotheque 2008–2011 R08086DS), Assistance Publique-Hôpitaux de Paris (Programme Hospitalier de Recherche Clinique (AOM05130/P051065 and AOM08198), by AIRG France, by Université Paris Descartes and Université Pierre et Marie Curie and by INSERM.

References

1. Warwicker P, Goodship TH, Donne RL, Pirson Y, Nicholls A, Ward RM, Turnpenny P, Goodship JA (1998) Genetic studies into inherited and sporadic hemolytic uremic syndrome. Kidney Int 53:836–844
2. de Cordoba SR, de Jorge EG (2008) Translational mini-review series on complement factor H: genetics and disease associations of human complement factor H. Clin Exp Immunol 151:1–13
3. Nilsson SC, Sim RB, Lea SM, Fremeaux-Bacchi V, Blom AM (2011) Complement factor I in health and disease. Mol Immunol 48: 1611–1620
4. Fremeaux-Bacchi V, Dragon-Durey MA, Blouin J, Vigneau C, Kuypers D, Boudailliez B, Loirat C, Rondeau E, Fridman WH (2004) Complement factor I: a susceptibility gene for atypical haemolytic uraemic syndrome. J Med Genet 41:e84
5. Bienaime F, Dragon-Durey MA, Regnier CH, Nilsson SC, Kwan WH, Blouin J, Jablonski M, Renault N, Rameix-Welti MA, Loirat C, Sautes-Fridman C, Villoutreix BO, Blom AM, Fremeaux-Bacchi V (2010) Mutations in components of complement influence the outcome of Factor I-associated atypical hemolytic uremic syndrome. Kidney Int 77:339–349
6. Richards A, Kemp EJ, Liszewski MK, Goodship JA, Lampe AK, Decorte R, Muslumanoglu MH, Kavukcu S, Filler G, Pirson Y, Wen LS, Atkinson JP, Goodship TH (2003) Mutations in human complement regulator, membrane cofactor protein (CD46), predispose to devel-

opment of familial hemolytic uremic syndrome. Proc Natl Acad Sci U S A 100:12966–12971

7. Noris M, Brioschi S, Caprioli J, Todeschini M, Bresin E, Porrati F, Gamba S, Remuzzi G (2003) Familial haemolytic uraemic syndrome and an MCP mutation. Lancet 362: 1542–1547
8. Roumenina LT, Frimat M, Miller EC, Provot F, Dragon-Durey MA, Bordereau P, Bigot S, Hue C, Satchell SC, Mathieson PW, Mousson C, Noel C, Sautes-Fridman C, Halbwachs-Mecarelli L, Atkinson JP, Lionet A, Fremeaux-Bacchi V (2012) A prevalent C3 mutation in aHUS patients causes a direct C3 convertase gain of function. Blood 119:4182–4191
9. Fremeaux-Bacchi V, Miller EC, Liszewski MK, Strain L, Blouin J, Brown AL, Moghal N, Kaplan BS, Weiss RA, Lhotta K, Kapur G, Mattoo T, Nivet H, Wong W, Gie S, Hurault de Ligny B, Fischbach M, Gupta R, Hauhart R, Meunier V, Loirat C, Dragon-Durey MA, Fridman WH, Janssen BJ, Goodship TH, Atkinson JP (2008) Mutations in complement C3 predispose to development of atypical hemolytic uremic syndrome. Blood 112: 4948–4952
10. Roumenina LT, Jablonski M, Hue C, Blouin J, Dimitrov JD, Dragon-Durey MA, Cayla M, Fridman WH, Macher MA, Ribes D, Moulonguet L, Rostaing L, Satchell SC, Mathieson PW, Sautes-Fridman C, Loirat C, Regnier CH, Halbwachs-Mecarelli L, Fremeaux-Bacchi V (2009) Hyperfunctional C3 convertase leads to complement deposition on endothelial cells and contributes to atypical hemolytic uremic syndrome. Blood 114:2837–2845
11. Goicoechea de Jorge E, Harris CL, Esparza-Gordillo J, Carreras L, Arranz EA, Garrido CA, Lopez-Trascasa M, Sanchez-Corral P, Morgan BP, Rodriguez de Cordoba S (2007) Gain-of-function mutations in complement factor B are associated with atypical hemolytic uremic syndrome. Proc Natl Acad Sci U S A 104: 240–245
12. Dragon-Durey MA, Sethi SK, Bagga A, Blanc C, Blouin J, Ranchin B, Andre JL, Takagi N, Cheong HI, Hari P, Le Quintrec M, Niaudet P, Loirat C, Fridman WH, Fremeaux-Bacchi V (2011) Clinical features of anti-factor H autoantibody-associated hemolytic uremic syndrome. J Am Soc Nephrol 21:2180–2187
13. Dragon-Durey MA, Loirat C, Cloarec S, Macher MA, Blouin J, Nivet H, Weiss L, Fridman WH, Fremeaux-Bacchi V (2005) Anti-Factor H autoantibodies associated with atypical hemolytic uremic syndrome. J Am Soc Nephrol 16:555–563
14. Roumenina LT, Loirat C, Dragon-Durey MA, Halbwachs-Mecarelli L, Sautes-Fridman C, Fremeaux-Bacchi V (2011) Alternative complement pathway assessment in patients with atypical HUS. J Immunol Methods 365:8–26
15. Noris M, Remuzzi G (2009) Atypical hemolytic-uremic syndrome. N Engl J Med 361:1676–1687
16. Salant DJ (2011) Targeting complement C5 in atypical hemolytic uremic syndrome. J Am Soc Nephrol 22:7–9
17. Servais A, Noel LH, Roumenina LT, Le Quintrec M, Ngo S, Dragon-Durey A, Macher MA, Zuber J, karras A, Provost F, Moulin B, Grunfeld JP, Niaudet P, Lesavre P, Fremeaux-Bacchi V (2012) Role of acquired and genetic complement abnormalities in dense deposit disease, glomerulonephritis with isolated C3 deposits, and membranoproliferative glomerulonephritis type I. Kidney Int 82(4):454–464
18. Jokiranta TS, Jaakola VP, Lehtinen MJ, Parepalo M, Meri S, Goldman A (2006) Structure of complement factor H carboxyl-terminus reveals molecular basis of atypical haemolytic uremic syndrome. EMBO J 25:1784–1794
19. Manuelian T, Hellwage J, Meri S, Caprioli J, Noris M, Heinen S, Jozsi M, Neumann HP, Remuzzi G, Zipfel PF (2003) Mutations in factor H reduce binding affinity to C3b and heparin and surface attachment to endothelial cells in hemolytic uremic syndrome. J Clin Invest 111:1181–1190
20. Kazatchkine MD, Fearon DT, Austen KF (1979) Human alternative complement pathway: membrane-associated sialic acid regulates the competition between B and beta1 H for cell-bound C3b. J Immunol 122:75–81
21. Jozsi M, Strobel S, Dahse HM, Liu WS, Hoyer PF, Oppermann M, Skerka C, Zipfel PF (2007) Anti factor H autoantibodies block C-terminal recognition function of factor H in hemolytic uremic syndrome. Blood 110:1516–1518
22. Heinen S, Sanchez-Corral P, Jackson MS, Strain L, Goodship JA, Kemp EJ, Skerka C, Jokiranta TS, Meyers K, Wagner E, Robitaille P, Esparza-Gordillo J, Rodriguez de Cordoba S, Zipfel PF, Goodship TH (2006) De novo gene conversion in the RCA gene cluster (1q32) causes mutations in complement factor H associated with atypical hemolytic uremic syndrome. Hum Mutat 27:292–293
23. Sanchez-Corral P, Gonzalez-Rubio C, Rodriguez de Cordoba S, Lopez-Trascasa M (2004) Functional analysis in serum from atypical hemolytic uremic syndrome patients reveals impaired protection of host cells associated with mutations in factor H. Mol Immunol 41:81–84
24. Stahl AL, Vaziri-Sani F, Heinen S, Kristoffersson AC, Gydell KH, Raafat R, Gutierrez A, Beringer O, Zipfel PF, Karpman D (2008) Factor H dysfunction in patients

with atypical hemolytic uremic syndrome contributes to complement deposition on platelets and their activation. Blood 111: 5307–5315
25. Krid S, Roumenina LT, Beury D, Charbit M, Boyer O, Fremeaux-Bacchi V, Niaudet P (2012) Renal transplantation under prophylactic eculizumab in atypical hemolytic uremic syndrome with CFH/CFHR1 hybrid protein. Am J Transplant 12:1938–1944
26. Johnson SA, Williams JM, Hakobyan S, Richards A, Perkins SJ, Marchbank KJ, Goodship TH, Morgan BP, Taylor CM, Savage CO (2010) Impact of compound heterozygous complement factor H mutations on development of atypical hemolytic uremic syndrome-A pedigree revisited. Mol Immunol 47:1585–1591
27. Ferreira VP, Herbert AP, Cortes C, McKee KA, Blaum BS, Esswein ST, Uhrin D, Barlow PN, Pangburn MK, Kavanagh D (2009) The binding of factor H to a complex of physiological polyanions and C3b on cells is impaired in atypical hemolytic uremic syndrome. J Immunol 182:7009–7018
28. Francis NJ, McNicholas B, Awan A, Waldron M, Reddan D, Sadlier D, Kavanagh D, Strain L, Marchbank KJ, Harris CL, Goodship TH (2012) A novel hybrid CFH/CFHR3 gene generated by a microhomology-mediated deletion in familial atypical hemolytic uremic syndrome. Blood 119:591–601

Chapter 20

Anti-Factor H Autoantibodies Assay

Marie-Agnès Dragon-Durey, Caroline Blanc, Lubka T. Roumenina, Nelly Poulain, Stéphanie Ngo, Pauline Bordereau, and Véronique Frémeaux-Bacchi

Abstract

Non-Shiga-toxin-associated hemolytic uremic syndrome (atypical HUS) is a rare form of thrombotic microangiopathy which associates hemolytic anemia, thrombocytopenia, and acute renal failure. In 10 % of cases the disease is linked to presence of autoantibodies directed against Factor H (FH), the main plasmatic alternative complement pathway regulatory protein. Their presence induces an acquired functional FH deficiency. The anti-FH autoantibodies screening must be performed at the very onset of the disease in all cases of HUS, in order, first, to make the proper diagnosis as early as possible, and second to support an appropriate therapy including early plasma exchanges and immunosuppressive treatments. Thus, anti-CFH IgG represents a diagnostic marker and the titer determination is useful for assessing disease evolution, because changes precede clinical symptoms, and for monitoring of treatment.

Presence of anti-FH IgG has been recently reported to be associated with other clinical context such as C3 glomerulopathies, but their pathogenicity in these conditions remains to be assessed.

Here we describe the ELISA assay allowing the detection of these autoantibodies and report the analysis which can be performed concomitantly to improve the diagnosis.

Key words Complement factor H, Autoantibodies, Complement factor H-related proteins, Atypical hemolytic uremic syndrome, C3 glomerulopathies

1 Introduction

Atypical (i.e., non-Shiga-toxin-associated) hemolytic uremic syndrome (aHUS) is a form of thrombotic microangiopathy in which acute renal failure is a predominant feature associated with hemolytic anemia and thrombocytopenia. This disease is considered as a prototypical alternative complement pathway dysregulation-associated disease due to genetic or acquired factors [1]. The autoimmune form of aHUS (AI-aHUS) was identified in 2005, defined by the presence of auto-antibodies directed against Factor H (FH), the main plasmatic alternative pathway regulatory protein [2]. This etiology account for 6–10 % of all aHUS forms. Most of the cases concern children [3].

Mihaela Gadjeva (ed.), *The Complement System: Methods and Protocols*, Methods in Molecular Biology, vol. 1100, DOI 10.1007/978-1-62703-724-2_20, © Springer Science+Business Media New York 2014

The occurrence of the disease at adulthood seems to be rare in comparison with the frequency in children because 86 % of the reported cases occurred from the age of 4–10 (median age: 7 years) [4]. This autoimmune disease affects equally males and females. Interestingly, AI-aHUS is highly associated with a particular genetic condition—a complete deficiency in a FH homologous protein Complement Factor H Related protein1 (CFHR1). This deficiency was found in 84 % of AI-HUS patients versus 2 % in the normal population [5]. It is due to unequal recombinations occurring in the genetic locus of the CFH family genes leading to homozygous deletion of the CFHR1 gene [6]. Despite this genetic background restriction, this etiology has been found in different ethnic groups [7].

This autoimmune form of aHUS has no specific clinical features as compared to the hereditary forms. However extra-renal complications such as liver and/or pancreas involvement or myocarditis may occur at the acute phase. Furthermore, this form is likely to relapse mainly during the first 6 months of follow-up or after renal transplantation. [3, 4] The long-term evolution is comparable to the hereditary forms of aHUS in term of ESDR (end stage renal disease) occurrence. However the early diagnosis and the anti-FH titer monitoring allowing the rapid establishment of specific treatments based on plasma exchanges and immunosuppressive therapy improves the prognosis.

The anti-FH antibodies' isotype is mainly IgG but exceptional IgA isotype has been reported [8]. Presence of anti-FH IgG induces a FH functional defect. Different tests may be performed to evaluate the functional consequences. A perturbation of FH decay accelerating activity has been reported in the first series of patients [2]. Reduced C3b binding when FH was pre-incubated with patients' derived IgG containing FH-autoantibodies has been found. Anti-FH IgG containing plasma have also been reported to induce enhanced hemolysis of non sensitized sheep red blood cells [8, 9], indicating a FH defect in protecting cell surfaces. Recent data suggest also that other FH functional defects implicating complement alternative pathway regulation may be induced by the auto-antibodies such as Factor I co factor activity.

Recently anti-FH IgG has been reported in association with other renal diseases such as the C3 glomerulopathies [10, 11]. However, their frequency and their functional consequences in this context remain to be established.

Here we describe the anti-FH assay procedure and we propose additional assays useful to ensure the diagnosis and evaluate the functional consequences.

2 Materials

2.1 Common Supplies

1. ELISA plates: 96 wells.
2. ELISA plate reader.

2.2 Buffers

1. Phosphate buffered saline (PBS) 10× PBS (0.1 M PBS, pH 7.2).
2. PBS/Tween: add 1 mL Tween 20 to 1 L PBS 1×.
3. Substrate solution for horseradish peroxidase revelation (*see* **Note 1**).
4. Stop solution: of the enzymatic revelation (*see* **Note 2**).

2.3 Antigens and Antibodies

1. Human purified Factor H.
2. Mouse anti-Human IgG–HRP.
3. Anti-FH antibody standard, anti-FH antibody positive and negative controls (*see* **Note 3**).

3 Methods

Prepare all solutions using ultrapure water and analytical grade reagents. Prepare and store all reagents at room temperature (unless indicated otherwise). Diligently follow all waste disposal regulations when disposing waste materials.

3.1 ELISA Coating with Factor H

1. Prepare a solution of purified Factor H at 10 μg/ml PBS (if the concentration of purified FH is 1 mg/ml, it must be diluted at 1/100 in PBS) and distribute 50 μl/well in half of the 96-well plate.
2. Homogenize by gently taping the plate.
3. Cover the microplate with plate seal and leave overnight at +4 °C.

3.2 Blocking

1. Dump coat solution.
2. Dispense 200 μl PBS/0.1 % Tween per well and cover the microplate with plate seal Incubate for 1 h at room temperature (RT).
3. Dump liquid.
4. Perform three washes with 250 μl wash solution (PBS/0.1 % Tween) per well. Dump wash solution and tarp hard on an absorbent paper on the bench to remove all liquid between each wash steps and at the end of the washes.

3.3 Sample Application

All samples (*see* **Note 4**) are dispensed in duplicate in the coated and in the non-coated parts of the plate (*see* Fig. 1):

1. The blank is performed by adding in duplicate 50 μl sample dilution buffer (PBS/0.1 % Tween).
2. The standard curve is prepared by adding twofold serial dilution of standard sample from 1/100 (10/1,000) to 1/3,200 (*see* Fig. 1).

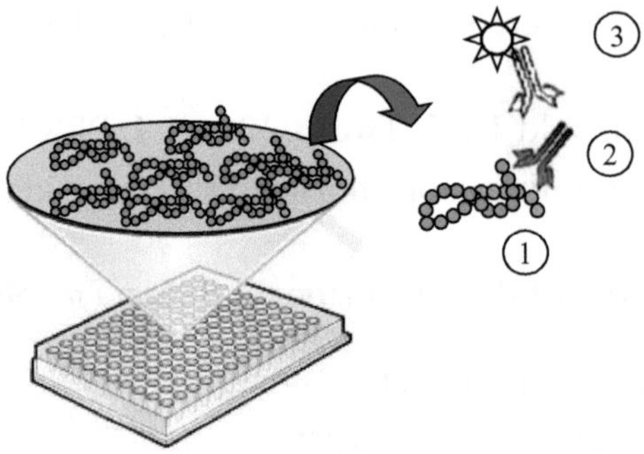

½ dilution
½ dilution
½ dilution
½ dilution

	1	2	3	4	5	6	7	8	9	10	11	12
A	Blk	Blk	NC	NC	PSn...	PSn...	Blk	Blk	NC	NC	PSn...	PSn...
B	Std1	Std1	PS1	PS1	PSn...	PSn...	Std	Std	PS1	PS1	PSn...	PSn...
C	Std2	Std2	PS2	PS2	PSn...	PSn...	Std	Std	PS2	PS2	PSn...	PSn...
D	Std3	Std3	PS3	PS3	PSn...	PSn...	Std	Std	PS3	PS3	PSn...	PSn...
E	Std4	Std4	PS4	PS4	PSn...	PSn...	Std	Std	PS4	PS4	PSn...	PSn...
F	Std5	Std5	PS5	PS5	PSn...	PSn...	Std	Std	PS5	PS5	PSn...	PSn...
G	Std6	Std6	PS6	PS6	PSn...	PSn...	Std	Std	PS6	PS6	PSn...	PSn...
H	PC	PC	PS7	PS7	PSn...	PSn...	PC	PC	PS7	PS7	PSn...	PSn...

Fig. 1 (**a**) *Principle of the technique.* It is a direct ELISA in which the target antigen [here Complement Factor H (1)] is coated in the wells of a microplate. Diluted plasma containing potentially autoantibodies (2) is dispensed in each well. After incubation and washing, a solution containing labeled anti human IgG antibody (3) is added and incubated. After additional washings, bound IgG are revealed using enzymatic colored reaction. (**b**) *Example of plate plane.* The plate is coated only partially (*in grey*) and the samples are dispensed in duplicate in both parts. *Blk* Blank, *Std* standard: the standard curve is obtained by serial dilutions of a reference sample, *PC* positive control, *NC* negative control, *Ps* patient's sample

3. Positive and negative controls are used; dispense 50 μl/well at appropriate dilutions.
4. Patients' samples are dispensed 50 μl/well of 1/50 diluted patients' samples (for example dilute 10 μl patient's sample with 490 μl of sample dilution buffer (PBS/0.1 % Tween)).
5. Dilute positive samples 500-fold then perform serial dilutions in order to obtain OD covered by the standard curve, dispense 50 μl/well.
6. Cover the microplate with plate seal and incubate for 1 h at room temperature (RT).
7. Dump liquid.
8. Perform three washes with 250 μl wash solution (PBS/0.1 % Tween) per well. Dump wash solution and tarp hard on bench

to remove all liquid between each wash and at the end of the washes.

3.4 ELISA Revelation

1. Dispense 50 µl per well of anti-IgG Ab labeled with horseradish peroxidase, diluted at 1/500 in PBS/0.1 % Tween and cover the microplate with plate seal.
2. Leave for 1 h at room temperature (RT).
3. Dump liquid.
4. Perform three washes with 250 µl wash solution (PBS/0.1 % Tween) per well. Dump wash solution and tarp hard to remove all liquid between each washing step and at the end of the washes.

3.5 ELISA Development

1. Dispense 50 µl of substrate solution (*see* **Note 1**) in each well and cover the microplate with plate seal.
2. Leave for 5–7 min in dark and at room temperature (a color appears when positive).
3. Stop the reaction by adding 25 µl of stop solution in each well.
4. Homogenize by gently taping the plate and read the plate on a microplate reader (*see* **Note 5**).
5. Calculate the anti-FH titer (*see* **Note 6**). Interprete the results according to the clinical data and the results of other complementary analysis (*see* **Notes 6–9**).

4 Notes

1. Substrate solution for horseradish peroxidase revelation with orthophenylene diamine: Prepare a substrate solution 10×: 11.2 g $NaH_2PO_4 \times 2H_2O + 650$ mg $C6H5Na_3 \times 2H_2O$, add distilled water for 50 ml final quantity.

   Substrate solution 1× will be prepared extemporaneously with 1 ml substrate solution 10×, 9 ml distilled water, one tablet 10 mg orthophenylene diamine (OPD), 80 µl of aqueous hydrogen peroxide 30 % RPE. The solution is mixed and kept in dark condition until use.

   Alternatively other usual HRP revelation system for ELISA may be used.
2. Stop solution of the enzymatic revelation: for a revelation with OPD use HCl 3 N: Prepare a stock solution with 150 ml HCl 10 N and 450 mL distilled water.
3. Standard and controls: We use plasma exchange products from anti-FH IgG positive patient as anti-FH antibody standard. We use plasma from patient with a moderate titer of anti-FH IgG Anti-FH antibody as positive control and plasma from healthy donors as negative control.

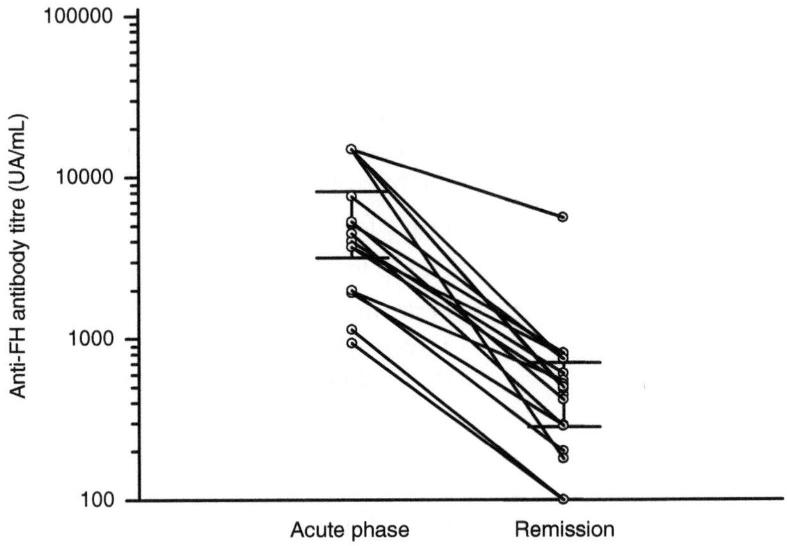

Fig. 2 Evolution of the IgG anti-FH titers during disease evolution. At disease remission and under immunosuppressive treatment the anti-FH IgG titers decrease significantly in most of patients, but remain positive

4. Samples: This assay may be performed using serum or plasma EDTA. Multiple freeze–thaw cycles of the samples may perturb the results mainly by decreasing the titer. Administration of plasma exchange and/or immunosuppressive therapy may decrease the anti-FH IgG titer.
5. ELISA plate reading: To read the plate with a revelation system using OPD, a 490 nm filter is used for reading and a 690 nm filter is used as reference.
6. Anti-FH titers calculation (Fig. 2):
   - The means of optical densities (OD) in duplicates are calculated.
   - The OD obtained in the blank and the non-coated wells must be subtracted to the mean of duplicates if they are superior to 0.100.
   - The titer is calculated according to the standard curve using a linear regression curve and a log/lin axis scales and the standard values as indicated below:
   - Standard 1/100 = 2,000 UA; 1/200 = 1,000 UA; 1/400 = 500 UA; 1/800 = 250 UA; 1/1,600 = 125 UA; 1/3,200 = 62.5 UA
   - If the OD obtained with a patient's sample are higher than the higher OD of the standard curve, the sample will must be

diluted in order to obtain an OD comprised between the higher and the lower OD of the standard curve. The dilution factor will be secondarily applied to the anti-FH titer.

- The positive threshold was calculated by the mean + 5 standard deviations of those obtained in 100 individual healthy donors' plasma and was determined at 100 UA/ml. Titers above this value are considered positive. This cut off should be determined by each laboratory with its specific experimental conditions and control population.

7. In a context of HUS, a biological complement exploration must be performed as soon as possible and preferably before a blood derived product administration.

   This exploration must contain measurement of antigenic levels of Factor H and Factor I by sensitive ELISA techniques and the determination of the peripheral blood cells membrane expression of CD46 (or MCP, Membrane cofactor protein) by flow cytometry, in order to investigate quantitative deficiency of one of these proteins. The exploration must also evaluate antigenic levels, as determined by nephelometry, of C3 and Factor B, which, if decreased, reflect systemic alternative pathway activation.

   In our experience of prospective screening for anti-FH IgG, we observe in more than 50 % of positive samples a systemic alternative pathway activation defined by decreased antigenic levels of C3 and Factor B (FB), associated sometimes with decreased FH levels. In all patients, these levels normalized at disease remission [4].

8. Other assays may complete the analysis:
   - CFHR1 deficiency determination by western blot [5] or by genetic analysis using specific PCR or multiplex ligand probe analysis [6],
   - Lysis of non-sensitized sheep erythrocytes (see Chapter 19),
   - Epitope mapping by ELISA using recombinant FH fragments [9, 12],
   - Research and quantification of factor H-anti-FH autoantibodies complexes by ELISA [8].

9. In a context of C3 glomerulopathy, an extensive complement exploration must also be performed comprising measurement of antigenic levels of Factor H and Factor I, determination of the peripheral blood cells membrane expression of CD46 by flow cytometry, evaluation of C3 and Factor B antigenic levels, and search for autoantibodies directed against alternative pathway C3 convertase (C3 nephritic factor) found in the majority of C3GN patients. The functional consequences of the anti-FH IgG in this context are not yet fully described.

Acknowledgement

This work was supported in part by grants from the Direction de la Recherche Clinique (DRC) of the Assistance Publique-Hôpitaux de Paris (APHP) (PHRC AOM05130; AOM08198; CIRC 06037) and by grants from Agence Nationale de la Recherche (ANR Genopath 2009–2012, 09geno031011).

References

1. Noris M, Remuzzi G (2009) Atypical hemolytic-uremic syndrome. N Engl J Med 361:1676–1687
2. Dragon-Durey MA, Loirat C, Cloarec S, Macher MA, Blouin J, Nivet H, Weiss L, Fridman WH, Fremeaux-Bacchi V (2005) Anti-Factor H autoantibodies associated with atypical hemolytic uremic syndrome. J Am Soc Nephrol 16:555–563
3. Dragon-Durey MA, Blanc C, Garnier A, Hofer J, Sethi SK, Zimmerhackl LB (2010) Anti-factor H autoantibody-associated hemolytic uremic syndrome: review of literature of the autoimmune form of HUS. Semin Thromb Hemost 36:633–640
4. Dragon-Durey MA, Sethi SK, Bagga A, Blanc C, Blouin J, Ranchin B, Andre JL, Takagi N, Cheong HI, Hari P, Le Quintrec M, Niaudet P, Loirat C, Fridman WH, Fremeaux-Bacchi V (2010) Clinical features of anti-factor H autoantibody-associated hemolytic uremic syndrome. J Am Soc Nephrol 21: 2180–2187
5. Jozsi M, Licht C, Strobel S, Zipfel SL, Richter H, Heinen S, Zipfel PF, Skerka C (2008) Factor H autoantibodies in atypical hemolytic uremic syndrome correlate with CFHR1/CFHR3 deficiency. Blood 111:1512–1514
6. Dragon-Durey MA, Blanc C, Marliot F, Loirat C, Blouin J, Sautes-Fridman C, Fridman WH, Fremeaux-Bacchi V (2009) The high frequency of complement factor H related CFHR1 gene deletion is restricted to specific subgroups of patients with atypical haemolytic uraemic syndrome. J Med Genet 46:447–450
7. Lee BH, Kwak SH, Shin JI, Lee SH, Choi HJ, Kang HG, Ha IS, Lee JS, Dragon-Durey MA, Choi Y, Cheong HI (2009) Atypical hemolytic uremic syndrome associated with complement factor H autoantibodies and CFHR1/CFHR3 deficiency. Pediatr Res 66:336–340
8. Strobel S, Hoyer PF, Mache CJ, Sulyok E, Liu WS, Richter H, Oppermann M, Zipfel PF, Jozsi M (2010) Functional analyses indicate a pathogenic role of factor H autoantibodies in atypical haemolytic uraemic syndrome. Nephrol Dial Transplant 25:136–144
9. Jozsi M, Strobel S, Dahse HM, Liu WS, Hoyer PF, Oppermann M, Skerka C, Zipfel PF (2007) Anti factor H autoantibodies block C-terminal recognition function of factor H in hemolytic uremic syndrome. Blood 110:1516–1518
10. Sethi S, Fervenza FC, Zhang Y, Nasr SH, Leung N, Vrana J, Cramer C, Nester CM, Smith RJ (2011) Proliferative glomerulonephritis secondary to dysfunction of the alternative pathway of complement. Clin J Am Soc Nephrol 6:1009–1017
11. Lorcy N, Rioux-Leclercq N, Lombard ML, Le Pogamp P, Vigneau C (2011) Three kidneys, two diseases, one antibody? Nephrol Dial Transplant 26:3811–3813
12. Moore I, Strain L, Pappworth I, Kavanagh D, Barlow PN, Herbert AP, Schmidt CQ, Staniforth SJ, Holmes LV, Ward R, Morgan L, Goodship TH, Marchbank KJ (2010) Association of factor H autoantibodies with deletions of CFHR1, CFHR3, CFHR4, and with mutations in CFH, CFI, CD46, and C3 in patients with atypical hemolytic uremic syndrome. Blood 115:379–387

Chapter 21

Purification of Native Surfactant Protein SP-A from Pooled Amniotic Fluid and Bronchoalveolar Lavage

Najmunisa Karbani, Eswari Dodagatta-Marri, Asif S. Qaseem, Priyaa Madhukaran, Patrick Waters, Anthony G. Tsolaki, Taruna Madan, and Uday Kishore

Abstract

Surfactant protein SP-A is a hydrophilic glycoprotein, similar to SP-D, which plays an important role in pulmonary surfactant homeostasis and innate immunity. SP-A is actively expressed in the alveolar type II cells and Clara cells. Their basic structure consists of triple-helical collagen region and a C-terminal carbohydrate recognition domain (CRD). By binding to the infectious microbes, SP-A (like SP-D) are involved in pathogen opsonization and agglutination and subsequent clearance of the microorganism, via recruitment of phagocytic cells via receptors for the collagen region. SP-A has also been localized at extrapulmonary sites such as salivary epithelium, amniotic fluid, prostate glands, and semen. The presence of SP-A in fetal and maternal tissue and amniotic fluid suggests it is involved in pregnancy and labor. Native SP-A can be purified from amniotic fluid and bronchiolar lavage fluid (BALF) via affinity chromatography. In addition, we also report here a procedure to express and purify a recombinant form of trimeric CRD in *Escherichia coli*. The availability of highly pure native SP-A and CRD region can be central to studies that examine the diverse roles that SP-A play in surfactant homeostasis, pulmonary infection and inflammation and pregnancy.

Key words Surfactant protein-A, SP-A, Purification, Amniotic fluid, BALF, Recombinant, Inflammation, Affinity chromatography

1 Introduction

The respiratory system gets exposed to inhaled toxins, infectious microbes, and allergens. Surfactant proteins are important for lowering surface tension to allow inhalation and expiration without difficulty and to mediate the innate immune response against pathogen causing diseases for the clearance of inhaled microorganisms to maintain lung sterility [1]. There are four surfactant proteins characterized so far including; SP-A, SP-B, SP-C, and SP-D. Surfactant protein A (SP-A) are phospholipid-binding proteins

Mihaela Gadjeva (ed.), *The Complement System: Methods and Protocols*, Methods in Molecular Biology, vol. 1100,
DOI 10.1007/978-1-62703-724-2_21,

synthesized by alveolar type II epithelial cells and stored as intracellular inclusion organelles called "lamellar bodies". During deep inhalation, the surfactants are secreted covering the alveolar space minimizing surface tension at the air-liquid interface to prevent lungs from collapsing. They are collagen-containing, calcium dependent C-type lectins belonging to the collectin family [2, 3]. SP-A is the most abundant protein amongst the other surfactant proteins, making up 90 % of the proteins out of SP-A, SP-B, SP-C, and SP-D. SP-A is expressed by two alleles; SP-A1 and SP-A2 which are localized on the long arm of chromosome 10 at position 10q21-24 forming a cluster with SP-D and MBL [4]. In comparison to SP-D, SP-A is tenfolds higher in level of expression and plays a major role in surfactant turnover and homeostasis [5, 6]. The primary structure of SP-A consists of an amino-terminus, triple-helical collagen-like domain of tripepetide Gly-X-Y repeats, a lectin connector neck region which stabilizes the trimers and a C-terminus C-type lectin carbohydrate recognition domain (CRD). SP-A forms a hexameric shape consisting of 18 polypeptide (6 trimerized) chains with seven amino acids at the N-terminal, 23 Gly-x-y repeats at the collagen region and 148 amino acids at the globular C-terminal [7, 8]. The overall structure of SP-A resembles that of C1q with bouquet-like conformation. The hexameric, hydrophobic protein of 630 KDa is made up of 6 × 105 kDa subunits. These subunits are made up of three polypeptide chains of 35 KDa each [9]. The three polypeptides are bound together by the disulfide bonds at the N-terminal region.

SP-A plays a major role in the pulmonary innate immunity. In the trimeric form, the CRD can recognize and bind to carbohydrates moieties and pattern associated molecular patterns (PAMPs) on the surfaces of viruses, bacteria, yeast, and fungi in a Ca^{2+}-dependent manner [10, 11]. They can also recognize and opsonize pathogenic microorganisms via CRD region for chemotaxis by interacting to receptors on immune molecules such as macrophages and neutrophils [12]. SP-A is known to exert both inflammatory as well as anti-inflammatory effects depending on the receptor it binds to. The interaction of SP-A via calcium-dependent CRD to signal inhibitory regulatory protein α (SIRPα) results in an anti-inflammatory effect and the binding of SP-A collagen domain to CD91/calreticulin activates the pro-inflammatory pathway [13].

SP-A proteins are lipid and carbohydrate recognition molecules which in most cases bind to glucose and mannose residues part of most microbial ligands. SP-A can recognize both gram-positive bacteria such as *Staphylococcus aureus* [12] and *Mycobacterium tuberculosis* [14] and gram-negative bacteria. In the case of *M. tuberculosis*, SP-A enhances the interaction of *M. tuberculosis* to alveolar macrophages [14, 15] suggesting its antimicrobial activity for its clearance. SP-A is relevant for yeast and fungi agglutination and phagocytosis. In cases of *Candida albicans* SP-A suppresses pro-inflammatory cytokine and chemokine production, i.e., TNF-α, IL-1β, MIP-α, and MCP-1 by alveolar macrophages and monocytes [16, 17].

By interacting with phagocytes, SP-A not only modulates the release of several cytokines, but also primes innate immune response against pathogens. In the situation of a viral infection caused by influenza A virus (IAV), the virus can enter the host lungs via its trimeric hemagglutinin (HA) molecule binding to sialic acid residues on the surface of epithelial cells of the lungs. SP-A benefits the host in two main ways: Firstly, the sialic acid present on the CRD of SP-A allows IAV to bind to promote agglutination inhibiting the infectivity [18]. Secondly, the binding of SP-A to IAV enhances virus to stimulate the respiratory burst of neutrophils [19].

SP-A is considered one of the primordial agents of innate immune defense. It can protect against allergenic challenges via allergen scavenging, inhibition of allergen-IgE cross-linking and histamine release, suppression of mast cells, basophils, B and T-cell proliferation, modulation of dendritic cells and macrophages, and Th cell polarization [20]. Subsequently, SP-A has been shown to bind to house dust mite extract *Dermatophagoides pteronyssinus; Derp* and 3-week culture filtrate (3wcf) as well as glycoprotein allergens; gp55 and gp45 of *Aspergillus fumigatus* in a carbohydrate specific and calcium dependent manner, blocking histamine release [21, 22]. This shows the significance of SP-A protection against in pulmonary hypersensitivity by resisting allergenic challenges and dampening hypersensitivity reactions in the lungs.

Using RT-PCR, SP-A is shown not to only synthesize in type II alveolar cells and Clara cells in the lungs, but extra-pulmonary sites of expression have also been shown. These include serum, amniotic fluid [23], sputum [24], thymus, prostate and mesentery [25], and also synoviocytes, lacrimal and salivary epithelia [26] as well as the human colon [27]. In pregnancy, the expression of SP-A is induced as early as 20 weeks gestation during fetal lung development. In the third trimester, there is a sudden surge of SP-A at 26 weeks rising six times more than SP-D between 26 and 40 weeks gestation [28], this could be linked to a possible signal to labor by preparing fetal lung maturation for survival in extra-uterine environment and pathogen clearance to prevent intra-amniotic infection.

In this chapter we describe protocols illustrating the purification of native SP-A from amniotic fluid and bronchoalveolar lavage fluid (BALF) adapted from Strong et al. [29], via Affinity Chromatography. We also describe the expression of a recombinant fragment of human SP-A (rhSP-A) in *Escherichia coli* and its purification via affinity chromatography. The rhSP-A contains the homotrimeric neck and CRD region inserted into the pET-101 vector. The bacterial cloning vector, pET-101 contains a T7 promoter site and an ampicillin resistant gene. pET-101 is then transfected into the competent plasmid, BL21 (λDE3) pLysS. This plasmid has a T7 lysozyme inserted to suppress the basal levels of T7 promoter by naturally inhibiting T7 RNA polymerase. The recombinant protein is localized in inclusion bodies due to over-expression. Following denaturation–renaturation cycles with urea gradient, the rhSP-A is finally purified using a maltose–sepharose matrix in affinity chromatography.

2 Materials

2.1 Purification of Native SP-A from Amniotic Fluid

1. 8 M Urea buffer I: 50 mM Tris–HCl, pH 7.4, 100 mM NaCl, 5 mM $CaCl_2$, 0.02 % NaN_3, 8 M urea.
2. Buffer I: 50 mM Tris–HCl, pH 7.4, 100 mM NaCl, 5 mM $CaCl_2$, 0.02 % NaN_3.

2.2 Affinity Chromatography for Native SP-A Purification

1. Affinity buffer I: 50 mM Tris–HCl, pH 7.4, 100 mM NaCl, 5 mM $CaCl_2$, 0.02 % NaN_3.
2. Affinity buffer I with 1 M NaCl: 50 mM Tris–HCl, pH 7.4, 1 M NaCl, 5 mM $CaCl_2$, 0.02 % NaN_3.
3. SP-A elution buffer with EDTA: 50 mM Tris–HCl, pH 7.4, 100 mM NaCl, 10 mM EDTA, 0.02 % NaN_3.

2.3 Purification of SP-A from BALF

1. Affinity buffer: 10 mM $CaCl_2$, 20 mM Tris–HCl, pH 7.5.
2. SP-A elution buffer: 10 mM EDTA, 20 mM Tris–HCl, pH 7.5.

2.4 BL21 (λDE3) pLysS: Competent Cell of Transformation and Expression

1. 1 L LB media: 10 g Tryptone, 10 g yeast, 5 g NaCl.
2. 100 mg/ml Ampicillin: 1 g Ampicillin in 10 ml of autoclaved dH_2O—filter-sterilized by passing through 0.2 μm filter.
3. 50 mg/ml Chloramphenicol: 0.5 g Chloramphenicol in 10 ml ethanol (100 %).
4. 1 M IPTG—2.83 g in 10 ml of autoclaved dH_2O—filter-sterilized by passing through 0.2 μm filter.

2.5 Cell Lysis and Inclusion Bodies Preparation in Order to Extract Recombinant SP-A Fragment Protein Containing Homotrimeric Neck and CRD Domain (rhSP-A)

1. 50 mg/ml Lysozyme: 0.5 g in 10 ml of autoclaved dH_2O use.
2. 100 mM Phenylmethylsulfonyl fluoride (PMSF) stock: 0.174 g PMSF dissolved in 10 ml isopropanol.
3. 50 ml/L Pellet Lysis buffer: 50 mM Tris–HCl, 200 mM NaCl, 5 mM EDTA, 0.1 %Triton-X, 1 mM PMSF, 0.50 mg/ml lysozyme (add PMSF and lysozyme (1:100 dilution of stock) fresh into lysis buffer just before use).

2.6 Denaturation of Inclusion Bodies and Renaturation of rhSP-A

1. 50 ml Resolubilization buffer with 6 M urea: 50 mM Tris–HCl, pH 7.5, 100 mM NaCl, 5 mM EDTA, 70 μl 2-mercaptoethanol (β-ME), 0.02 % NaN_3, 6 M urea.
2. 1 L 4 M-Urea buffer: 50 mM Tris–HCl, pH 7.5, 100 mM NaCl, 5 mM EDTA, 0.02 % NaN_3, 4 M urea.
3. 1 L 2 M-Urea buffer: 50 mM Tris–HCl, pH 7.5, 100 mM NaCl, 5 mM EDTA, 0.02 % NaN_3, 2 M urea
4. 1 L 1 M-Urea buffer: 50 mM Tris–HCl, pH 7.5, 100 mM NaCl, 5 mM EDTA, 0.02 % NaN_3, 1 M urea.
5. 1 L Final dialysis buffer: 50 mM Tris–HCl, pH 7.5, 100 mM NaCl, 5 mM EDTA, 0.02 % NaN_3.
6. 1 L Calcium buffer/Affinity buffer: 20 mM Tris–HCl pH 7.5, 100 mM NaCl, 5 mM $CaCl_2$, 0.02 % NaN_3.

2.7 Purification of rhSP-A via Affinity Chromatography Using Maltose–Sepharose Purification Column

1. 1 L Affinity buffer: 50 mM Tris–HCl, pH 7.5, 100 mM NaCl, 5 mM $CaCl_2$, 0.02 % NaN_3.
2. 500 ml High salt buffer: 1 M NaCl, 50 mM Tris–HCl, pH 7.4, 5 mM $CaCl_2$, 0.02 % NaN_3.
3. SP-A elution buffer containing 5 mM EDTA: 50 mM Tris–HCl, pH 7.4, 100 mM NaCl, 5 mM EDTA, 0.02 % NaN_3.

2.8 Sodium Dodecyl Sulfate Polyacrylamide Gel Electrophoresis

1. SDS-gel: 30 % Bis-acrylamide, 1.5 M Tris–HCl, pH 8.8 (resolving gel), 1.0 M Tris–HCl, pH 6.8 (stacking gel), 10 % dodecylsulfate (SDS), 10 % ammonium persulfate (APS), TEMED.
2. 1× Running buffer (1 L): 3 g Tris base, 14.4 g glycine, 10 ml SDS (10 %), 990 ml dH_2O.
3. 2× SDS sample buffer (10 ml): 1.25 ml 0.5 M Tris–HCl, pH 6.8, 2 ml 50 % glycerol, 2 ml 10 % SDS, 0.5 ml β-ME, 0.5 % Bromophenol blue, 4 ml dH_2O.
4. Coomassie blue stain (1 L): 100 ml Glacial acetic acid, 400 ml methanol, 1 g Coomassie Blue R250, and 500 ml dH_2O.
5. De-stain solution (1 L): 100 ml Glacial acetic acid, 400 ml methanol, and 500 ml dH_2O.

2.9 Western Blot Buffers

1× Transfer buffer (1 L): 2.9 g Glycine, 5.8 g Tris base, 0.37 g SDS, 200 ml methanol, 800 ml dH_2O.

3 Methods

3.1 Purification of SP-A from Human Amniotic Fluid

Amniotic fluid is normally collected following vaginal rupturing of the fetal membranes or during spontaneous rupturing. The collected amniotic fluid is usually stored at −80 °C after equilibration with 5 mM $CaCl_2$ until it is required for purification.

1. Thaw 1 L of pooled amniotic fluid completely by incubating at 37 °C (usually it takes 5–6 h) with occasional mixing. *See* **Note 1**.
2. Pass amniotic fluid through 3 mm Whatman filter paper three times for a clearer suspension and to avoid future clogging of maltose-sepharose column.
3. Pass amniotic fluid through a cell strainer to remove fat and other large aggregates/debris.
4. Centrifuge at 13,800 × *g* for 40 min at 4 °C to separate SP-A rich pellet from the supernatant that is rich in SP-D.
5. Add 20 ml of 8 M urea buffer I to the pellet for further SP-A extraction. The urea helps to extract and unfold the protein which is then folded back to correct conformation by urea gradient dialysis.
6. Stir for 1 h at 4 °C using a magnetic stirrer to allow solubilization of SP-A.
7. Centrifuge the suspension at 13,800 × *g* in a microcentrifuge for 20 min at 4 °C and collect the supernatant.
8. Transfer the supernatant into a dialysis membrane and dialyze against 1 L of Buffer I containing no urea inside a measuring cylinder to remove urea from SP-A. Leave cylinder on a magnetic stirrer overnight at 4 °C.
9. Next day, collect dialysate (~20 ml) in a centrifugation tube and spin at 10,000 × *g* for 20 min at 4 °C and discard the pellet. Solubilized and correctly folded SP-A should be in the supernatant.
10. Proceed to affinity chromatography.

3.2 Affinity Chromatography

1. Wash 5 ml bed volume maltose-sepharose with 50 ml autoclaved distilled water (the preparation of maltose-sepharose is described in Chapter 22), followed by equilibration with four bed volumes of Affinity Buffer I.
2. Add the equilibrated maltose-sepharose into the supernatant containing SP-A and allow it to mix on a magnetic stirrer for 30 min at room temperature. This allows binding of soluble SP-A to maltose-sepharose.
3. Pass this supernatant containing maltose-sepharose bound to SP-A through the column three times in order to allow the bed to settle.
4. Wash the column after collecting all the flow through with five bed volumes of Affinity Buffer I containing 1 M NaCl
5. Elute 20 × 1 ml fractions of SP-A with Buffer I containing 10 mM EDTA. Collect all 1 ml fractions over ice (*see* **Note 2**).
6. 25 μl of each fraction is separated on a 12 % SDS-PAGE (*see* Table 1) to assess protein and its purity (Fig. 1).

Table 1
Components and volume for preparing 12 and 15 % SDS-PAGE

Resolving gel	12 %	15 %	Stacking gel	
Components	**Volume (ml)**		**Components**	**Volume (ml)**
dH_2O	3.3	2.3	dH_2O	3.4
30 % Bis-acrylamide mix	4	5	30 % Bis-acrylamide mix	0.83
1.5 M Tris–HCl, pH 8.8	2.5	2.5	1.0 M Tris–HCl, pH 6.8	0.63
10 % SDS	0.1	0.1	10 % SDS	0.05
10 % APS	0.1	0.1	10 % APS	0.05
TEMED	0.015	0.015	TEMED	0.014

Prepare the stacking and resolving gel separately and add resolving gel first to the casting plates. After this has polymerized, add TEMED to the stacking gel and mix. Add this on top of the resolving gel inserting a comb to create wells after polymerization. The gel is then ready to be placed in a holder and into the tank containing 1× running buffer for wells to be filled with samples and protein marker. Set voltage to 100 V for 90 min for proteins to be separated according to size and charge

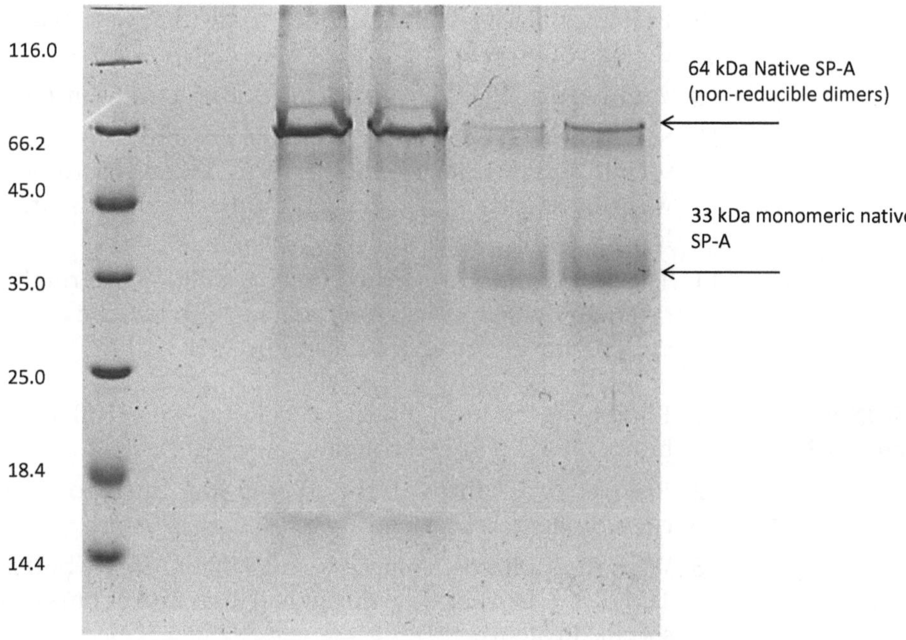

Fig. 1 SDS-PAGE (10 % w/v) analysis of purified native SP-A under reducing conditions purified from BAL fluid. Majority of SP-A is the monomeric polypeptide chain of SP-A (33 kDa) and the lighter band corresponds to the non-reducible dimer proportion of SP-A. There are slight traces of the SP-A in its oligomeric form. This is confirmed by western blotting

3.3 SDS-PAGE: 12 % and 15 %

To prepare a 12 % or 15 % SDS-PAGE, follow the instructions below:

1. In two separate 50 ml beakers label one "resolving gel" and the other "stacking gel".
   For a standard size gel, 10 ml of resolving gel and 5 ml of stacking gel is sufficient.
2. Assemble the clean glass plates onto the glass holder and stand and check for no leakages.
3. Prepare resolving gel for either 12 % or 15 % (Table 1). *See* **Note 3**.
4. Once the TEMED has been added to the resolving gel the polymerization reaction will have begun, mix well then add the resolving gel to the plates (*see* **Note 4**).
5. After 20 min the gel will have polymerized. Add 10 % APS and TEMED to the stacking gel and pipette directly on top of the resolving gel, inserting the comb to form wells as the gel polymerizes.
6. Mix the protein samples with equal amounts of 2 × SDS sample buffer and heat to 95 °C for 10 min for protein denaturation.
7. The sample is then cooled to room temperature and centrifuged at 13,800 × *g* for 1 min before loading one sample per well.
8. Protein standard marker is added to the first well to determine the size of protein.
9. Add 1× running buffer to the tank as instructed by manufacturer.
10. Set the power pack connected to the gel apparatus to 100 V for 90 min to allow the proteins to be separated according to size, with the smaller molecules separating through the gel matrix faster with the larger molecules trailing behind.
11. The gel is then placed in staining solution overnight to be taken up by the proteins and destained to remove background staining for the protein bands to become visible.

3.4 Purification of SP-A from BALF

1. Equilibrate maltose-sepharose column with 100 ml Affinity buffer. Discard flow through.
2. Pass the BALF through the column four times to ensure efficient binding.
3. Wash the sepharose column with 10 ml of Affinity buffer I with 1 M NaCl. Discard flow through. This removes unbound nonspecific proteins.
4. Elute the proteins with 20 ml SP-A eluting buffer containing EDTA in 1 ml fractions over ice (Fig. 2).

3.5 Competent Cell Preparation of BL21 (λDE3) pLysS for Recombinant SP-A Production

1. Inoculate a single colony of BL21 (λDE3) pLysS in 5 ml LB containing 5 μl of chloramphenicol (50 mg/ml).
2. Incubate overnight (~16 h) in a 37 °C shaker at 700 × *g*. Primary inoculum is now ready.

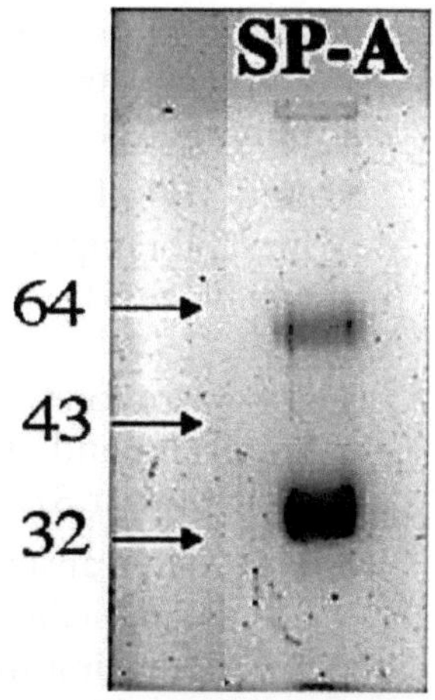

Fig. 2 Western blot to detect native SP-A from amniotic fluid. Initially 1 and 2 μg proteins were separate on a SDS-PAGE and transferred at 320 amp for 90 min. The membrane was blocked with 5 % milk-powder/PBS buffer and probed with anti-human SP-A in a 1:5,000 dilution. The primary antibody was detected with a HRP conjugated Protein A in a 1:5,000 dilution. The bands were visible after DAB reacting with HRP to display protein bands; monomers and dimers of SP-A at 33 kDa and 64 kDa, respectively

3. Next day, transfer 1 ml of primary inoculum into 25 ml LB containing chloramphenicol.
4. Incubate for 2–3 h in the shaking incubator for cells to grow to log phase indicated by 0.3 against plain LB medium at $OD_{600\ nm}$.
5. Centrifuge the sample at 1,800 × *g* for 10 min to collect BL21 (λDE3) pLysS cells to pellet.
6. Discard supernatant in disinfectant and resuspend pellet in 12.5 ml 0.1 M $CaCl_2$.
7. Incubate pellet on ice for 1 h to make cells competent.
8. Centrifuge cells again at low speed centrifugation 1,800 × *g* for 5 min to pellet the cells.
9. Discard supernatant and resuspend cells in 2 ml 0.1 M $CaCl_2$.
10. The cells are now ready for transformation.

3.6 Transformation of Recombinant SP-A-Trimeric (pUK-A1) in BL21 (λDE3) pLysS

1. Take 200 μl of competent cells and add to a 15 ml Falcon tube.
2. Add 2 μl of plasmid directly to the competent cells and incubate on ice for 1 h.
3. Heat shock the cells to take up the plasmid at 42 °C for 90 s.
4. Transfer the culture to ice for 5 min.

5. Add 800 μl of LB to the sample to make 1 ml total volume, and incubate at 37 °C for approximately 45 min to allow one full cell cycle to take place to increase transformed cells.
6. Add 100 μl of transformed cultured to an LB agar + ampicillin/chloramphenicol plate and incubate overnight at 37 °C (*see* **Note 5**).

3.7 Pilot-Scale Expression

1. Inoculate four separate colonies in 5 ml LB containing 5 μl of ampicillin and chloramphenicol to grow overnight in shaking incubator at 37 °C.
2. Next day, transfer 500 μl of primary culture into 10 ml LB with 10 μl ampicillin and chloramphenicol and incubate in the 37 °C shaking incubator to grow to log phase, indicated by a reading of 0.6–0.8 at 600 nm against plain LB medium.
3. When optimum OD has been reached, take 1 ml of un-induced sample and add 5 μl of 1 M IPTG to make a final concentration of 0.5 μM to the 10 ml culture.
4. Incubate both induced and un-induced in a 37 °C shaking incubator for a further 3 h to allow induction to take place and to over-express protein of interest.
5. After 3 h, take 1 ml of un-induced and induced samples and centrifuge at 13,800 × *g* for 15 min to pellet cells.
6. Discard supernatant.
7. Add 100 μl of 2× treatment buffer and denature proteins to separate 10 μl of each sample on a 15 % SDS-PAGE (*see* Table 1) (*see* **Note 6**).
8. After observing gel, the colony giving best expression can be streaked on a LB agar plate containing ampicillin and chloramphenicol using the primary inoculum.
9. This plate of colonies can be used to make multiple large-scale batches before reseeding the plate of colonies the following month.
10. Proceed to large-scale expression.

3.8 Large-Scale Expression

1. Inoculate one colony from SP-A-trimeric culture plate into 25 ml LB medium with 25 μl ampicillin and chloramphenicol.
2. Incubate in a 37 °C shaking incubator for 16 h.
3. Transfer 25 ml of the primary culture into 1 L LB medium with 1,000 μl ampicillin and chloramphenicol.
4. Incubate this secondary culture at 37 °C shaker for approximately 3 h until the OD reaches between 0.6 and 0.8.
5. Pipette 1 ml sample from culture for negative control ("un-induced sample").

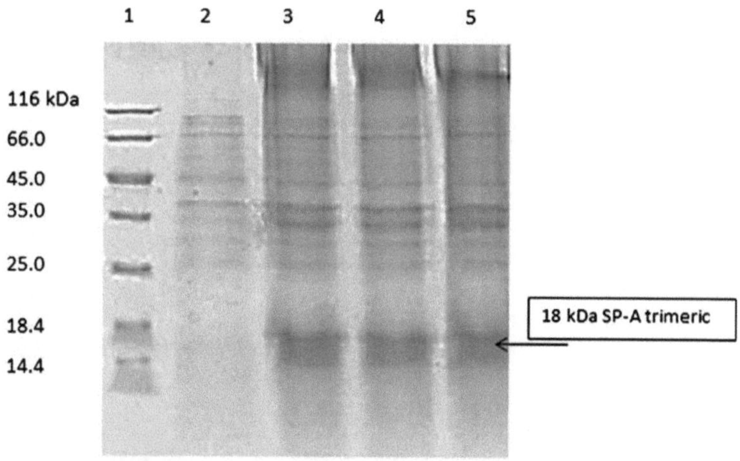

Fig. 3 SDS-PAGE after large-scale expression of SP-A-trimeric. Expression of recombinant SP-A showing un-induced (*lane 2*) and induced (*lane 3–5*) of 3 × 1 L batches. *Lane 1*: Protein marker contains molecular weight ranging from lowest to highest: 14.4, 18.4, 25.0, 35.0, 45.0, 66.2, 116.0, *Lane 2*: un-induced, *Lane 3–5*: induced batches 1–3. 10 μl of sample including 2× treatment buffer was loaded to each well

6. To the rest of the sample, "induce" add 500 μl 0.5 mM IPTG from 1 M stock and re-incubated in the 37 °C shaker for 3 h with "un-induced" sample.
7. After 3 h, take 1 ml from "induced" sample and centrifuge along with 1 ml "un-induced" sample at high speed 13,800 × *g* for 15 min.
8. Discard supernatant and add 100 μl of 2× treatment buffer to the pellet. Denature at 95 °C and separate on a 15 % SDS-PAGE (Table 1) to determine protein expression (Fig. 3).
9. Centrifuge the entire 1 L "induced" culture at 13,800 × *g* at 4°C, for 15 min to collect pellet containing proteins in inclusion bodies.
10. The pellet can be stored at −20 °C or used straight away for lysing and sonication.

3.9 Lysing Inclusion Bodies to Extract Protein

1. If pellet was stored at −20 °C, it should be thawed on ice.
2. Resuspend the pellet in 50 ml lysis buffer and stir at 4 °C.
3. Whilst stirring, add PMSF to 1 mM and 0.5 mg/ml lysozyme to the lysis buffer. Allow to stir for ~2 h (until there are no visible lumps).
4. Keep suspension on ice and sonicate at 4 kHz for 30 s with 2 min interval between each cycle to allow sonicator to cool down, repeating for 15 cycles.

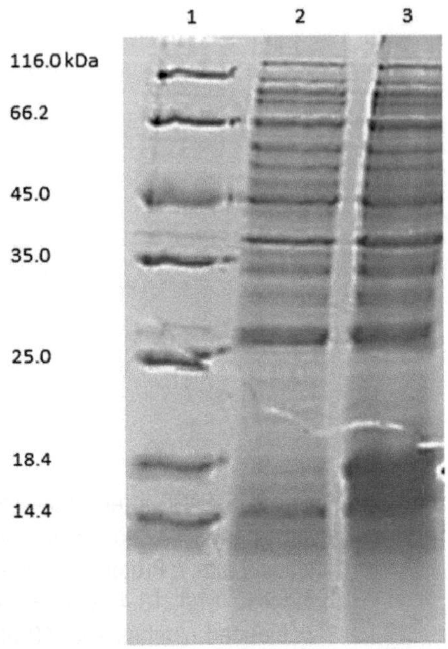

Fig. 4 15 % SDS-PAGE after lysis, sonication. Pellets containing SP-A in inclusion bodies are lysed and sonicated. After centrifugation of sample, protein is present in pellet before solubilsation. *Lane 1*: Protein marker contains molecular weight ranging from lowest to highest: 14.4, 18.4, 25.0, 35.0, 45.0, 66.2, 116.0, *Lane 2*: supernatant after centrifugation of lysed and sonicated sample, *Lane 3*: pellet after centrifugation of lysed and sonicated sample. 10 μl of sample including 2× treatment buffer was loaded to each well

5. Centrifuge sample to collect the protein rich pellet out of inclusion bodies at 13,800 × *g* for 15 min at 4 °C.
6. Collect 50 μl sample of supernatant and pellet to separate on a 12 % SDS-PAGE (Table 1) to confirm protein is visible in pellet (Fig. 4) (*see* **Note 7**).

3.10 Denaturing and Refolding Recombinant Proteins

1. To the pellet, add 50 ml resolubilization buffer containing 6 M urea.
2. Incubated pellet at 4 °C whilst on a magnetic flea containing resolubilization buffer for exactly 1 h.
3. Centrifuge sample at 13,800 × *g*, at 4 °C, for 15 min to separate the debris rich pellet and supernatant containing protein. Take a sample of the supernatant to separate on an SDS-PAGE to ensure protein is in the supernatant and has been extracted out of pellet.

3.11 Stepwise Dialysis to Refold Protein and Remove Urea Traces

1. Transfer the supernatant into a dialysis bag and add to a 1 L measuring cylinder containing 1 L 4 M-urea buffer and fresh β-ME.
2. Dialyze the sample for 2 h on a magnetic stirrer at 4 °C.

3. Transfer the dialysis bag to another 1 L cylinder containing 2 M-urea buffer with fresh β-ME.
4. Repeat **step 2**.
5. Transfer the dialysis bag to another 1 L cylinder containing 1 M-urea buffer with fresh β-ME and repeat **step 2**.
6. Transfer the dialysis bag to another 1 L cylinder containing 0 M-urea final dialysis buffer.
7. Dialyze sample overnight at 4 °C whilst stirring.
8. The next day, clarify dialysate by centrifugation at 13,800 × *g*, at 4 °C, for 15 min.
9. Transfer the supernatant into a new dialysis bag and dialyze against 1 L of calcium buffer for 3 h to completely remove traces of urea.
10. Clarify dialysate by centrifugation at 13,800 × *g*, at 4 °C, for 15 min.
11. The sample is now ready for affinity chromatography.

3.12 Recombinant SP-A Purification by Affinity Chromatography

1. Wash maltose-sepharose column thoroughly with 100 ml autoclaved dH_2O.
2. Equilibrate the maltose-sepharose column with 75 ml affinity buffer (with 5 mM $CaCl_2$).
3. Pass the supernatant through the maltose-sepharose column four times.
4. Wash column with 20 ml high-salt buffer (1 M NaCl) to remove any debris and unbound proteins.
5. Elute proteins with 20 ml elution buffer in 1 ml fractions over ice.
6. Estimate protein concentration at OD_{280}, using elution buffer as a reference.
7. Separate proteins on a 12 % SDS-PAGE (Table 1) to determine protein estimation and purity (Fig. 5).

3.13 Western Blot

1. Initially, prepare a 12 % SDS-PAGE (Table 1) and separate desired protein of interest to be probed.
2. After the dye front has reached the end of the gel, remove gel and equilibrate in 1× transfer buffer along with fibro pads, nitrocellulose membrane and filter paper for 10 min.
3. Assemble the sandwich in the following order: fibro pads, 2× filter paper, gel, membrane, 2× filter paper and fibro pads (*see* **Note 8**).
4. After closing the cassette, place inside the holder and into the tank containing 1× transfer buffer with the black side of cassette facing the black side of holder.

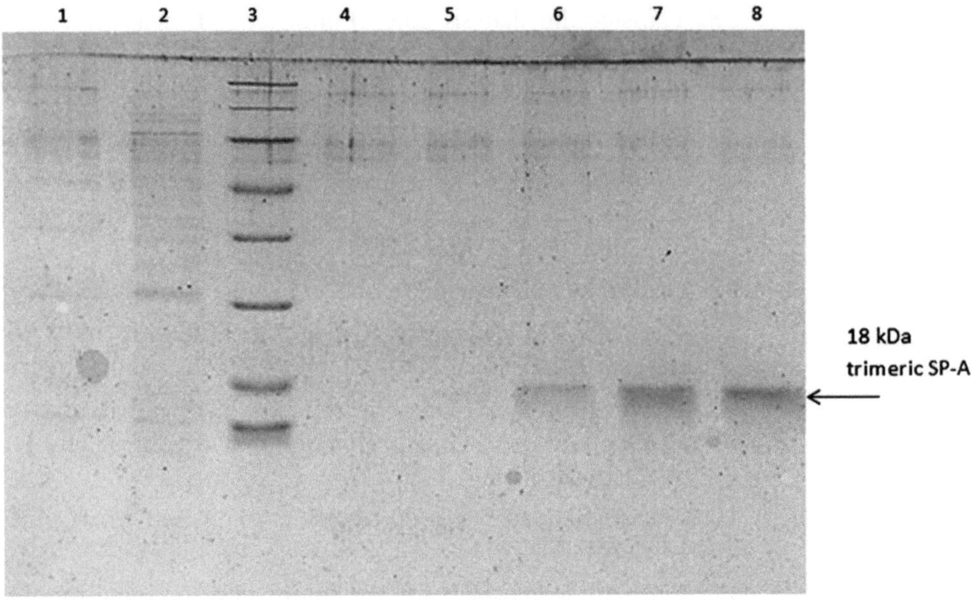

Fig. 5 12 % SDS-PAGE of purified SP-A samples after affinity chromatography. The eluted samples were separated on a protein gel to determine size and purity. As controls the flow through after passing sample and flow through after washing column with affinity buffer was loaded to check for protein loss and contaminant removal. *Lane 1*: flow through from sample containing recombinant trimeric SP-A, *Lane 2*: flow through after washing column with affinity buffer containing 1 M NaCl, *Lane 3*: Protein marker contains molecular weight ranging from lowest to highest: 14.4 kDa, 18.4 kDa, 25.0 kDa, 35.0 kDa, 45.0 kDa, 66.2 kDa, 116.0 kDa, *Lane 4–8*: eluted samples 1–5 containing pure protein. 20 μl of sample including 2× treatment buffer was loaded to each well

5. For transfer to take place, set power pack to 340 amp for 90 min for proteins to be transferred to the nitrocellulose membrane.
6. Block the membrane with 5 % nonfat milk powder/PBS buffer overnight at room temperature to prevent nonspecific binding.
7. The next day, decant the blocking buffer and wash membrane with 20 ml 1× PBS for 10 min.
8. Add 10 ml of 1:500 dilution of primary antibody (rabbit anti-human SP-A) (1 mg/ml) to the membrane and incubate for 2 h at room temperature on a rocker.
9. Decant the antibody and wash the membrane thrice with PBS containing 0.05 % Tween-20, for 10 min each removing old wash buffer each time.
10. Add 10 ml of 1:1,000 dilution of secondary antibody (protein A-HRP) (1 mg/ml) over the membrane and leave for a 1 h incubating at room temperature on a rocker.

11. Again, decant the antibody and wash the membrane with PBS Tween 20, 0.05 % thrice for 10 min each.
12. Whilst the final wash is taking place, prepare two tablets of DAB (sigma) dissolved in dH_2O as recommended by manufacturer.
13. After removing wash buffer, pour DAB over the membrane and incubate for 2–10 min until sufficient color develops for bands to be visible.

4 Notes

1. Proteins can be cleaved by proteases if left for too long at room temperature.
2. If the concentration is low then the samples can be pooled and concentrated using polyethylene glycol.
3. Keep at least 1 cm distance from the wells to the resolving gel to allow proteins to stack evenly before being separated through the resolving gel.
4. Do not add TEMED until just before adding to the glass plates as this will start the polymerization reaction.
5. Add the rest of the culture (i.e., 900 μl) to 5 ml LB and grow overnight to streak next day. This is done as a backup, in case the number of transformed colonies is very low.
6. Un-induced sample is used as a control to detect SP-A. SP-A should be expressed in induced sample only, which is indicated as a thick band most highly expressed at ~18 kDa.
7. Supernatant can be stored at −20 °C in case there was still some protein that needed further extraction.
8. Ensure that there are no air bubbles in between the gel and membrane as this will affect the transfer of proteins.

References

1. Crouch E, Wright JR (2001) Surfactant proteins A and D and pulmonary host defense. Annu Rev Physiol 63:521–554
2. Lu J et al (2002) Collectins and ficolins: sugar pattern recognition molecules of the mammalian innate immune system. Biochim Biophys Acta 1572(2–3):387–400
3. Holmskov U, Thiel S, Jensenius JC (2003) Collections and ficolins: humoral lectins of the innate immune defense. Annu Rev Immunol 21:547–578
4. Sorensen GL, Husby S, Holmskov U (2007) Surfactant protein A and surfactant protein D variation in pulmonary disease. Immunobiology 212(4–5):381–416
5. Ogasawara Y et al (1994) Chimeras of surfactant proteins A and D identify the carbohydrate recognition domains as essential for phospholipid interaction. J Biol Chem 269(47):29785–29792
6. Haagsman HP, van Golde LM (1991) Synthesis and assembly of lung surfactant. Annu Rev Physiol 53:441–464
7. Tenner AJ et al (1989) Human pulmonary surfactant protein (SP-A), a protein structurally homologous to C1q, can enhance FcR- and CR1-mediated phagocytosis. J Biol Chem 264(23):13923–13928
8. Wright JR (2005) Immunoregulatory functions of surfactant proteins. Nat Rev Immunol 5(1):58–68

9. Voss T et al (1988) Macromolecular organization of natural and recombinant lung surfactant protein SP 28–36. Structural homology with the complement factor C1q. J Mol Biol 201(1):219–227
10. King RJ et al (1986) Interaction between the 35 kDa apolipoprotein of pulmonary surfactant and saturated phosphatidylcholines. Effects of temperature. Biochim Biophys Acta 879(1):1–13
11. Hawgood S et al (1987) Nucleotide and amino acid sequences of pulmonary surfactant protein SP 18 and evidence for cooperation between SP 18 and SP 28–36 in surfactant lipid adsorption. Proc Natl Acad Sci U S A 84(1):66–70
12. Geertsma MF et al (1994) Binding of surfactant protein A to C1q receptors mediates phagocytosis of *Staphylococcus aureus* by monocytes. Am J Physiol 267(5 Pt 1):L578–L584
13. Gardai SJ et al (2003) By binding SIRPalpha or calreticulin/CD91, lung collectins act as dual function surveillance molecules to suppress or enhance inflammation. Cell 115(1):13–23
14. Gaynor CD et al (1995) Pulmonary surfactant protein A mediates enhanced phagocytosis of *Mycobacterium tuberculosis* by a direct interaction with human macrophages. J Immunol 155 (11):5343–5351
15. Pasula R et al (1997) Surfactant protein A (SP-A) mediates attachment of *Mycobacterium tuberculosis* to murine alveolar macrophages. Am J Respir Cell Mol Biol 17(2):209–217
16. Rosseau S et al (1997) Phagocytosis of viable *Candida albicans* by alveolar macrophages: lack of opsonin function of surfactant protein A. J Infect Dis 175(2):421–428
17. Rosseau S et al (1999) Surfactant protein A down-regulates proinflammatory cytokine production evoked by *Candida albicans* in human alveolar macrophages and monocytes. J Immunol 163(8):4495–4502
18. Benne CA et al (1995) Interactions of surfactant protein A with influenza A viruses: binding and neutralization. J Infect Dis 171(2): 335–341
19. Hartshorn KL et al (1997) Mechanisms of anti-influenza activity of surfactant proteins A and D: comparison with serum collectins. Am J Physiol 273(6 Pt 1):L1156–L1166
20. Kishor U et al (2002) Protective roles of pulmonary surfactant proteins, SP-A and SP-D, against lung allergy and infection caused by *Aspergillus fumigatus*. Immunobiology 205 (4–5):610–618
21. Wang JY et al (1996) Interaction of human lung surfactant proteins A and D with mite (*Dermatophagoides pteronyssinus*) allergens. Clin Exp Immunol 106(2):367–373
22. Wang JY et al (1998) Inhibitory effect of pulmonary surfactant proteins A and D on allergen-induced lymphocyte proliferation and histamine release in children with asthma. Am J Respir Crit Care Med 158(2):510–518
23. Miyamura K et al (1994) Surfactant proteins A (SP-A) and D (SP-D): levels in human amniotic fluid and localization in the fetal membranes. Biochim Biophys Acta 1210(3): 303–307
24. Masuda T et al (1991) Surfactant apoprotein-A concentration in sputum for diagnosis of pulmonary alveolar proteinosis. Lancet 337 (8741): 580–582
25. Chailley-Heu B et al (1997) Expression of hydrophilic surfactant proteins by mesentery cells in rat and man. Biochem J 328(Pt 1): 251–256
26. Dobbie JW (1996) Surfactant protein A and lamellar bodies: a homologous secretory function of peritoneum, synovium, and lung. Perit Dial Int 16(6):574–581
27. Eliakim R et al (1997) Isolation and characterization of surfactant-like particles in rat and human colon. Am J Physiol 272(3 Pt 1): G425–G434
28. Khoor A et al (1993) Developmental expression of SP-A and SP-A mRNA in the proximal and distal respiratory epithelium in the human fetus and newborn. J Histochem Cytochem 41(9):1311–1319
29. Strong P et al (1998) A novel method of purifying lung surfactant proteins A and D from the lung lavage of alveolar proteinosis patients and from pooled amniotic fluid. J Immunol Methods 220(1–2):139–149

Chapter 22

Purification of Surfactant Protein D (SP-D) from Pooled Amniotic Fluid and Bronchoalveolar Lavage

Eswari Dodagatta-Marri, Asif S. Qaseem, Najmunisa Karbani, Anthony G. Tsolaki, Patrick Waters, Taruna Madan, and Uday Kishore

Abstract

Surfactant protein SP-D is a multimeric collagenous lectin, called *collectin*. SP-D is a multifunctional, pattern recognition innate immune molecule, which binds in a calcium dependent manner to an array of carbohydrates and lipids, thus offering resistance to invading pathogens, allergen challenge, and pulmonary inflammation. SP-D is predominantly found in the endoplasmic reticulum of type 2 pneumocytes and in the secretory granules of Clara or non-ciliated bronchiolar cells. The highest expression of SP-D is observed in the distal airways and alveoli. There is also an extra pulmonary existence of SP-D. The common sources of native full-length human SP-D are bronchoalveolar lavage (BAL) washings from normal or preferably patients suffering from alveolar proteinosis who overproduce SP-D in the lungs. Amniotic fluid collected at the term during parturition is another reasonable source. Here, we describe a simple and rapid method of purifying native SP-D away from SP-A which is also present in the same source. We also describe procedures of expressing and purifying a recombinant fragment of human SP-D (rhSP-D) comprising trimeric neck and carbohydrate recognition domains that has been shown to have therapeutic effects in murine models of allergy and infection.

Key words Surfactant protein-D, SP-D, Purification, Amniotic fluid, Recombinant SP-D, Inflammation, Affinity chromatography

1 Introduction

The respiratory surface in the lungs inevitably interacts with a variety of inhaled toxins, microbes and other particulate matter. Host defense mechanisms within the lungs must facilitate clearance of inhaled pathogens and particles, while minimizing an inflammatory response that could damage the thin delicate gaseous-exchange lining of the alveoli and distal airways. Pulmonary surfactant is a complex of lipids and proteins that are physiologically essential. There are of four types of surfactant proteins; SP-A [1], SP-B [2], SP-C [3], and SP-D, which constitute 5.3, 0.7, 0.4, and 0.6 % of

Mihaela Gadjeva (ed.), *The Complement System: Methods and Protocols*, Methods in Molecular Biology, vol. 1100,
DOI 10.1007/978-1-62703-724-2_22, © Springer Science+Business Media New York 2014

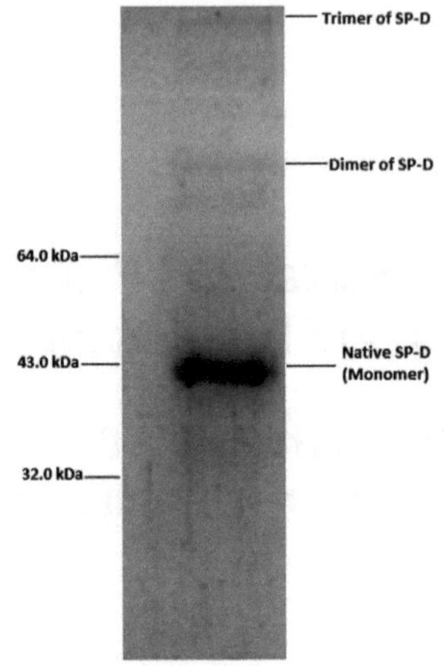

Fig. 1 SDS–PAGE (10 % w/v) analysis of purified SP-D under reducing conditions. SP-D is composed of a 43 kDa polypeptide chain, with *faint bands* corresponding to dimers and trimers of the 43 kDa chain can also been seen

total surfactant, respectively [4–7]. The gene encoding the SP-D protein is localized at the genomic region of 10q22.2–23.1 near the MBL gene [8] of chromosome 10 in humans. The SP-D polypeptide chain is 355 residues long, with N-terminal 25 non-collagen residues, 177 collagenous residues and 153 residues of the C-terminal lectin domain [9] (Fig. 1). The lectin domain is the globular head region of the protein which binds to pathogen-associated molecular patterns (PAMPs), whilst the collagenous region initiates phagocytosis [10].

Both SP-A and SP-D bind to carbohydrate structures on the surfaces of pathogens, such as viruses [11], bacteria [12], yeast [13], fungi [14], pollen, apoptotic and necrotic cells [15–18]. SP-D also directly binds to type II cell apical membranes [19] and alveolar macrophages [20]. Most of SP-D is found in the aqueous bronchoalveolar lavage fluid (BALF), which binds to phosphotidylinositol (PI) and glucosylceramide, which are sugar moieties present in surfactants [21]. As a potent opsonin, SP-D interacts with a range of pathogens and engineers clearance mechanism including aggregation/agglutination, growth inhibition, enhancement of phagocytosis by phagocytic cells, and production of superoxidative burst and nitric oxide [22].

SP-D has also been implicated in protecting lungs against allergenic challenge [23]. SP-D can bind allergens derived from house dust mite [24] and *Aspergillus fumigatus* [25] inhibit specific IgE binding to allergens and dampen histamine release by sensitized basophils [14]. The interaction with allergens is mediated via CRD region. Thus, the rhSP-D composed of trimeric neck and CRD region only, produced in *Escherichia coli*, has been shown to be protective in murine models of lung allergy [26–28].

A significant level of SP-D has been detected immunohistochemically in human trachea, brain, testis, salivary gland, heart, prostate, kidneys, small intestine, pancreas, and placenta. Lower levels of expression have also been detected in spleen, adrenal gland, uterus, and mammary glands [29–31]. SP-A, on the other hand, is found to be at low levels in the human and rat small and large intestines [32], mesentery, and colon [33–35]. SP-A is found in human prostate, thymus, amniotic fluid and epithelium, and salivary glands in very low quantities [34]. SP-A has also been detected in the entire human lacrimal apparatus including lacrimal gland, nasolacrimal ducts, conjunctiva, cornea, and human tear fluid [35].

Here, we describe a step-by-step method to purify human SP-D from pooled amniotic fluid and BAL fluid. The BAL washings from pulmonary alveolar proteinosis patients are excellent source of native SP-D [36]. The fact that SP-D binds to maltose reasonably well, via its CRD region, has been exploited for purification that involves use of maltose agarose or sepharose as an affinity matrix.

2 Materials

2.1 Protein Purification Buffers

1. Low salt affinity buffer: 50 mM Tris–HCl, pH 7.4, 100 mM NaCl, 5 mM $CaCl_2$.
2. High salt affinity buffer: 50 mM Tris–HCl, pH 7.4, 1 M NaCl, 10 mM $CaCl_2$.
3. Elution buffer: 50 mM Tris–HCl, pH 7.4, 50 mM $MnCl_2$ and 0.02 % NaN_3.
4. EDTA buffer: for $MnCl_2$ removal 50 mM Tris–HCl, pH 7.4, 100 mM NaCl, 5 mM EDTA and 0.02 % NaN_3.
5. Buffer I + 8 M urea: 50 mM Tris–HCl, pH 7.4, 100 mM NaCl, 5 mM $CaCl_2$, 0.02 % NaN_3 and 8 M urea.
6. Buffer I: 50 mM Tris–HCl, pH 7.4, 100 mM NaCl, 5 mM $CaCl_2$ 0.02 % NaN_3.

2.2 Ion Exchange Chromatography

1. High salt affinity buffer: 50 mM Tris–HCl, pH 7.4, 1 M NaCl, 5 mM $CaCl_2$,0.02 % NaN_3.
2. Low salt affinity buffer: 50 mM Tris–HCl, pH 7.4, 100 mM NaCl, 5 mM $CaCl_2$ 0.02 % NaN_3.
3. SP-D eluting buffer with maltose: 50 mM Tris–HCl, pH 7.4, 100 mM NaCl, 25 mM maltose, 0.02 % NaN_3.

2.3 SDS-PAGE

1. SDS-gel: 30 % Bis-acrylamide, 1.5 M Tris–HCl, pH 8.8 (resolving gel), 1.0 M Tris–HCl, pH 6.8 (stacking gel), 10 % SDS, 10 % APS, TEMED.
2. 1× Running buffer (1 l): 3 g Tris base, 14.4 g glycine, 10 ml SDS (10 %), 990 ml dH_2O.
3. 2× SDS sample buffer (10 ml): 1.25 ml 0.5 M Tris–HCl, pH 6.8, 2 ml 50 % glycerol, 2 ml 10 % SDS, 0.5 ml β-mercaptoethanol, 0.5 % Bromophenol blue, 4 ml dH_2O.
4. Coomassie blue stain (1 L): 100 ml Glacial acetic acid, 400 ml methanol, 1 g Coomassie blue R250, and 500 ml dH_2O.
5. De-stain solution (1 L): 100 ml Glacial acetic acid, 400 ml methanol, and 500 ml dH_2O.

2.4 Western Blot Buffers

1. 1× Transfer buffer: 2.9 g Glycine, 5.8 g Tris base, 0.37 g SDS, 200 ml methanol, 800 ml dH_2O.

2.5 Maltose–Sepharose

1. Divinylsulfone (DVS).
2. Sepharose 4B.
3. 0.5 M Sodium carbonate.
4. 0.5 M Sodium bicarbonate.
5. 20 % D-maltose in 0.5 M sodium carbonate.

2.6 Bis(Sulfosuccinimidyl)Suberate Cross-linking

1. HEPES buffer [10 mM HEPES (pH 7.5), 100 mM NaCl, 1 mM EDTA].
2. DMSO (Dimethyl sulfoxide).

3 Methods

3.1 Purification of Surfactant protein D

3.1.1 Separation of SP-D from Amniotic Fluid

1. Amniotic fluid can be collected following vaginal rupturing of the fetal membranes which is carried out to induce or facilitate the progress of labor or during spontaneous rupturing from pregnant women at term following appropriate ethical approval. This is usually stored at −80 °C until required for purification.
2. Thaw amniotic fluid from −80 °C at 37 °C for 5–6 h or overnight at 4 °C. Make sure (whilst at 37 °C) that it is regularly mixed to keep temperature consistent to avoid overheating of proteins.
3. Pool all amniotic fluid to allow purification of protein in large amounts.
4. Centrifuge the pooled amniotic fluid in a table top bench centrifuge at 10,000 ×*g* for 40 min at 4 °C to separate SP-A, mainly in the pellet, from the supernatant containing SP-D.
5. The amniotic fluid is then passed through a cell strainer to remove fat and other large aggregates. This will remove phospholipids and large unwanted material.

6. To further separate other cellular material, the amniotic fluid is passed through muslin cloth three times for a clearer suspension and to avoid future clogging of maltose–sepharose column during affinity chromatography.
7. The amniotic fluid is calcified to 5 mM $CaCl_2$ to increase the volume and decrease viscosity ($CaCl_2$ is added drop-by-drop whilst monitoring pH to 7.5).
8. Stir at 4 °C for 1 h. This allows aggregation of the calcium dependent proteins SP-A and SP-D.
9. Proceed to affinity chromatography.

3.1.2 Affinity Chromatography

1. Maltose–sepharose (see the preparation of affinity matrix below) is washed with 100 ml autoclaved distilled water and then equilibrated with four bed volumes of low salt affinity buffer I (*see* Subheading 2.1, **item 1**).
2. The maltose–sepharose bed is then transferred to the amniotic fluid supernatant obtained from the previous step to allow SP-D to bind to the maltose–sepharose for efficient purification. This is left to stir at 4 °C for a further 1 h.
3. Pass the amniotic fluid containing the maltose–sepharose through the column and allow the maltose–sepharose to settle, collect the flow through and pass through the column thrice in total.
4. Remove nonspecifically bound proteins with four bed volumes of affinity buffer containing 1 M NaCl (see Subheading 2.1, **item 2**).
5. 10 × 1 ml fractions of SP-D are eluted with elution buffer I over ice (see Note 1).
6. Optical density of each fraction is read at 280 nm using elution buffer without $MnCl_2$ as a reference (*see* **Notes 2** and **3**) (Fig. 2).

3.1.3 Removal of BSA and Manganese Chloride and Concentration of SP-D Protein

7. 100 μl of each fraction is used for TCA precipitation and this is separated on a 15 % SDS–PAGE to visualize protein concentration and purity.
8. The fractions with the highest concentrations are pooled and dialysis bag is immersed in 1 L EDTA buffer to remove $MnCl_2$ (*see* Subheading 2.1, **item 4**).
9. The dialysis bag is left in a cylinder on a magnetic stirrer overnight at 4 °C (*see* **Note 4**).
10. The dialysis bag is then placed in a beaker containing polyethylene glycol MW 6,000–10,000 (Sigma) for 2 h until the volume of the dialysate is reduced by half.
11. The content from the dialysis bag can then be aliquoted into 1 ml fractions for storage at −20 °C. 2× 100 μl fractions will be required for protein estimation using BCA assay (see below).

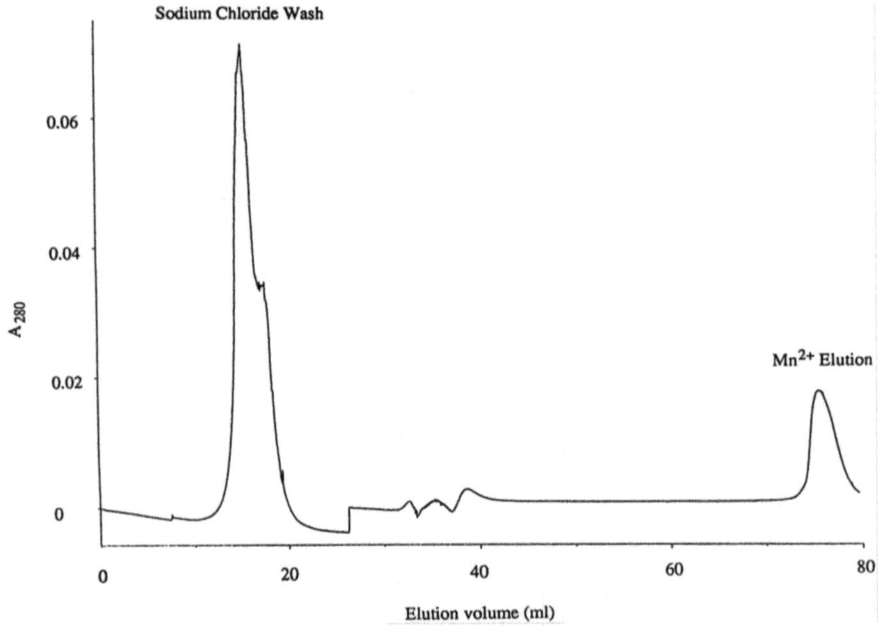

Fig. 2 NaCl wash and elution of SP-D with $MnCl_2$ from the maltosyl–agarose column. Several proteins, including HSA and histone degradation products bind nonspecifically to maltosyl–agarose and are readily eluted with high salt wash in the presence of calcium while SP-D remains bound. SP-D is specifically eluted by replacing $CaCl_2$ with $MnCl_2$ when changing to elution buffer containing 50 mM $MnCl_2$ after 25 ml of the sodium chloride high salt wash, as outlined in Subheading 2

3.1.4 Gel Filtration Chromatography

To further clean the purified SP-D away from minor contaminants SP-A and DNA etc., gel filtration chromatography can be performed.

12. Prepare Superose 6 preparative column; add concentrated SP-D preparation onto the column.
13. Equilibrate with name of the buffer (20 mM Tris–HCl, 100 mM NaCl, 1 mM EDTA).
14. SP-D elutes as a single peak with molecular weight of >1,000 kDa and SP-A elutes as broad peak with molecular weight of 670 kDa.
15. Other contaminants that co-purify with the proteins on the affinity column elute late, close to the inclusion volume of the column.
16. The fractions with good protein concentrations can be pooled and concentrated adopting the method described above with polyethylene glycol.

3.2 Preparation of Competent Cells

1. Inoculate a single colony of *E. coli* BL21 (λDE3) pLysS (Invitrogen) in 10 ml of Luria broth (LB) media with 10 μl of chloramphenicol (stock: 50 mg/ml dissolved in ethanol) overnight at 37 °C shaker.
2. Following morning, remove 500 μl from BL21 (λDE3) pLysS culture and inoculate into a 50 ml Falcon tube containing 25 ml of LB medium with 25 μl of chloramphenicol.

3. Incubate at 37 °C on a shaker (200 rpm) and measure optical density (A_{600}) every hour until it reaches a value between 0.3 and 0.4 (early log Phase).
4. Centrifuge the culture at 2,000 × *g* for 5 min.
5. After centrifugation, discard the supernatant, and add 12.5 ml of sterile 0.1 M $CaCl_2$ to the cell pellet.
6. Resuspend the cells and place them in the temporary state of competence at ice for 1 h.
7. After 1 h, centrifuge the cells for 5 min at 2,000 × *g*.
8. Discard the supernatant, and resuspend the pellet in 2 ml of 0.1 M $CaCl_2$ and store in ice, the cells are now ready to be transformed.

3.3 Transformation of Cells

1. Remove 200 μl of cells from the competent cells prepared earlier, and place inside a 10 ml Falcon tube containing 1–2 μl of (pUK-D1) construct.
2. Place the mixture on ice for 1 h.
3. Give a heat shock to the mixture at 42 °C for 90 s.
4. Following heat shock, place the cells on ice for a further 5 min, and then resuspend in 800 μl of LB.
5. Place the mixture inside a 37 °C incubator for approximately 45 min.
6. After incubation, streak the cells on an LB agar plate containing (Amp/Chl) and leave inside a 37 °C incubator to grow overnight.

3.3.1 Protein Expression

1. Grow a single colony of transformed (pUK-D1) cells in 25 ml LB along with 100 μg/ml ampicillin + 50 μg/ml chloramphenicol overnight in a shaker at 37 °C.
2. On the following morning, inoculate the overnight primary culture of 25 ml bacterial culture into 1 L LB along with 100 μg/ml ampicillin + 50 μg/ml chloramphenicol and grow inside a 37 °C shaker, until the absorbance A_{600} reaches 0.6–0.8.
3. After the cells reach log phase (A_{600} at 0.6–0.8) induce with 0.4 mM IPTG for 3 h and harvest the cells by centrifugation at 9,000 × *g* for 15 min.
4. Following centrifugation, discard the supernatant and store the pellet at −20 °C for further processing (Fig. 3).

3.3.2 Cell Lysis

1. Resuspend the cell pellet obtained after IPTG induction in ice cold lysis buffer containing (50 mM Tris–HCl, 200 mM NaCl, 5 mM EDTA, 0.1 % v/v Triton X-100, 0.1 mM PMSF, pH 7.5, 50 μg/ml lysozyme) and vortex for 1 h in cold room at 4 °C and then sonicate the sample (ten cycles at 30 s each).

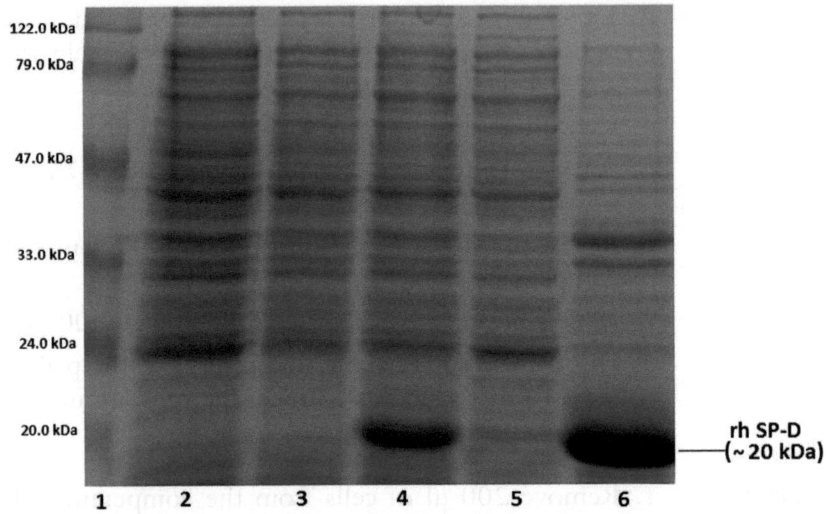

Fig. 3 SDS–PAGE (12 % w/v) analyses of rhSP-D at various stages of expression and purification. A recombinant fragment of human SP-D containing homotrimeric neck and CRD regions (rhSP-D) was expressed as inclusion bodies using *Escherichia coli* BL21 (λDE3) pLysS as hosts under T7 promoter. 3 h after induction with 0.4 mM IPTG, the rhSP-D accumulated as an over-expressed protein of 20 kDa (*lane 4*) compared with uninduced cells (*lane 2*) and induced cells at zero hr (*lane 3*). Bacterial cells were sonicated and the inclusion bodies (*lane 6*) containing insoluble rhSP-D were recovered in the pellet. The supernatant of the sonicate (*lane 5*) did not contain rhSP-D

3.3.3 Dialysis

1. Harvest the sonicate by centrifugation at 9,000 × *g* for 15 min and solubilize the recovered rh SP-D in the inclusion bodies in 100 ml buffer I (50 mM Tris–HCl pH 7.5, 100 mM NaCl) containing 10 mM 2-mercaptoethanol and 8 M Urea.
2. Carry out a step wise dialysis of the resolubilized material against buffer I containing 4 M urea, 2 M urea, 1 M urea and no urea, each for 2 h.
3. Centrifuge the dialysate at 9,000 × *g* for 15 min to clarify, and then dialyze with calcium buffer (20 mM Tris–HCl pH 7.5, 100 mM NaCl, 10 mM $CaCl_2$, 0.05 % sodium azide) for 3 h to completely remove urea from the dialysate (Fig. 4, *lane 1*).

3.3.4 Protein Purification by Affininty Chromotography

1. The rhSP-D is purified by affinity chromatography using maltose–sepharose column.
2. Rinse the maltose–sepharose column with distilled water prior to use. After thorough rinsing of the column with dH_2O, pass 50 ml of affinity column buffer containing (50 mM Tris–HCl pH 7.5, 100 mM NaCl, 5 mM $CaCl_2$, sodium azide-0.05 %) through the column.
3. After rinsing the column pass the protein sample through the column once.
4. Wash the column with affinity column buffer.

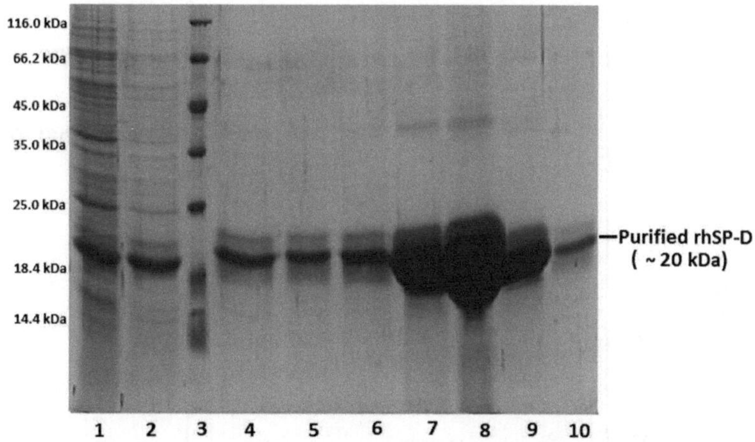

Fig. 4 SDS–PAGE (12 % w/v) analyses of rhSP-D of purification. Insoluble rh SP-D were refolded via a denaturation and renaturation procedure and the soluble fraction was further purified using Q-sepharose ion-exchange chromatography. The refolded protein (*lane 1*) was passed through maltose-agarose. A significant proportion of the refolded rh SP-D did not bind to the column (*lane 2*). *Lane 3* is standard protein marker. The peak fractions containing rhSP-D were subsequently affinity purified on a maltose–agarose column (*lanes 4–10*)

5. Elute the bound protein by using elution buffer containing 5 mM EDTA (25 ml) (50 mM Tris–HCl pH 7.5, 100 mM NaCl, 5 mM EDTA, 0.05 % sodium azide) (Fig. 4). The affinity eluted protein ran as a trimer on a Superose-12 gel filteration column (Fig. 5).

3.4 Endotoxin Removal from Recombinant SP-D

1. 5 ml of Polymyxin B agarose gel (Sigma) is packed in a 20 ml column.
2. Wash with 50 ml of 1 % sodium deoxycholate and then further rinse with 50 ml of autoclaved distilled water to completely remove 1 % sodium deoxycholate.
3. After rinsing the column, the protein is loaded onto the column, and left to incubate at room temperature for half an hour for the protein to bind completely.
4. After the incubation period the protein is eluted and collected in 1.0-ml fractions.
5. The LPS free rhSP-D protein is then checked for purity by running it on 15 % SDS gel to ensure the removal of LPS.
6. The endotoxin level was examined by QCL-1000 Limulus amebocyte lysate system (BioWhittaker, Walkersville, MD, USA) and was found to be ~4 pg μg^{-1} of rhSP-D.
7. The protein is further quantified by measuring the absorbance at 280 nm of the eluted and the concentration of the sample was determined via Spectrophotometry.

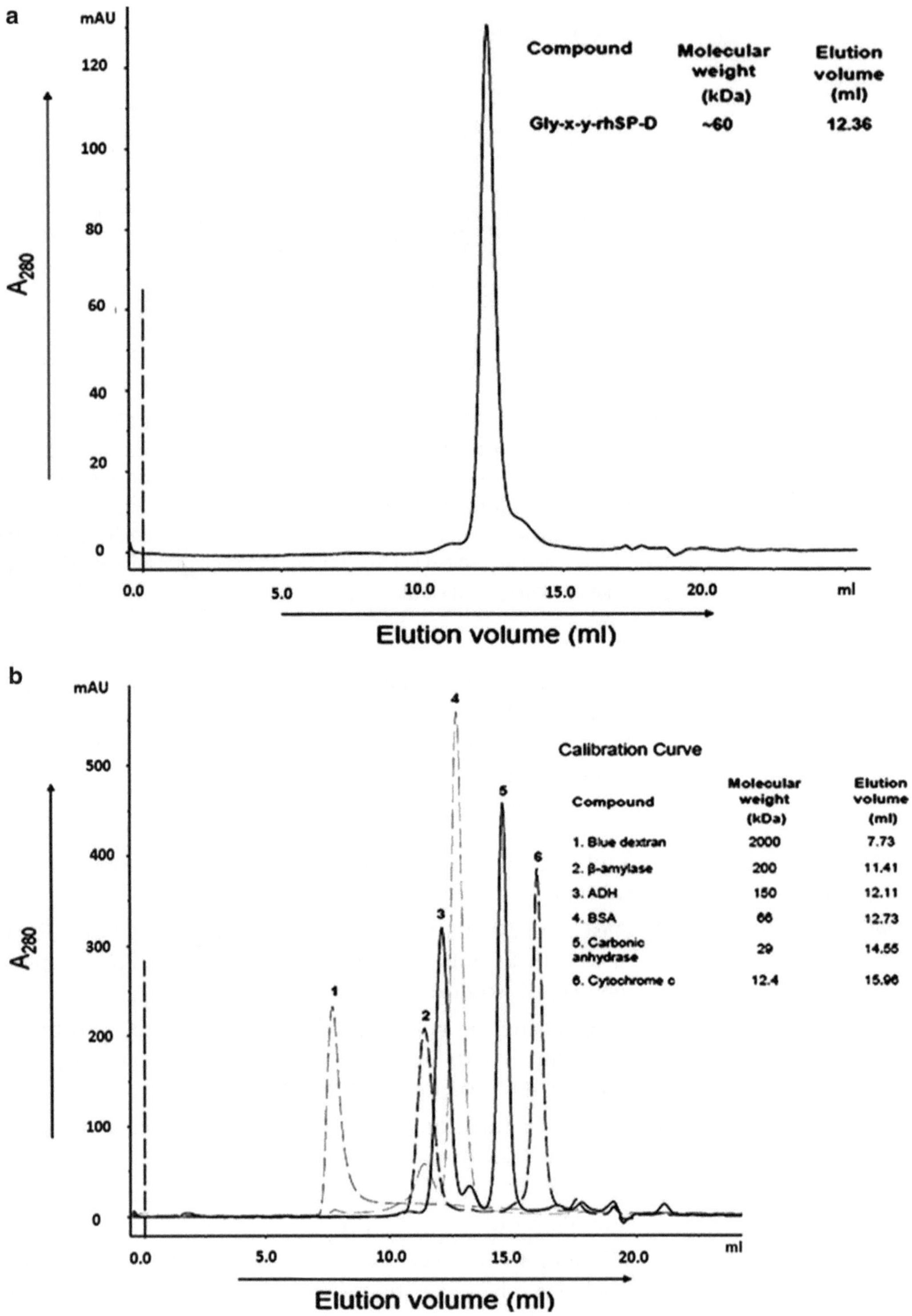

Fig. 5 (**a**) Elution profile of rhSP-D from an FPLC Superose 12 column (HR 10/30). The column was eluted with Tris-buffered saline–EDTA buffer at a flow rate of 0.3 ml/min. (**b**) Calibration of the column was carried out using the following marker proteins: blue dextran (2,000 kDa), β-amylase (200 kDa), alcohol dehydrogenase (150 kDa), carbonic anhydrase (29 kDa), and cytochrome C (12.4 kDa)

3.5 Preparation of Maltose–Sepharose Column

Preparation of D-maltose-sepharose 4B by divinylsulfone activation method: (immobilizing hydroxyl-containing compounds) Sepharose is first activated with the bifunctional reagent divinyl sulfone (DVS) (Sigma) and then coupled under basic conditions to the hydroxyls of D-mannose. Reductive amination, epoxy and DVS activation provide three excellent alternatives for the obtaining an optimal affinity support.

Immobilization: (DVS to activate sepharose) (*see* **Note 5**).

1. Activate sepharose 4B (100 ml settled gel with DVS); DVS is a bifunctional cross-linking reagent, used to activate agarose and other hydroxyl matrices (*see* **Note 6**).
2. DVS introduces reactive vinyl groups into the matrix that will couple to amines, alcohols, sulfhydryls, and phenols (see Note 7).
3. DVS activated gels are more reactive than epoxy-activated gels, and therefore coupling proceeds rapidly and completely (*see* **Note 8**).

3.5.1 Activation

1. Wash sepharose 4B (100 ml) settled gel with 1 L water in a sintered glass funnel, suction dry to a wet cake and transfer to a 500 ml beaker.
2. Suspend the gel in 100 ml 0.5 M sodium carbonate and stir the suspension.
3. Slowly add, drop wise, DVS (10 ml) with constant stirring over a 15 min period. After addition is completed, stir gel suspension for 1 h at room temperature.
4. Extensively wash the activated gel with water until the filtrate is no longer acidic (*see* **Note 9**).

3.5.2 Immobilization

1. Wash the DVS-activated sepharose 4B with 1 L water, suction dry to a moist cake and add to a D-maltose solution (20 % D-maltose in 0.5 M sodium carbonate).
2. Stir the reaction mixture at room temperature for 24 h.
3. Filter and wash the gel successively with 2 L each of water and 0.5 M sodium bicarbonate containing 5 ml β-mercaptoethanol.
4. Mix at room temperature for 2 h to block the excess vinyl groups.
5. Finally wash the gel with 2 L of water.
6. D-maltose-sepharose 4B can be stored in 0.02 % sodium azide at 4 °C.

3.6 Bis(Sulfosuccinimidyl)Suberate (BS_3) Cross-linking

1. Prepare a 25 mM solution of BS3, by dissolving 2 mg BS3 in 140 μl of DMSO.
2. Using a 20-fold excess approach (20:1 cross-linker–protein), add BS3 cross-linker solution to the protein sample so that the final cross-linker concentration is between 0.5 and 5 mM.

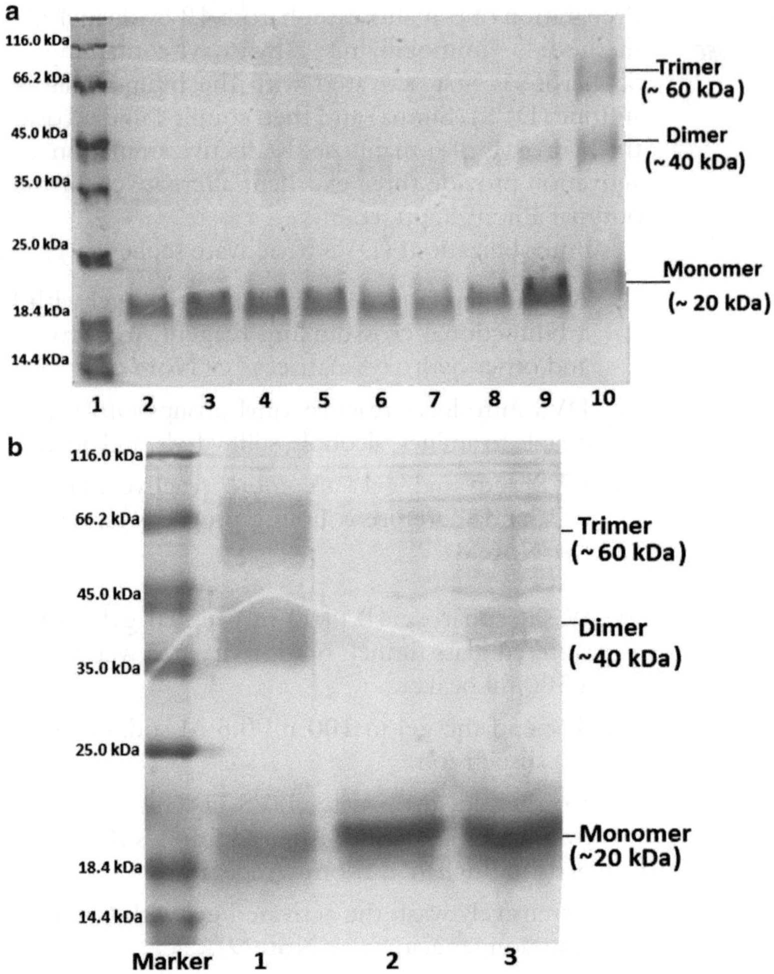

Fig. 6 (**a**) SDS–PAGE (12 % w/v) bis (sulfosuccinimidyl) suberate (BS3) cross-linking of recombinant fragment of human SP-D containing trimeric neck containing CRD region (rhSP-D). Treatment of rhSP-D with 0.01 mM BS3 at different time intervals of 0, 1, 2, 4, 6, 8, 16, 32 min, respectively (*lanes 3–9*) and the *lane 10* showing 1 mM BS3. (**b**) SDS–PAGE (12 % w/v) bis (sulfosuccinimidyl) suberate (BS3) cross-linking of recombinant fragment of human SP-D containing trimeric neck containing CRD region (rhSP-D). Treatment of rhSP-D with three different concentrations of BS3: 0.1 mM (*lane 1*), 0.01 mM (*lane 2*), and 1 mM (*lane 3*)

3. Incubated rhSP-D with different concentrations (1 mM, 0.1 mM, and 0.01 mM BS3).
4. Allow the sample to react at room temperature for 45 min to 1 h. Allow slightly longer if reaction must be done on ice (this reaction rate is only slightly slower at low temperatures).
5. Quench and unreacted BS3 with 25 to 60 mM Tris–HCl (pH 7.5) and allow reacting for 10–15 min at room temperature.
6. Run the SDS-PAGE for the detection of cross-linking (Figs. 6 and 7).

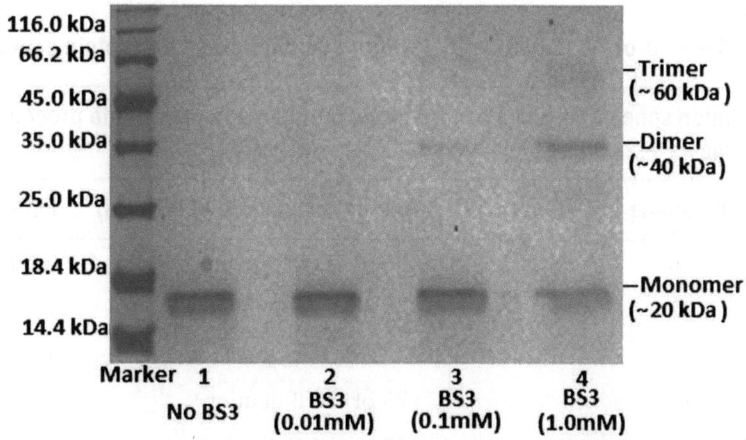

Fig. 7 SDS–PAGE (12 % w/v) bis (sulfosuccinimidyl) suberate (BS3) cross-linking of recombinant fragment of human SP-D containing trimeric neck containing CRD region (rhSP-D). Treatment of rhSP-D with three different concentrations of BS3: 0.01 mM (*lane 3*), 0.1 mM (*lane 4*), and 1 mM (*lane 5*), and untreated rhSP-D (*lane 2*)

3.7 TCA Assay

1. Take 200 μl of protein and mix with equal volumes of 20 % TCA (trichloroacetic acid) in a 2 ml Eppendorf tube, keep on ice for 20 min. if concentrations are low then keep 5 min on ice and 15 min at −20 °C.
2. Centrifuge for 15 min at 20,000 × g at 4 °C, decant the supernatant and add 200 μl of 70 % ethanol, flick and mix content, centrifuge for 15 min at 20,000 × g at 4 °C and decant supernatant.
3. Allow excess ethanol to air dry for 5–10 min. Do not allow excessive drying as this makes the pellet difficult to dissolve.
4. Add 30 μl of 2× protein treatment buffer and pipette up and down for equal mixing.
5. Denature protein on heating block for 10 min at 95 °C.
6. Add each sample to a well of SDS-PAGE.

3.8 Bicinchoninic Acid Protein Assay

BCA assay is carried out according to manufacturer's instructions. See below for protocol using BCA (Thermo Scientific).

1. To carry out protein estimation, it is important to perform a standard curve by preparing protein standards using the BSA of 2 mg/ml provided in the kit.
2. Nine vials are labeled A-I and BSA is diluted to range from 20 μg to 2 mg/ml according to Tables 1 and 2 using PBS as a diluent.
3. Prepare working reagent by mixing reagent A and reagent B at a 1:50 dilution. 2 ml of working reagent is required per sample including for the protein standards which is repeated twice.

Table 1
Dilution of protein standards to perform standard curve for protein estimation

Dilution scheme for standard test tube protocol and microplate procedure (working range = 20–2,000 μg/ml)			
Vial	**Volume of diluent (μl)**	**Volume and source of BSA (μl)**	**Final BSA concentration (μg/ml)**
A	0	300 of stock	2,000
B	125	375 of stock	1,500
C	325	325 of stock	1,000
D	175	175 of vial B dilution	750
E	325	325 of vial C dilution	500
F	325	325 of vial E dilution	250
G	325	325 of vial F dilution	125
H	400	100 of vial G dilution	25
I	400	0	0 = Blank

Table 2
Components and volumes for preparing 12 and 15 % SDS-PAGE

Resolving gel	12 %	15 %	Stacking gel	
Components	**Volume (ml)**		**Components**	**Volume (ml)**
dH_2O	3.3	2.3	dH_2O	3.4
30 % Bis-acrylamide mix	4	5	30 % Bis-acrylamide mix	0.83
1.5 M Tris–HCl, pH 8.8	2.5	2.5	1.0 M Tris–HCl, pH 6.8	0.63
10 % SDS	0.1	0.1	10 % SDS	0.05
10 % APS	0.1	0.1	10 % APS	0.05
TEMED	0.015	0.015	TEMED	0.014

The following formula can be used to calculate the total working reagent required (no. of standards + no. of unknown samples) × (2 replicates) × (2 ml volume of working reagent per sample).

4. Label 2× test tubes for each sample containing 100 μl of sample + 2 ml working reagent.
5. This is incubated at 37 °C for 30 min. The reagent will turn from purple to green, depending on the protein concentration. The higher the concentration the greener the solution.

6. The test tubes are then cooled down to room temperature, however measuring the absorbance within the first 10 min.
7. Using a spectrophotometer at 562 nm, each sample optical density is detected and the average of the duplicate sample is taken for a more accurate measurement of protein. The working reagent is used as a reference.
8. A standard curve can be made using the standard protein samples and the optical density detected for the unknown samples can be used to detect the approximate protein content in the sample.

3.9 SDS-PAGE: 12 % and 15 %

Protocol:

To prepare a 12 % or 15 % SDS-PAGE, follow the instructions below:

1. In two separate 50 ml beakers label one "resolving gel" and the other "stacking gel".
2. For a standard size gel, 10 ml of resolving gel and 5 ml of stacking gel is sufficient.
3. Assemble the clean glass plates onto the glass holder and stand and check for no leakages.
4. Prepare the following for either 12 % or 15 % resolving gel then the standard stacking gel. Do not add TEMED until required just before adding to the glass plates.
5. Once the TEMED has been added the polymerization reaction will have begun, therefore add the resolving gel immediately.
6. After 20 min the gel will have polymerized and then 10 % APS and TEMED can be added to the stacking gel and loaded on top of the resolving gel with the comb inserted for the gel to polymerize and form wells.
7. The gel with the glass plates can be assembled into the gel holder with the anode and cathode conductors and a buffer dam can be added to the opposite side to allow current to flow.
8. The protein samples for separation are mixed with equal amounts of 2× SDS sample buffer and heated to 95 °C for 10 min for denaturation.
9. The sample is then cooled to room temperature and microfuged at 12,000 × *g* for 1 min before loading one sample per well.
10. Protein standard marker is added to the first well to determine unknown protein sample size.
11. 1× Running buffer is added to the tank as instructed by manufacturer.
12. Set the power pack connected to the gel apparatus to 100 V for 90 min to allow the proteins to be separated according to

size, with the smaller molecules passing through the gel matrix quickly with the larger molecules trailing behind.

13. The gel is then placed in staining solution overnight and destained the next day for the protein bands to be visible.

4 Notes

1. Add $MnCl_2$ fresh on the day you need to use it as $MnCl_2$ oxidizes.
2. Due to color changes over time of $MnCl_2$ giving improper protein estimations.
3. Both supernatant and flow through and buffers should always be on ice.
4. Note if the color is still dark; allow dialysis to continue for up to 48 h.
5. Since DVS is highly toxic, all operations involved in activation and coupling should be done in the fume hood.
6. DVS activated gels are very useful for immobilizing sugars through hydroxyl groups.
7. Immobilized ligands prepared by the DVS method are unstable at alkaline pH (not stable above pH-8.0-amine linked gels and above pH-9.0- or 10.0-hydroxyl-linked gels).
8. Primary stability of this procedure is caused by the liability of the ether bond formed between DVS and the matrix at the time of activation.
9. Gel can be used to couple to ligands or stored for further use. For storage, extensively wash the activated gel with acetone and keep as suspension in acetone at 4 °C.

References

1. King RJ, Klass DJ, Gikas EG, Clements JA (1973) An uncommon phosphatidylcholine specific for surface-active material in canine lung. Am J Physiol 224(4):788–795
2. Glasser SW, Korfhagen TR, Weaver T, Pilot-Matias T, Fox JL, Whitsett JA (1987) cDNA and deduced amino acid sequence of human pulmonary surfactant-associated proteolipid SPL(Phe). Proc Natl Acad Sci U S A 84(12):4007–4011
3. Warr RG, Hawgood S, Buckley DI, Crisp TM, Schilling J, Benson BJ et al (1987) Low molecular weight human pulmonary surfactant protein (SP5): isolation, characterization, and cDNA and amino acid sequences. Proc Natl Acad Sci U S A 84(22):7915–7919
4. Weaver TE, Whitsett JA (1991) Function and regulation of expression of pulmonary surfactant-associated proteins. Biochem J 273(Pt 2):249–264
5. Kishore U, Reid KB (2001) Structures and functions of mammalian collectins. Results Probl Cell Differ 33:225–248
6. Weaver TE (1998) Synthesis, processing and secretion of surfactant proteins B and C. Biochim Biophys Acta 1408(2–3):173–179
7. Pérez-Gil J, Keough KM (1998) Interfacial properties of surfactant proteins. Biochim Biophys Acta 1408(2–3):203–217
8. Crouch E, Rust K, Veile R, Donis-Keller H, Grosso L (1993) Genomic organization of

human surfactant protein D (SP-D). SP-D is encoded on chromosome 10q22.2-23.1. J Biol Chem 268(4):2976–2983
9. Lu J, Willis AC, Reid KB (1992) Purification, characterization and cDNA cloning of human lung surfactant protein D. Biochem J 284(Pt 3):795–802
10. Gardai SJ, Xiao YQ, Dickinson M, Nick JA, Voelker DR, Greene KE et al (2003) By binding SIRPalpha or calreticulin/CD91, lung collectins act as dual function surveillance molecules to suppress or enhance inflammation. Cell 115(1):13–23
11. Hartshorn KL, Crouch EC, White MR, Eggleton P, Tauber AI, Chang D et al (1994) Evidence for a protective role of pulmonary surfactant protein D (SP-D) against influenza A viruses. J Clin Invest 94(1):311–319
12. Kuan SF, Rust K, Crouch E (1992) Interactions of surfactant protein D with bacterial lipopolysaccharides. Surfactant protein D is an *Escherichia coli*-binding protein in bronchoalveolar lavage. J Clin Invest 90(1):97–106
13. Schelenz S, Malhotra R, Sim RB, Holmskov U, Bancroft GJ (1995) Binding of host collectins to the pathogenic yeast *Cryptococcus neoformans*: human surfactant protein D acts as an agglutinin for acapsular yeast cells. Infect Immun 63(9):3360–3366
14. Madan T, Kishore U, Shah A, Eggleton P, Strong P, Wang JY et al (1997) Lung surfactant proteins A and D can inhibit specific IgE binding to the allergens of *Aspergillus fumigatus* and block allergen-induced histamine release from human basophils. Clin Exp Immunol 110(2):241–249
15. Kishore U, Strong P, Perdikoulis MV, Reid KB (2001) A recombinant homotrimer, composed of the alpha helical neck region of human surfactant protein D and C1q B chain globular domain, is an inhibitor of the classical complement pathway. J Immunol 166(1):559–565
16. Wright JR (2005) Immunoregulatory functions of surfactant proteins. Nat Rev Immunol 5(1):58–68
17. Kishore U, Greenhough TJ, Waters P, Shrive AK, Ghai R, Kamran MF et al (2006) Surfactant proteins SP-A and SP-D: structure, function and receptors. Mol Immunol 43(9):1293–1315
18. Mahajan L, Madan T, Kamal N, Singh VK, Sim RB, Telang SD et al (2008) Recombinant surfactant protein-D selectively increases apoptosis in eosinophils of allergic asthmatics and enhances uptake of apoptotic eosinophils by macrophages. Int Immunol 20(8):993–1007
19. Herbein JF, Savov J, Wright JR (2000) Binding and uptake of surfactant protein D by freshly isolated rat alveolar type II cells. Am J Physiol Lung Cell Mol Physiol 278(4):L830–L839
20. Miyamura K, Leigh LE, Lu J, Hopkin J, López Bernal A, Reid KB (1994) Surfactant protein D binding to alveolar macrophages. Biochem J 300(Pt 1):237–242
21. Ogasawara Y, Kuroki Y, Akino T (1992) Pulmonary surfactant protein D specifically binds to phosphatidylinositol. J Biol Chem 267(29):21244–21249
22. Barnes P, Liew F (1995) Nitric oxide and asthmatic inflammation. Immunol Today 16(3): 128–130
23. Erpenbeck VJ, Schmidt R, Günther A, Krug N, Hohlfeld JM (2006) Surfactant protein levels in bronchoalveolar lavage after segmental allergen challenge in patients with asthma. Allergy 61(5):598–604
24. Wang JY, Kishore U, Lim BL, Strong P, Reid KB (1996) Interaction of human lung surfactant proteins A and D with mite (*Dermatophagoides pteronyssinus*) allergens. Clin Exp Immunol 106:367–373
25. Madan T, Reid KB, Singh M, Sarma PU, Kishore U (2005) Susceptibility of mice genetically deficient in the surfactant protein (SP)-A or SP-D gene to pulmonary hypersensitivity induced by antigens and allergens of *Aspergillus fumigatus*. J Immunol 174(11): 6943–6954
26. Madan T, Kishore U, Singh M, Strong P, Hussain EM, Reid KB et al (2001) Protective role of lung surfactant protein D in a murine model of invasive pulmonary aspergillosis. Infect Immun 69(4):2728–2731
27. Singh M, Madan T, Waters P, Parida SK, Sarma PU, Kishore U (2003) Protective effects of a recombinant fragment of human surfactant protein D in a murine model of pulmonary hypersensitivity induced by dust mite allergens. Immunol Lett 86(3):299–307
28. Fisher JH, Mason R (1995) Expression of pulmonary surfactant protein D in rat gastric mucosa. Am J Respir Cell Mol Biol 12(1):13–18
29. Madsen J, Kliem A, Tornoe I, Skjodt K, Koch C, Holmskov U (2000) Localization of lung surfactant protein D on mucosal surfaces in human tissues. J Immunol 164(11):5866–5870
30. Herías MV, Hogenkamp A, van Asten AJ, Tersteeg MH, van Eijk M, Haagsman HP (2007) Expression sites of the collectin SP-D suggest its importance in first line host defence: power of combining in situ hybridisation. RT-PCR and immunohistochemistry. Mol Immunol 44(13):3324–3332
31. Lin Z, deMello D, Phelps D, Koltun W, Page M, Floros J (2001) Both human SP-A1 and

Sp-A2 genes are expressed in small and large intestine. Pediatr Pathol Mol Med 5:367–386
32. Chailley-Heu B, Rubio S, Rougier J, Ducroc R, Barlier-Mur A, Ronco P et al (1997) Expression of hydrophilic surfactant proteins by mesentery cells in rat and man. Biochem J 328:251–256
33. Rubio S, Lacaze-Masmonteil T, Chailley-Heu B, Kahn A, Bourbon J, Ducroc R (1995) Pulmonary surfactant protein A (SP-A) is expressed by epithelial cells of small and large intestine. J Biol Chem 270:12162–12169
34. Madsen J, Tornoe I, Nielsen O, Koch C, Steinhilber W, Holmskov U (2003) Expression and localization of lung surfactant protein A in human tissues. Am J Respir Cell Mol Biol 29:591–597
35. Brauer L, Kindler C, Jäger K, Sel S, Nölle B, Pleyer U et al (2007) Detection of surfactant proteins A and D in human tear fluid and the human lacrimal system. Invest Ophthalmol Vis Sci 48:3945–3953
36. Honda Y, Kuroki Y, Matsuura E, Nagae H, Takahashi H, Akino T et al (1995) Pulmonary surfactant protein D in sera and bronchoalveolar lavage fluids. Am J Respir Crit Care Med 152(6 Pt 1):1860–1866

Chapter 23

Functional Analysis of C5a Effector Responses In Vitro and In Vivo

Christian M. Karsten, Yves Laumonnier, and Jörg Köhl

Abstract

C5a is a powerful proinflammatory and immunomodulatory mediator as evidenced by its involvement in infectious, allergic, and autoimmune diseases as well as in cancer. C5a exerts most of its biologic functions through binding and activation of the G protein-coupled C5a receptor (C5aR). C5aR activation promotes complex signaling pathways eventually resulting in increased intracellular calcium $(Ca^{2+})_i$ concentration. One of the prototypic effector functions associated with C5aR activation is the reconfiguration of the cell cytoskeleton resulting in increased cell motility and ligand-specific cell migration. Here, we describe three assays to assess C5a-mediated effector functions: (1) increase in $(Ca^{2+})_i$ in bone marrow-derived neutrophils using the intracellular fluorescent Ca^{2+}-sensitive indicator Fluo-4 AM and flow cytometry-based methods; (2) in vitro migration of murine, bone marrow-derived neutrophils using a modified Boyden chamber; and (3) in vivo migration of neutrophils from the circulation into the peritoneal cavity. To control for the specificity of the C5a-mediated effects, C5aR-deficient mice, neutralizing C5aR-specific antibodies and potent pharmacologic C5aR inhibitors are available.

Key words Flow cytometry, Intracellular calcium, Chemotaxis, CD88, C5a receptor, Neutrophils

1 Introduction

The anaphylatoxins (AT) C3a and C5a are proinflammatory and immunoregulatory mediators of the innate immune system. They are generated by proteolytic cleavage of C3 and C5 through specific C3 or C5 convertases formed in response to local or systemic activation of the complement system. Further, endogenous humoral or cellular proteases of the clotting cascade and activated neutrophils or macrophages as well as exogenous, microbial-derived proteases can promote specific C3 and C5 cleavage to release the ATs. The ATs are potent inflammatory mediators targeting a broad spectrum of immune and non-immune cells [1]. In addition to their pro-inflammatory properties, ATs regulate

Christian M. Karsten and Yves Laumonnier contributed equally to this work.

Mihaela Gadjeva (ed.), *The Complement System: Methods and Protocols*, Methods in Molecular Biology, vol. 1100,
DOI 10.1007/978-1-62703-724-2_23, © Springer Science+Business Media New York 2014

tissue regeneration [2, 3] and tissue fibrosis [2, 4, 5] as well as brain development [6]. The biologic functions are mediated through the activation of their cognate G-protein coupled receptors. C5a binds to two distinct receptors, namely, the C5a receptor (C5aR/CD88) [7, 8] and the C5a receptor-like 2 (C5L2) [9, 10]. C3a binds to a distinct C3aR [11, 12]. Here, we focus on effector functions mediated by the C5aR (CD88).

The C5aR is primarily expressed on cells of the myeloid lineage such as monocytes/macrophages, neutrophils, basophils, eosinophils, and mast cells [13–16], conventional and plasmacytoid dendritic cells [17, 18]. Some data suggest that the C5aR is also expressed on B cells [19] and T cells [20, 21]. Further, more recent reports show expression on NK and NKT cells [22] as well as in γδT-cells [23]. C5aR is also expressed in a variety of non-immune cells [24].

Binding of C5a to its receptor drives the activation of heterotrimeric G-proteins, i.e., the pertussis toxin-sensitive $G\alpha_{i2}$ [25] and the insensitive $G\alpha_{16}$ [26]. This initial event triggers intracellular Ca^{2+} $(Ca^{2+})_i$ mobilization [27] and activates the PI-3 kinase (PI3K)-dependent AKT and the Mitogen Activated Protein Kinases ERK 1/2 pathways [28]. It is well appreciated that PI3K/AKT and ERK1/2 participate in chemoattractant-mediated cell migration. Consistently, C5a has been shown to be a potent chemoattractant for neutrophils both in vitro and in vivo [29]. C5a-dependent recruitment and activation of myeloid cells is an important inflammatory and immunoregulatory mechanism in infection, autoimmune and allergic diseases [1] as well as in cancer [30]. Here, we describe three assays to assess C5a-mediated neutrophil migration in vitro and in vivo and C5a-mediated increase in $(Ca^{2+})_i$. Methods to determine C5a-mediated enzyme release from myeloid cells and ATP from platelets, to assess C3a and C5a concentrations in body fluids and to express and purify ATs have been described previously [31].

2 Materials

All solutions should be prepared with ultrapure water and analytical grade reagents. Prepare all buffers at room temperature. Reagents used to prepare cell culture should be sterilized by autoclaving at 120 °C for 20 min.

2.1 General Solutions

1. Hank's balanced salt solution HBSS (137.93 mM NaCl, 5.33 mM KCl, 0.338 mM Na_2HPO_4, 0.44 mM KH_2PO_4, 4.17 mM $NaHCO_3$, 0.493 mM $MgCl_2 \cdot 6H_2O$, 0.407 mM $MgSO_4 \cdot 7H_2O$, 1.26 $CaCl_2$, 5.56 mM D-Glucose).
2. Phosphate buffered saline PBS (137 mM NaCl, 2.7 mM KCl, 10 mM Na_2HPO_4, 2 mM KH_2PO_4). Control the pH, adjust to pH 7.4 if necessary.
3. Red blood cell lysis buffer: 155 mM NH_4Cl, 10 mM $NaHCO_3$, 0.1 mM EDTA.

4. Human recombinant C5a (Hycult biotech) dissolved in pyrogen free water (Aqua ad injectabilia, B. Braun) at a final concentration of 830 μM (*see* **Note 1**).

2.2 Materials for Cell Preparation

1. Cell strainer, 40 μm mesh (BD Bioscience).
2. Syringe with 26G needle (BD Bioscience).
3. 50 ml Polypropylene tube (BD Bioscience).

2.3 Solutions for Cell Surface Staining

1. Bovine serum albumin (Grade III, Sigma).
2. 4′,6-Diamidino-2-phenylindole (Sigma).
3. Fc Block anti-CD16/32mAb, clone 2.4G2 (eBioscience).
4. Anti-Ly6G antibody, clone 1A8, labeled with allophycocyanin (APC) (eBioscience) and corresponding isotype control (*see* **Note 2**).

2.4 Solutions for Ca^{2+} Measurements

1. Fluorescent calcium indicator Fluo-4 AM, 1 mM stock solution in dimethylsulfoxide (DMSO, Invitrogen Molecular Probes) (*see* **Note 3**).
2. Calcium ionophore ionomycin, 100 μM in DMSO stock solution (Sigma) (*see* **Note 4**).

2.5 Materials and Solutions for Chemotaxis

1. Chemotaxis-Buffer: HBSS with 2 % BSA.
2. Staining and fixation kit (eBioscience).
3. Hemacolor® staining solutions (Merck).
4. Vecta Mounting Medium (Vector).
5. Chemotaxis chamber (Neuroprobe AP48) with filter wiper (P48W), clamps for holding the filters (Neuroprobe, P48CL and P48CS).
6. PCTE (Polycarbonate track-tech) membrane with 3 μm pore width (Neuroprobe).
7. 24-Well plate (Tissue culture plate, flat bottom suspension cells, Sarstedt).
8. BD Truecount absolute counting tubes (BD Bioscience).

2.6 Software to Analyze the C5a-Mediated Increase in $(Ca^{2+})_i$

FlowJo (Tree Star, Inc.).

FCS Express version 4 or higher (De Novo Software).

3 Methods

3.1 Preparation of Bone Marrow Cells

1. Remove long bones (femurs and tibias) from C57BL/6J mouse. To flush the bones, use a sterile syringe containing 5 ml of sterile PBS connected to a 26 G needle. Cut the end of the bones with a scissor to make the marrow accessible for flushing. Place a 40 μm strainer on a 50 ml polypropylene tube and flush the bones holding them over the strainer until the complete marrow is flushed out and the bone turns opalescent

white. Carefully disperse the marrow over the strainer using the plunger of a 5 ml syringe. Wash the plunger with the remaining volume of PBS.

2. Centrifuge the cells for 5 min (400 × g) at RT.
3. Discard the supernatant, resuspend the cells in 3 ml of red blood cell lysis buffer and incubate for 3 min at RT. Then add PBS to a total volume of 20 ml to stop the lysis. Centrifuge the cells for 5 min (400 × g) at RT, discard the supernatant and resuspend the cells in 20 ml of PBS. Take 20 μl of this cell suspension to determine the cell number (the typical yield ranges between 3 and 3.5×10^7 cells) and stain the cells with trypan blue to assess the cell viability. Centrifuge the cells again for 5 min at RT (400 × g). Resuspend the cells in the appropriate buffer (for Ca^{2+} measurement, *see* Subheading 2.2; for chemotaxis, see Subheading 2.3).
4. Adjust the cells to 1×10^7/ml and add 1 μg Fc block antibody per 100 μl cell suspension. Incubate for 15 min at 4 °C.
5. Add 0.5 μg anti-Ly6G antibody per 100 μl cell suspension and incubate in the dark for another 15 min at 4 °C (*see* **Note 5**).
6. Centrifuge the cells for 5 min (400 × g) at RT and resuspend them in 500 μl PBS.
7. The cells are now ready for functional testing (for Ca^{2+} measurement, *see* Subheading 2.2; for chemotaxis, *see* Subheading 2.3).

3.2 C5a-Mediated Increase in Intracellular Calcium $(Ca^{2+})_i$ in Bone Marrow-Derived Neutrophils

1. To determine a dose–response curve of C5a-mediated increase in $(Ca^{2+})_i$, we routinely use five different C5a concentrations ranging from 0.1 to 4 nM C5a and run duplicate samples. As this procedure will require 1×10^7 cells, adjust the labeled bone marrow cells to a concentration of 1×10^7 cells/ml in PBS.
2. Add 10 μL of Fluo-4 AM to reach a final concentration of 10 μM, mix well and incubate in the dark for 30 min at RT (*see* **Notes 6–8**).
3. Add 500 μl PBS and centrifuge the cells for 5 min (400 × *g*) at RT. Repeat this procedure once.
4. Incubate for another 30 min in the dark at RT (*see* **Note 9**).
5. Take 50 μl of the cell suspension and add DAPI to a final concentration of 3 μM to define the percentage of dead cells.
6. Measure the fluorescence in the FITC channel for 30 s to record the baseline.
7. Remove the sample tube from the flow cytometer. Quickly add C5a (0.1, 0.25, 1, 2, or 4 nM, see Note 10). Reconnect the sample to the sample line and resume the measurement.
8. Measure the sample for 3 min.
9. Remove the sample tube from the flow cytometer. Add 1 μL of ionomycin, vortex briefly. Reconnect the sample and resume the measurement.
10. Measure for another 3 min.

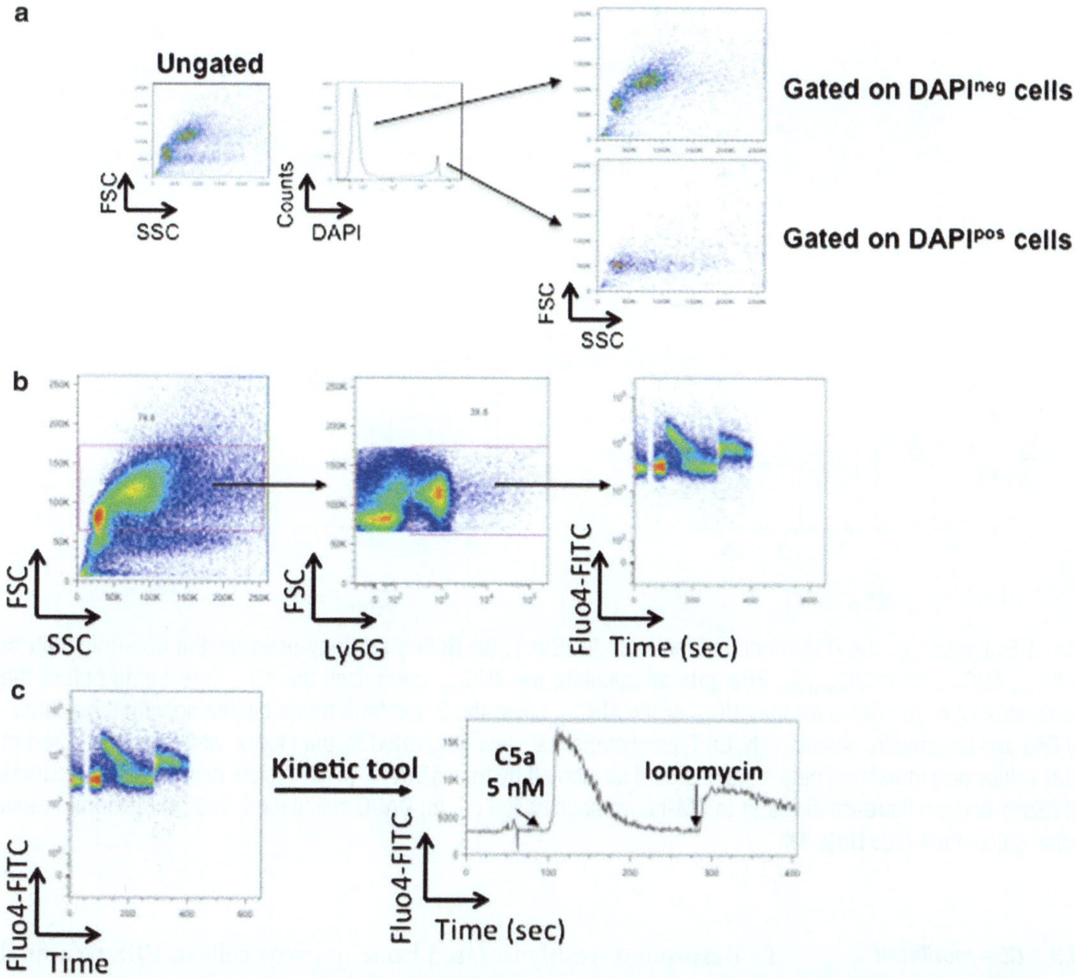

Fig. 1 C5a-mediated increase in $(Ca^{2+})_i$ in bone marrow-derived neutrophils. Bone marrow cells were isolated as described in Subheading 2.1 and stained for Ly6G expression (clone 1A8-APC, eBioscience 5 μg/ml). After washing and loading with Fluo-4 AM (described in Subheading 2.2), cells were first stimulated with C5a (4 nM) and then with ionomycin (1 μM). (**a**) Typical FSC/SSC dot plot obtained with mouse bone marrow cells. The frequency and position of dead cells in the FSC/SSC plot is determined by DAPI staining. As the FSC signal of $DAPI^{pos}$ cells is <60, you may directly gate on cells that are FSC <60 without additional DAPI staining. (**b**) *Left panel*, gating on BM cells that are FSC >60 to exclude dead cells; *middle panel*, gating on $Ly6G^{hi}$ FCS^{hi} cells allows the selection of living neutrophils; *right panel*, recording of the Fluo-4 AM signal in the $Ly6G^{hi}$ FSC^{hi} population in response to C5a. (**c**) Transformation of the Fluo-4 AM signal in $Ly6G^{hi}$ FSC^{hi} cells in response to C5a or ionomycin treatment into a curve by the FloJo software. Depicted is a dot plot, in which the Fluo-4 AM signal is emitted in the FITC-channel (*y-axis*) and plotted against the time (*x-axis*)

11. To determine the C5a-mediated increase of $(Ca^{2+})_i$ in bone marrow neutrophils (Figs. 1 and 2), first gate on BM cells that are FSC >60 (Fig. 1b, left panel) as such cells represent the $DAPI^{neg}$ living cells, whereas dead BM cells ($DAPI^{pos}$) are FSC <60 (Fig. 1a, c and 2; *see* **Notes 11–13**).

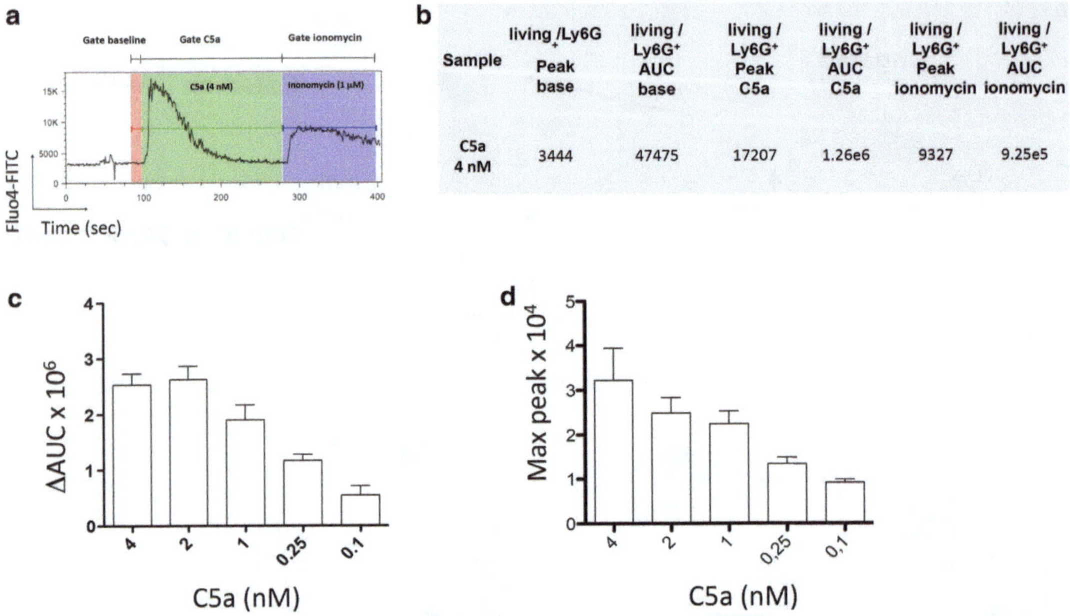

Sample	living /Ly6G+ Peak base	living / Ly6G+ AUC base	living / Ly6G+ Peak C5a	living / Ly6G+ AUC C5a	living / Ly6G+ Peak ionomycin	living / Ly6G+ AUC ionomycin
C5a 4 nM	3444	47475	17207	1.26e6	9327	9.25e5

Fig. 2 Evaluation of the C5a-mediated increase in $(Ca^{2+})_i$. (**a**) Gating strategy used for the determination of AUC_{base}, AUC_{C5a}, and $AUC_{ionomycin}$. The gate to calculate the AUC_{base} comprises the 15 s time frame before the addition of C5a. The gates for the AUC_{c5a} or the AUC_{iono} cover the 3 min time frame beginning with the addition of C5a and ionomycin, respectively. (**b**) Typical statistical view generated by the FlowJo software; the different AUC values and maximum peaks are depicted as labeled by the software. (**c–d**) Typical dose–response curves of C5a-mediated increase in $(Ca^{2+})_i$ in BM-neutrophils based on: (**c**) DAUC calculation; and (**d**) maximum peak value calculation (*see* **Note 14**)

3.3 C5a-mediated Chemotaxis of Bone Marrow-Derived Neutrophils

3.3.1 Assembly of the Chemotaxis Chamber and Chemotaxis Assay

1. Resuspend freshly isolated bone marrow cells in PBS to a final concentration of 6×10^6 cells/ml. Let the cells rest for 30 min at 37 °C in the CO_2 incubator (24-well plate; 0.5 ml per well).
2. Fill the wells of the lower part of the chamber (Fig. 3) (*see* **Note 14**) with the C5a solution (12.5 nM, diluted in chemotaxis buffer). The wells can hold a maximum volume of 26 μl. It is critical to avoid the formation of air bubbles while filling the bottom well, as such bubbles will prevent C5a-driven cell migration by blocking the contact between the chemoattractant and the membrane. A positive meniscus should be visible after administration of the chemoattractant to ensure that it is in contact with the membrane after assembly of the chamber. Include an appropriate negative control (i.e., chemotaxis buffer) for your experiment.
3. Use forceps to handle the membranes. Mark one corner of the membrane for orientation (*see* **Note 15**). Make sure that the membrane will cover all wells filled with fluid. Lift the membrane at both ends and let the middle part touch the lower chamber. Slowly lower both ends of the membranes until the entire membrane is attached to the low chamber covering all wells (*see* **Note 16**).

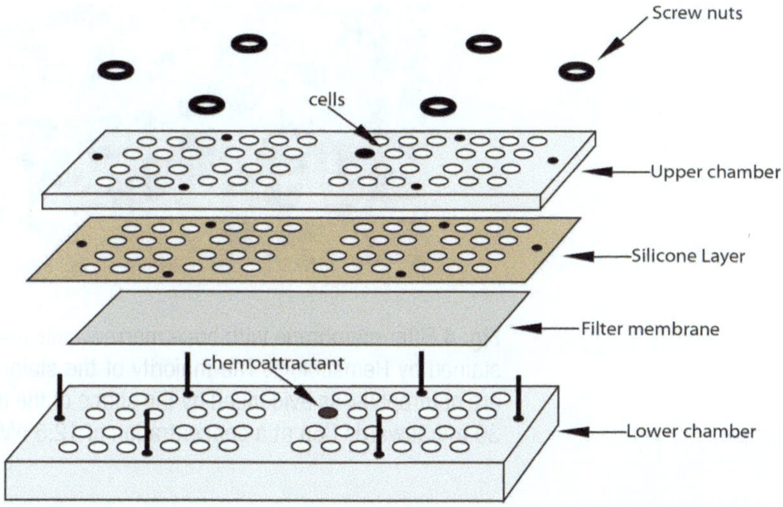

Fig. 3 Composition of the chemotaxis chamber. The chemotaxis chamber comprises four different components: (1) the upper chamber; (2) the silicone layer; (3) the filter membrane; and (4) the lower chamber. The wells of the upper chamber hold the cells, whereas the lower chamber contains the chemoattractant. Cells that have migrated through the filter membrane are stained at the *bottom* side using the Hemacolor® Kit and enumerated by microscopic evaluating of at least ten high power fields

4. Assemble the upper chamber and the silicone layer, and push them firmly down on the lower chamber (Fig. 3). When the upper chamber comes into contact with the lower chamber, do not release the pressure, until you have tightened the screws. The upper wells can be filled with a maximum of 50 μl cell suspension. Do not use higher volumes, as this may result in fluid spillover and contamination of adjacent wells.
5. Add 50 μl of your prepared cell suspension (for neutrophils use a total of 300,000 cells/well) to the wells. Avoid air bubbles, as this will limit the access of your cells to the chemoattractant (*see* **Note 17**).
6. Place the chemotaxis chamber into the CO_2 incubator (37 °C, 5 % CO_2). Incubation times may vary, depending on the cell type and the chemoattractant. For chemotaxis of neutrophils with C5a as chemoattractant, please incubate for 30 min. To determine the appropriate incubation time, *see* **Note 18**.

3.3.2 Disassembly of the Chemotaxis Chamber and Enumeration of Migrated Neutrophils

1. After removing the chamber from the incubator, discard the fluid from the upper wells by inverting the chamber and shaking it over a piece of paper towel.
2. Disassemble the chamber by unscrewing the screw nuts while constantly keeping the pressure on the upper lid with your free hand.
3. Invert the whole chamber and push it toward a paper towel to disassemble the lower and the upper chamber. Do not touch

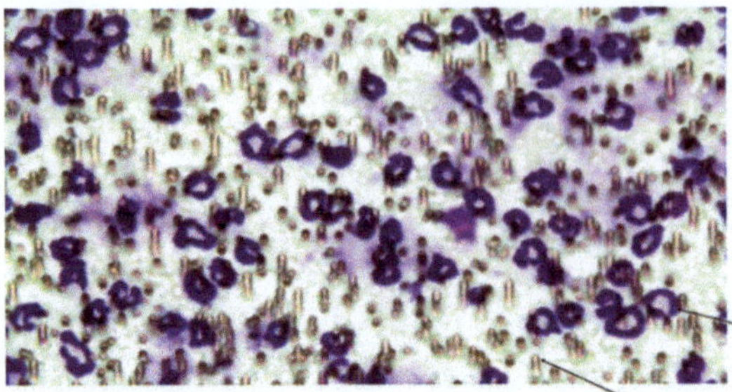

Fig. 4 Filter membrane with bone marrow cells migrated in response to C5a and stained by Hemacolor®. The majority of the stained cells (*marked by an arrow*) are neutrophils, as evidenced by the shape of the nucleus. The cells migrated for 30 min towards C5a at a concentration of 12.5 nM

the filter on top of the silicone gasket and the upper chamber, as this might contaminate the filter and distort your results.

4. Use forceps and clamps to remove the membrane from the silicone gasket. Hold the membrane with the forceps and rinse the side, which was originally facing the wells containing the cells (i.e., the side facing to the upper chamber) three times with PBS. We routinely use a petri dish as sink for the rinse flow. After each washing step, use the membrane wiper to mechanically remove cells from the bottom side of the membrane. Make sure that only migrated cells remain on the membrane. Let it air-dry for at least 30 min.
5. For cell staining, flip the membrane so that the cells are facing down. Fill a petri dish with fixation solution. Use clamps and wipe the membrane 20 times in fixation solution. Let it air-dry for at least 30 min.
6. Stain the membrane using Hemacolor® staining solutions (1 and 2) according to the manufacturer's recommendations.
7. Mount the membrane with cells facing down on a microscope slide and let it dry for 30 min. Use Vector shield mounting medium to preserve your membrane.
8. Determine the number of migrated cells using a light microscope. Count at least ten fields in the designated area to avoid non-representative results due to uneven cell distribution (Figs. 4 and 5)

3.4 C5a-Mediated Cell Migration In Vivo

1. Prepare 1 ml of a 2 μM C5a solution dissolved in PBS. Inject mice with a total of 200 nM (200 μl each) i.p. Inject 200 μl PBS as control.
2. Sacrifice the mice 6 h after the C5a injection. Lavage the peritoneum by injecting 5 ml of ice-cold PBS into the peritoneal cavity using a 24 G needle. Gently massage the belly and subsequently aspirate the fluid using the same syringe (the typical yield is 4 ml).
3. Centrifuge cells for 5 min ($400 \times g$) at RT.

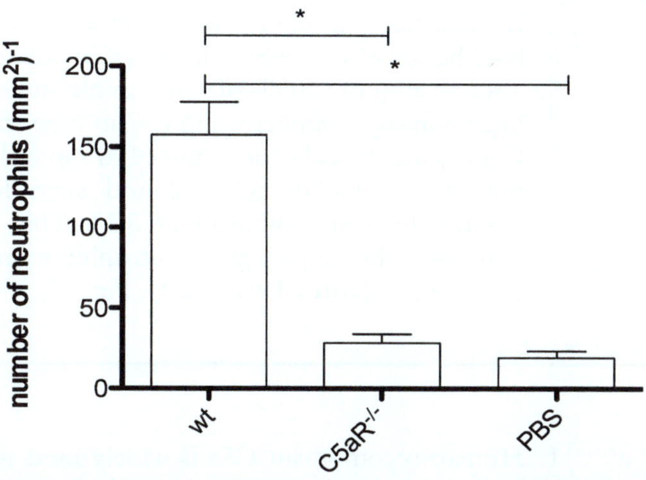

Fig. 5 C5a-mediated chemotaxis of BM neutrophils is dependent on C5aR signaling. BM-derived cells were used at a density of 6×10^6 cells/ml. C5a (12.5 nM) was diluted in chemotaxis medium and placed in the bottom wells of the modified Boyden chamber (Fig. 6). 50 μl of the cell suspension were placed in the top wells and incubated for 30 min at 37 °C. Subsequently, membranes were removed and the cells on the bottom side (side with migrated cells, originally facing the C5a containing well) were stained with Hemacolor®. Depicted is the number of migrated cells per mm^2 from wt and C5aR mice as calculated from the evaluation of ten high-power fields. PBS-treated cells served as control. Values shown are means of triplicate samples ± sem ($n = 3$)

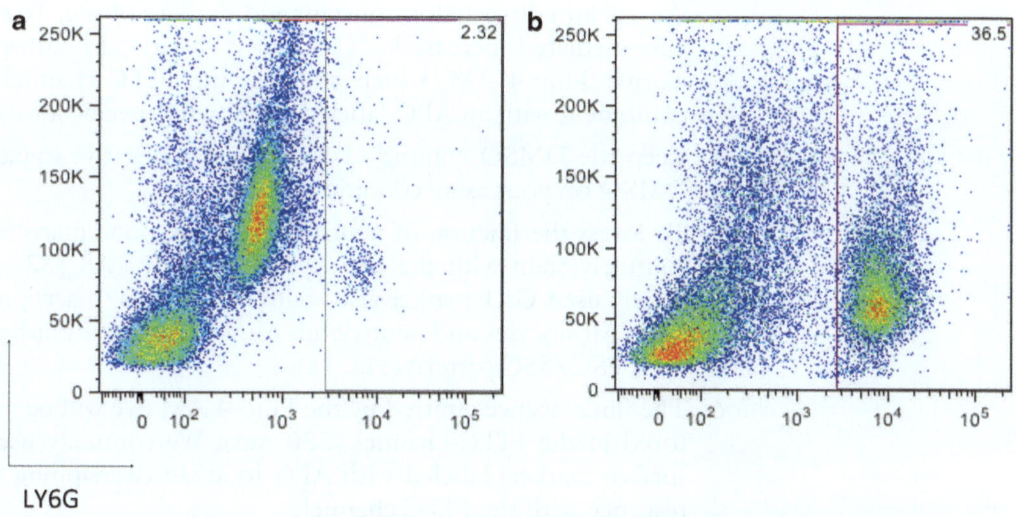

Fig. 6 Intraperitoneal injection of C5a drives neutrophil migration into the peritoneal cavity. Mice were injected i.p. with 200 μl PBS (**a**) or 200 nM C5a (**b**) in 200 μl PBS. After 6 h, cells from the peritoneum were harvested by lavage, stained for LY6G expression (2.4), and analyzed by flow cytometry. The two representative *dot plots* show strong neutrophilic infiltration of the peritoneum in response to C5a administration (**b**) as evidenced by a high frequency of $Ly6G^{hi}$ cells

4. In case that your sample is contaminated with red blood cells, lyse the red blood cells as described in Subheading 3.1, **step 2**.
5. Take an aliquot (20 μl) of your sample and enumerate the cells in a counting chamber using trypan blue staining.
6. Centrifuge the cells for 5 min ($400 \times g$) at RT. Adjust the cell number to 1×10^6 cells/ml and stain for neutrophils as described above (Subheading 3.1). This will allow you to determine the frequency of neutrophils migrated into the peritoneum (*see* **Notes 19** and **20**) (Fig. 6).

4 Notes

1. Human recombinant C5a is widely used to stimulate rodent cells, as the binding affinity is similar to mouse C5a [32]. Due to its high pK value, C5a tends to stick to plastic surfaces. Always use low binding tubes (e.g., Eppendorf LoBind® tubes) and pipette tips (e.g., epT.I.P.S.®LoRetention) to avoid substantial loss of C5a during the dilution procedures.
2. The phycoerythrin (PE) label is not recommended because the strong Ca^{2+}-derived FITC signal overlaps with the PE signal.
3. The choice of the calcium indicator depends on the experimental settings and the sensitivity required. The choice of dye depends on the excitation and emission wavelengths, the calcium dissociation constant and the ease of use. To study C5a-mediated increase in $(Ca^{2+})_i$ in BM-derived neutrophils, we use Fluo-4 AM, which emits in the FITC channel and combine it with an APC-labeled anti-Ly6G-specific antibody.
4. Keep the DMSO volume <1 % to avoid a negative impact of DMSO on your assay conditions.
5. To assess the fraction of neutrophils in the bone marrow, we routinely stain with the anti-Ly6G antibody 1A8 [33]. The widely used Gr-1 marker also stains monocytes/macrophages [34]. Monocytes and neutrophils can also be distinguished by their FSC/SSC pattern (Fig. 1a).
6. The fluorescence emitted by the Fluo-4 AM dye will be monitored in the FITC channel (530 nm). We routinely use cell surface markers labeled with APC to avoid overlapping fluorescence with the FITC channel.
7. The lipophilic transport of the acetylmethylester of Fluo-4 AM is temperature sensitive. Please consider adjustment of your incubation time if you work in a lab without air conditioning.
8. The most eminent problem resulting from fluorescent calcium indicator dye loading is the presence of dead cells in the assay.

Fluo-4 AM is transported through the cell membrane only when the lipophilic acetoxymethylester moieties are preserved as they cover the negative charges of the carboxyl groups involved in Ca^{2+} binding. Removal of the acetoxymethylester is caused by de-esterification. In case of cell death, excessive amounts of esterase are released leading to a marked decrease in the availability of the fluorescent dye and subsequent decrease in indicator dye loading.

9. Once inside the cells, Fluo-4 AM is converted into Fluo-4, acetic acid, and formaldehyde by intracellular esterase during the incubation time.
10. Do not vortex your sample as this procedure can drive calcium mobilization and distort your results.
11. The fluorescence signal of the Fluo-4 AM indicator dye can overlap with the DAPI signal resulting in a miscalculation of the frequency of dead cells. This is why we directly gate on BM cells with an FSC signal >60 and avoid gating on $DAPI^{neg}$ cells. Alternatively, you may want to use a viability dye that does not overlap with the emission spectrum of the Fluo-4 AM indicator dye.
12. Dead cells usually represent 4–6 % of total cells. Next, gate on $Ly6G^{hi}$ neutrophils as shown in Fig. 1b, middle panel. Now record the Fluo-4 AM $(Ca^{2+})_i$ signal of the $Ly6G^{hi}$ living cells in the FITC channel (Fig. 1b, right panel). Use appropriate evaluation software that allows for a time-dependent analysis of the data (e.g., FlowJo or FCS Express). We routinely determine: (1) the area under the curve (AUC) recorded during the 3 min measurement; and (2) the maximum peak of the calcium-dependent fluorescence emission within the first 20 s after the addition of C5a. The two parameters provide complementary information regarding the kinetic of the intracellular Ca^{2+} flux and the amplitude of the response, respectively.
13. To visualize the kinetic of C5a-mediated increase in $(Ca^{2+})_i$, plot the time (*x*-axis) versus the FITC-signal (*y*-axis) as shown in Fig. 1c. To further quantify the C5a-mediated increase in $(Ca^{2+})_i$, use the kinetic tool provided by your evaluation software. This tool will allow you to calculate the area under the curve (AUC, Fig. 2a). You can directly assess the value for the maximum peak by opening the statistics related to this plot. The AUC is calculated as a function of the fluorescence signal recorded within a defined time frame. We routinely use the following time frames: 30 s for the baseline (AUC_{base}) and 3 min for the C5a-stimulated (AUC_{c5a}) or the ionomycin-treated sample (AUC_{iono}) (Fig. 2a). Ionomycin is used as a fluorescent dye loading control. The individual AUCs are directly calculated by the software and will appear in the statistical table associated with the plot (Fig. 2b). To compare the

increase in $(Ca^{2+})_i$ induced by the individual C5a concentrations, subtract the AUC_{base} from the AUC_{c5a} resulting in the ΔAUC. Figure 2c shows typical dose–response curves for C5a-mediated increases in $(Ca^{2+})_i$ based on ΔAUC (left panel) or maximum peak (right panel) calculations.

14. Activation of C5aR in neutrophils leads to a strong Ca^{2+} influx into the cells that may last up to 3 min. In our hands, the dose–response relationship based on the maximum peak calculation is best reflected when you determine the maximum peak value 20 s after the addition of C5a.
15. The chamber and all materials involved in the chemotaxis assay should be pre-warmed in the CO_2 incubator to 37 °C.
16. Mark the membrane, e.g., by cutting off one corner to keep track of the orientation.
17. Please note that some adjustment after dropping the membrane is tolerable; however, too much movement of the already attached membrane will lead to cross-contamination of adjacent wells.
18. To avoid air bubbles while filling the upper wells, please hold the pipette in a steep angle so that the end of the pipette tip rests against the wall of the chamber just above the filter, and the side of the tip rests against the top rim of the well. The content of the pipette has to be ejected rapidly. Wells with air bubbles (seen by a untypically large meniscus) can be emptied using a paper towel (e.g., Kimwipe) and a pipette tip and refilled for further use.
19. To determine the appropriate incubation time, the manufacturer recommends the use of blind-well chambers that are removed from the incubator sequentially every 5 min. Filters are stained and analyzed. This procedure allows determining the time needed by unstimulated cells to migrate through the filter.
20. To convert the neutrophil frequency measured by the flow cytometer into the neutrophil numbers present in the peritoneum, we routinely use two methods. First, we relate the neutrophil frequency to the cell number determined during **step 5**. For example, if we have determined a frequency of 5 % neutrophils and the cell count in **step 5** has been 100,000 cells, the total neutrophil number in the peritoneum will be 5,000. This is a so-called multiple platform test, since not all data are collected with the same machine. We also use a single platform approach. This method comprises counting beads. Routinely, we use BD Truecount absolute counting tubes (BD Bioscience). Following the recommendations of the supplier will allow you to accurately calculate the cell number in your sample.

References

1. Klos A, Tenner AJ, Johswich KO et al (2009) The role of the anaphylatoxins in health and disease. Mol Immunol 46:2753–2766
2. Strey CW, Markiewski M, Mastellos D et al (2003) The proinflammatory mediators C3a and C5a are essential for liver regeneration. J Exp Med 198:913–923
3. Mastellos D, Papadimitriou JC, Franchini S et al (2001) A novel role of complement: mice deficient in the fifth component of complement (C5) exhibit impaired liver regeneration. J Immunol 166:2479–2486
4. Hillebrandt S, Wasmuth HE, Weiskirchen R et al (2005) Complement factor 5 is a quantitative trait gene that modifies liver fibrogenesis in mice and humans. Nat Genet 37:835–843
5. Addis-Lieser E, Köhl J, Chiaramonte MG (2005) Opposing regulatory roles of complement factor 5 in the development of bleomycin-induced pulmonary fibrosis. J Immunol 175:1894–1902
6. Benard M, Gonzalez BJ, Schouft MT et al (2004) Characterization of C3a and C5a receptors in rat cerebellar granule neurons during maturation: neuroprotective effect of C5a against apoptotic cell death. J Biol Chem 279:43487–96
7. Gerard NP, Gerard C (1991) The chemotactic receptor for human C5a anaphylatoxin. Nature 349:614–617
8. Boulay F, Mery L, Tardif M et al (1991) Expression cloning of a receptor for C5a anaphylatoxin on differentiated HL-60 cells. Biochemistry 30:2993–2999
9. Cain SA, Monk PN (2002) The orphan receptor C5L2 has high affinity binding sites for complement fragments C5a and C5a des-Arg(74). J Biol Chem 277:7165–7169
10. Okinaga S, Slattery D, Humbles A et al (2003) C5L2, a nonsignaling C5A binding protein. Biochemistry 42:9406–9415
11. Crass T, Raffetseder U, Martin U et al (1996) Expression cloning of the human C3a anaphylatoxin receptor (C3aR) from differentiated U-937 cells. Eur J Immunol 26:1944–1950
12. Ames RS, Li Y, Sarau HM et al (1996) Molecular cloning and characterization of the human anaphylatoxin C3a receptor. J Biol Chem 271:20231–20234
13. Chenoweth DE, Goodman MG (1983) The C5a receptor of neutrophils and macrophages. Agents Actions Suppl 12:252–273
14. Chenoweth DE, Hugli TE (1978) Demonstration of specific C5a receptor on intact human polymorphonuclear leukocytes. Proc Natl Acad Sci U S A 75:3943–3947
15. Gerard NP, Hodges MK, Drazen JM et al (1989) Characterization of a receptor for C5a anaphylatoxin on human eosinophils. J Biol Chem 264:1760–1766
16. Werfel T, Oppermann M, Begemann G et al (1997) C5a receptors are detectable on mast cells in normal human skin and in psoriatic plaques but not in weal and flare reactions or in uticaria pigmentosa by immunohistochemistry. Arch Dermatol Res 289:83–86
17. Köhl J, Baelder R, Lewkowich IP et al (2006) A regulatory role for the C5a anaphylatoxin in type 2 immunity in asthma. J Clin Invest 116:783–796
18. Zhang X, Lewkowich IP, Köhl G et al (2009) A protective role for C5a in the development of allergic asthma associated with altered levels of B7-H1 and B7-DC on plasmacytoid dendritic cells. J Immunol 182: 5123–5130
19. Ottonello L, Corcione A, Tortolina G et al (1999) rC5a directs the in vitro migration of human memory and naive tonsillar B lymphocytes: implications for B cell trafficking in secondary lymphoid tissues. J Immunol 162: 6510–6517
20. Lalli PN, Strainic MG, Yang M et al (2008) Locally produced C5a binds to T cell-expressed C5aR to enhance effector T-cell expansion by limiting antigen-induced apoptosis 153. Blood 112:1759–1766
21. Strainic MG, Liu J, Huang D et al (2008) Locally produced complement fragments C5a and C3a provide both costimulatory and survival signals to naive CD4+ T cells. Immunity 28:425–435
22. Fusakio ME, Mohammed JP, Laumonnier Y et al (2011) C5a regulates NKT and NK cell functions in sepsis. J Immunol 187: 5805–5812
23. Han G, Geng S, Li Y et al (2011) GammadeltaT-cell function in sepsis is modulated by C5a receptor signalling. Immunology 133: 340–349
24. Monk PN, Scola AM, Madala P et al (2007) Function, structure and therapeutic potential of complement C5a receptors. Br J Pharmacol 152:429–448
25. Skokowa J, Ali SR, Felda O et al (2005) Macrophages induce the inflammatory response in the pulmonary Arthus reaction through G alpha i2 activation that controls C5aR and Fc receptor cooperation. J Immunol 174:3041–3050
26. Amatruda TT, Gerard NP, Gerard C et al (1993) Specific interactions of chemoattractant

factor receptors with G- proteins. J Biol Chem 268:10139–10144
27. Monk PN, Partridge LJ (1993) Characterization of a complement-fragment-C5a-stimulated calcium- influx mechanism in U937 monocytic cells. Biochem J 295:679–684
28. Hawlisch H, Belkaid Y, Baelder R et al (2005) C5a negatively regulates toll-like receptor 4-induced immune responses. Immunity 22:415–426
29. Fernandez HN, Henson PM, Otani A et al (1978) Chemotactic response to human C3a and C5a anaphylatoxins. I. Evaluation of C3a and C5a leukotaxis in vitro and under stimulated in vivo conditions. J Immunol 120:109–115
30. Markiewski MM, Deangelis RA, Benencia F et al (2008) Modulation of the antitumor immune response by complement. Nat Immunol 9:1225–1235
31. Köhl J (1997) In: Dodds AW, Sim RB (eds) Complement: a practical approach. Oxford University Press, Oxford, pp 135–163
32. Gerard C, Bao L, Orozco O et al (1992) Structural diversity in the extracellular faces of peptidergic G-protein-coupled receptors. Molecular cloning of the mouse C5a anaphylatoxin receptor. J Immunol 149:2600–2606
33. Daley JM, Thomay AA, Connolly MD et al (2008) Use of Ly6G-specific monoclonal antibody to deplete neutrophils in mice. J Leukoc Biol 83:64–70
34. Zhang X, Majlessi L, Deriaud E et al (2009) Coactivation of Syk kinase and MyD88 adaptor protein pathways by bacteria promotes regulatory properties of neutrophils. Immunity 31:761–771

Chapter 24

Detection of Complement Receptors 1 and 2 on Mouse Splenic B Cells Using Flow Cytometry

Luke R. Donius and John H. Weis

Abstract

The complement receptor 2 (*Cr2*) gene is exclusively expressed in B cells and follicular dendritic cells (FDC) in mice and in humans. However, mice also express an alternative splice variant, CR1, of the *Cr2* gene. CR2 and CR1 are receptors for the complement component 3 (C3) cleavage fragments C3d(g) and iC3b. Additionally, CR1 is a receptor for C3b and regulates complement convertase activity. CR1 and CR2 have various functions including antigen retention by FDC, regulation of surface complement convertases, and canonically as the B cell coreceptor in which CR2 acts to lower the threshold for B cell activation. Detection of CR1 and CR2 can be utilized to identify B cells and, depending on expression level, to delineate various B cell populations. This protocol describes methods for detecting CR1/2 expression on splenic B cell subsets via flow cytometry.

Key words Complement receptor 1, Complement receptor 2, CR1, CR2, CD21, CD35, B cell coreceptor, B cell activation, Flow cytometry, Marginal zone B cell, Follicular mature B cell, Transitional 1 B cell, Transitional 2 B cell

1 Introduction

Complement receptor 2 (CR2) and the alternative isoform CR1 are cellular receptors that bind enzymatic products of complement protein C3: C3d(g) and iC3b for CR2 as well as C3b and C4b for CR1 [1]. (It should be noted that CR1 and CR2 are also known by their cluster of differentiation (CD) designations, CD35 and CD21, respectively. Both names are used commonly and will be used in the following protocol.) CR2 reduces the threshold for B cell stimulation [2, 3], facilitates transport of immune complexes to immune follicles [4, 5], and retains immune complexes in immune follicles [6, 7]. CR1 has an additional role as a surface regulator of C3 convertases [1, 8, 9]. CR1 and CR2 are important markers for B cells and FDC and are a critical bridge for complement-driven immune modulation of the humoral immune

Mihaela Gadjeva (ed.), *The Complement System: Methods and Protocols*, Methods in Molecular Biology, vol. 1100,
DOI 10.1007/978-1-62703-724-2_24, © Springer Science+Business Media New York 2014

response [6, 10, 11]. Identification of CR1 and CR2 is common for identifying B cells and aiding in delineation of B cell subsets [12]. Antibody detection of CR1/2 by flow cytometry is a common method of detection and is an often included identification of B cell subsets. The protocol described in the chapter *Detection of Complement Receptors 1 and 2* describes methods for detecting CR2 and CR1 on the surface of cells via flow cytometry.

2 Materials

1. FACS (Fluorescent Activated Cell Sorting) buffer: 0.1 % bovine serum albumin, 1× PBS, pH 7.4.
2. 75 × 12 mm Conical bottom tube.
3. 12 × 75 mm 5 ml Polystyrene round-bottom tube.
4. Red blood cell lysis buffer (ACK buffer): Combine 8.3 g NH_4Cl, $KHCO_3$ and 200 μl of 0.5 M EDTA pH 7.4 in 800 ml deionized H_2O. Adjust pH to 7.4 and bring solution to 1 L total volume with deionized H_2O.
5. Tube rack for holding 12 × 75 mm diameter tubes on ice.
6. Tabletop centrifuge with temperature control capable of maintaining 4 °C.
7. Rat anti-mouse CR2 (CD21/35) antibody, FITC conjugated, clone 7G6 (BD Pharmingen, San Diego, CA, USA).
8. Rat anti-mouse CD24 antibody, PE-Cy7 conjugated, clone M1/69 (eBioscience San Diego, CA, USA).
9. Rat anti-mouse CD23 antibody, Phycoerythrin (PE) conjugated, clone B3B4 (eBioscience San Diego, CA, USA).
10. Anti-human/mouse CD45R (B220) PerCP-Cy5.5- conjugated antibody, clone RA3-6B2.
11. Fc receptor block, anti-mouse CD16/32, purified antibody, clone 93.
12. 100 μm cell strainer.
13. 1 mM Stock solution of DAPI in deionized H_2O.
14. Flow cytometer capable of exciting/detecting at 495/519 nm (FITC), 358/461 nm (DAPI), 480;565/578 nm (PE), 482/694 nm (PerCP-Cy5.5), 480;565/767 nm (PE-Cy7).

3 Methods

1. To assess cells for CR2 expression, obtain a single-cell suspension in FACS buffer from a source of interest. Cells commonly assessed in this manner are cells from the peripheral blood, the

spleen, the peritoneal cavity, and the bone marrow (*see* **Note 1** and **2**). This protocol describes the preparation and antibody staining of splenocytes, although cells from any of the preceding sources could be assessed in a similar manner.

2. Centrifuge the cells at 300 × *g* for 5 min at 4 °C and aspirate the supernatant.
3. Resuspend the cell pellet in 1 ml of 4 °C chilled ACK lysis buffer with gentle pipetting to lyse red blood cells and incubate for 5 min.
4. Centrifuge the cells at 300 × *g* for 5 min at 4 °C and aspirate the supernatant.
5. Resuspend the pellet in 10 ml of 4 °C chilled FACS buffer and place on ice.
6. Count the cells in the sample to determine the total cells per milliliter. Transfer 2×10^6 cells to a 75 × 12 mm conical bottom tube (*see* **Note 3**). Place the tube on ice and proceed with preparing the antibody mix for staining the cells.
7. Prepare the antibody mix of FITC-conjugated Rat anti-mouse CD21/35 (CR2) antibody diluted 1:200 (2.5 μg/ml) (*see* **Note 4**), PE-conjugated anti-mouse CD23 antibody diluted 1:200 (1 μg/ml), PE-Cy7-conjugated anti-mouse CD24 antibody diluted 1:600 (0.3 μg/ml), Rat anti-mouse CD16/32 antibody diluted 1:1,000 (0.5 μg/ml) (*see* **Note 5**), and PerCP-Cy5.5-conjugated B220 antibody diluted 1:200 (1 μg/ml) in FACS buffer (100 μl/sample).
8. Centrifuge the cells at 300 × *g* for 5 min at 4 °C and aspirate the supernatant.
9. Resuspend each sample of cells in 100 μl of the prepared antibody mix. Incubate the sample on ice in the dark for 20 min.
10. Dilute each sample with 1 ml of FACS buffer, centrifuge the cells at 300 × *g* for 5 min at 4 °C, and aspirate the supernatant.
11. Resuspend the cells in 1 ml of FACS buffer (*see* **Note 6**) and filter through a 100 μm cell strainer into round -bottom tube. Add 3 μl of DAPI (3 μM final concentration), gently vortex, and let sit for 5 min. Acquire fluorescence staining data using a flow cytometer (*see* **Note 7**).
12. Identification of transitional 1, transitional 2, marginal zone, and follicular mature B cells is done by gating on the DAPI negative (live) and B220 positive (B cells), and then separating the groups by CD23 expression (positive are the transitional 2 and follicular mature B cells and negatives are the transitional 1 and marginal zone B cells). Gating the B cells within the CD23 positive or CD23 negative groups by CD21/35 and CD24 expression can then be used to transitional 1 B cells

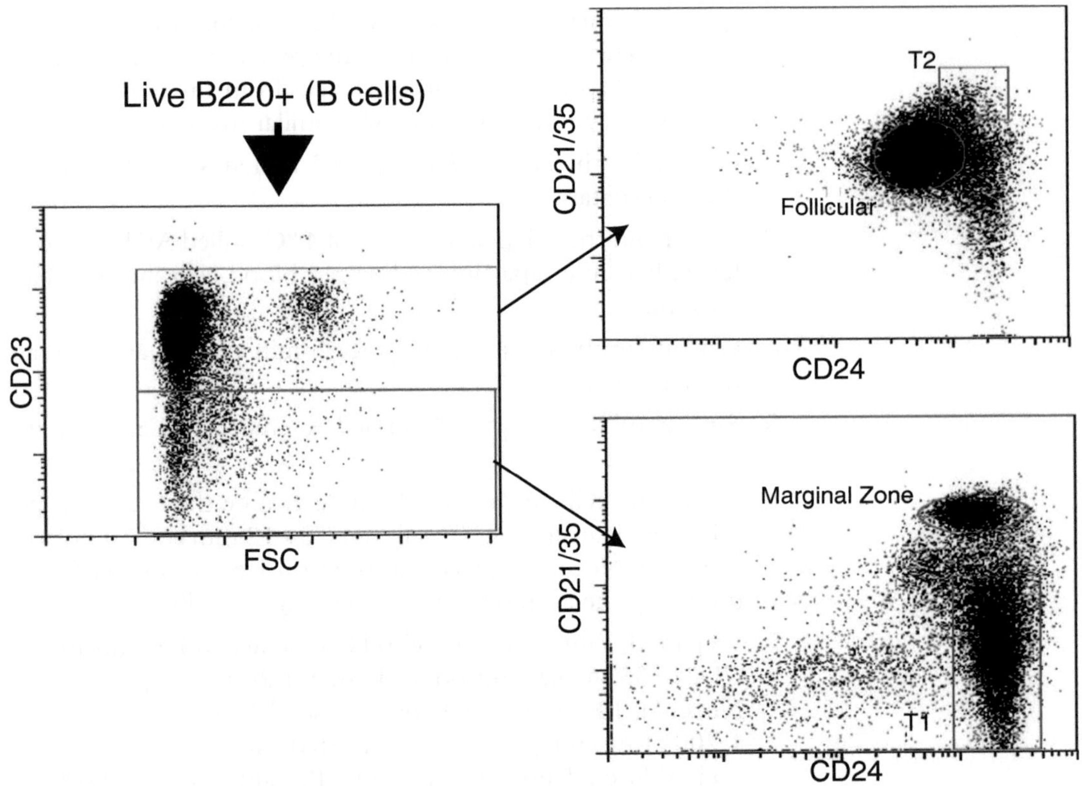

Fig. 1 Surface expression of CD23, CD24, and CD21/35 on the total live B220+ cells in the spleen can be used to identify splenic B cell subsets. These subsets include mature follicular B cells and marginal zone B cells as well as the immature B cell populations transitional 1 (T1) and T2

($CD23^-/CD21/35^{Lo}/CD24^+$), marginal zone B cells ($CD23^-/CD21/35^{Hi}/CD24^+$), transitional 2 B cells ($CD23^+/CD21/35^{Hi}/CD24^{Hi}$), and follicular mature B cells ($CD23^+/CD21/35^{Lo}/CD24^{Lo}$) (Fig. 1).

4 Notes

1. In order to assess cells for CR2 expression using this method the cells must be able to be processed through a flow cytometer. Lymphocytes are ideal for analysis by flow cytometry. However, of the two major cell types in the spleen that express CR1/2, B cells, and FDC, this protocol will result only in analysis of the former. FDC can be analyzed but FDC isolation protocols should be sought out in order to efficiently collect them.
2. This protocol has been written for detection of CR2 on the surface of mouse cells. A similar procedure could be used on human/primate cells with antibodies that recognize human epitopes.

3. Ideally this protocol describes antibody staining of 2×10^6 cells. However, a range of $1–5 \times 10^6$ cells per sample may be labeled. Consistency between samples is the most important factor.
4. The CR2 monoclonal antibody clone 7G6 has been shown to bind both CR2 (CD21) and the isoform CR1 (CD35) [13]. No antibody is currently known to recognize only CR2. However, the anti-CD35 antibody (clone 8C12), available through BD Pharmingen, exclusively binds CR1.
5. Rat anti-CD16/32 is necessary to block the Fc Receptors so that cells expressing these receptors do not bind antibody via the Fc region in an epitope-independent manner.
6. The final resuspended volume of the cells to be analyzed by flow cytometry can be reduced in order to reduce data collection time if the total cell number is low.
7. All fluorescent parameters must be defined for the flow cytometer by single-color positive controls and an unstained negative control. All channels used must be compensated to eliminate cross-fluorescence in multiple detectors. Consult the manual or expert users for information on proper operation of your specific flow cytometer.

References

1. Molina H, Kinoshita T, Webster CB, Holers VM (1994) Analysis of C3b/C3d binding sites and factor I cofactor regions within mouse complement receptors 1 and 2. J Immunol 153:789–795
2. Carter RH, Spycher MO, Ng YC, Hoffman R, Fearon DT (1988) Synergistic interaction between complement receptor type 2 and membrane IgM on B lymphocytes. J Immunol 141:457–463
3. Luxembourg AT, Cooper NR (1994) Modulation of signaling via the B cell antigen receptor by CD21, the receptor for C3dg and EBV. J Immunol 153:4448–4457
4. Whipple EC, Shanahan RS, Ditto AH, Taylor RP, Lindorfer MA (2004) Analyses of the in vivo trafficking of stoichiometric doses of an anti-complement receptor 1/2 monoclonal antibody infused intravenously in mice. J Immunol 173(4):2297–2306
5. Suzuki K, Grigorova I, Phan TG, Kelly LM, Cyster JG (2009) Visualizing B cell capture of cognate antigen from follicular dendritic cells. J Exp Med 206:1485–1493
6. Haas KM, Hasegawa M, Steeber DA, Poe JC, Zabel MD, Bock CB, Karp DR, Briles DE, Weis J, Tedder TF (2002) Complement receptors CD21/35 link innate and protective immunity during *Streptococcus pneumoniae* infection by regulating IgG3 antibody responses. Immunity 17:713–723
7. Mattsson J, Yrlid U, Stensson A, Schön K, Karlsson MCI, Ravetch JV, Lycke NY (2011) Complement activation and complement receptors on follicular dendritic cells are critical for the function of a targeted adjuvant. J Immunol 187(7):3641–3652
8. Krych-Goldberg M, Atkinson JP (2001) Structure-function relationships of complement receptor type 1. Immunol Rev 180:112–122
9. Seregin SS, Aldhamen YA, Appledorn DM, Schuldt NJ, McBride AJ, Bujold M, Godbehere SS, Amalfitano A (2009) CR1/2 is an important suppressor of Adenovirus-induced innate immune responses and is required for induction of neutralizing antibodies. Gene Ther 16:1245–1259
10. Jacobson A, Weis J, Weis J (2008) Complement receptors 1 and 2 influence the immune environment in a B cell receptor-independent manner. J Immunol 180(7):5057–5066
11. Carroll MC, Isenman DE (2012) Regulation of humoral immunity by complement. Immunity 37:199–207
12. Su TT, Rawlings DJ (2002) Transitional B lymphocyte subsets operate as distinct checkpoints in murine splenic B cell development. J Immunol 168:2101–2110

13. Molina H, Wong W, Kinoshita T, Brenner C, Foley S, Holers VM (1992) Distinct receptor and regulatory properties of recombinant mouse complement receptor 1 (CR1) and Crry, the two genetic homologues of human CR1. J Exp Med 175:121–129

Chapter 25

Quantification of Complement Receptor 2 Calcium Signaling Enhancement Using Flow Cytometry

Luke R. Donius and John H. Weis

Abstract

The complement receptor 2 (*Cr2*) gene is exclusively expressed in B cells and follicular dendritic cells (FDC) in mice and in humans. CR2 is a receptor for the complement component 3 (C3) cleavage fragments C3d(g) and iC3b. On B cells CR2 acts as the B cell co-receptor in which ligand binding of CR2 effectively lowers the threshold for B cell activation. This protocol describes methods for the functional analysis of calcium signaling enhancement provided by CR2 co-receptor activity.

Key words Complement receptor 1, Complement receptor 2, CR1, CR2, CD21, CD35, B cell co-receptor, B cell activation, Flow cytometry

1 Introduction

Complement receptor 2 (CR2) and the alternative isoform CR1 are receptors that bind enzymatic products of complement protein C3: C3d(g) and iC3b for CR2 as well as C3b and C4b for CR1 [1]. (It should be noted that CR1 and CR2 are also known by their cluster of differentiation (CD) designations, CD35 and CD21, respectively. Both names are used commonly and will be used in the following protocol.) Binding of C3 opsonized antigen by CR1/2 is documented to be utilized in reduction of the threshold for B cell stimulation [2, 3], transportation of immune complexes to follicles [4], and retention of immune complexes in follicles [5, 6]. CR1 has an additional role as a regulator of C3 convertases [1, 7, 8]. CR1 and CR2 are important markers for B cells and FDC and are a critical bridge for complement-driven immune modulation of the humoral immune response [5, 9, 10]. The function of CR2 as the B cell co-receptor is the textbook role that is attributed to CR2 [3]. The protocol described in the following chapter, Chap. 25: *Functional Analysis of*

Mihaela Gadjeva (ed.), *The Complement System: Methods and Protocols*, Methods in Molecular Biology, vol. 1100,
DOI 10.1007/978-1-62703-724-2_25, © Springer Science+Business Media New York 2014

Complement Receptor 2, describes methods for stimulating CR2 and monitoring the enhancement of B cell receptor (BCR) Ca^{2+} mobilization by flow cytometry.

2 Materials

2.1 Generation of Anti-CD21/35-Coated Latex Beads

1. 1.5 ml Microcentrifuge tubes, 39 × 10 mm.
2. 100 nm Carboxylate Modified Latex (CML) Beads (Life Technologies, Carlsbad, CA, USA).
3. 0.5 M 2-(*N*-morpholino)ethanesulfonic acid (MES) buffer: Dissolve MES to 0.5 M in deionized H_2O, pH 7 with 1 N potassium hydroxide (KOH).
4. Pierce BCA Protein Assay Kit (Thermo Scientific Rockford, IL, USA).
5. *N*-(3-Dimethylaminopropyl)-*N′*-ethylcarbodiimide hydrochloride (EDC).
6. *N*-hydroxysulfosuccinimide (Sulfa-NHS).
7. 0.05 M MES buffer: Dissolve MES to 0.05 M in deionized H_2O, pH 7 with 1 N KOH.
8. 4-(2-hydroxyethyl)-1-piperazineethanesulfonic acid (HEPES) buffer: 0.05 M HEPES, pH 7.4 with 10 N sodium hydroxide (NaOH).
9. Storage buffer: 0.05 M HEPES, pH 7.4, 1 % BSA, 0.05 % sodium azide.
10. Tabletop centrifuge with temperature control.
11. Goat F(ab)$_2$ anti-rat IgG Fc antibody (Jackson ImmunoResearch West Baltimore Pike, PA, USA).
12. Rat anti-CD21/35 antibody clone 7G6 (IgG2b) (BD Pharmingen San Diego, CA, USA).
13. Rat IgG2b isotype control.
14. Antibody binding buffer: 10 mM HEPES, 20 % fetal calf serum (FCS), pH 7.4.
15. Wash buffer: RPMI 1640, 10 % FCS.

2.2 Preparation of B Cells for Flow Cytometry

1. 15 ml Screw cap conical tubes.
2. RPMI 1640.
3. 100 μm Cell strainer.
4. Fluorescent activated cell sorting (FACS) buffer: 0.1 % bovine serum albumin (BSA) in 1× PBS, pH 7.4.
5. Pipet aid.

6. 10 ml Pipet.
7. 15 ml Conical tube.
8. Fluo-4, acetoxymethyl (AM) ester, 1 mM solution in DMSO, cell permeant (Life Technologies Carlsbad, CA, USA).
9. Cell staining buffer: 0.1 % BSA, RPMI 1640.
10. Anti-human/mouse CD45R (B220) phycoerythrin (PE) conjugated antibody, clone RA3-6B2 (eBioscience San Diego, CA, USA).
11. Fc receptor block, anti-mouse CD16/32, purified antibody, clone 93 (eBioscience San Diego, CA, USA).
12. 75 × 12 mm Conical bottom tube.
13. 12 × 75 mm 5 ml polystyrene round-bottom tube.
14. 1 mM Stock solution of DAPI in deionized H_2O.

2.3 Calcium Flux Measurement

1. Flow cytometer capable of exciting/detecting at 494/506 nm (Fluo-4 AM), 358/461 nm (DAPI), and 480;565/578 nm (PE).
2. $F(ab)_2$ goat anti-mouse IgM (Jackson ImmunoResearch, West Grove, PA, USA).
3. 10 % Bleach in deionized H2O.
4. Ionomycin, free acid, *Streptomyces conglobatus* (EMD4Biosciences Billerica, MA, USA).

3 Methods

3.1 Generation of Anti-CD21/35-Coated Latex Beads

1. Add to a 1.5 ml microcentrifuge tube a 450 μl aliquot of CML Beads (4.6×10^{13} beads/ml), sonicate for 3 min, and then centrifuge them at 13,400 × *g* for 5 min.
2. Discard the supernatant, and resuspend the pellet in 50 μl of 0.5 M MES with 2 mg of EDC and 2 mg of Sulfa-NHS. Incubate this mixture for 20 min at room temperature.
3. Wash the CML beads three times with 0.5 M MES at 16,100 g for 3 min each time.
4. After the third wash resuspend the activated beads with 500 μl of goat $F(ab)_2$ anti-rat IgG Fc antibody at 0.6 mg/ml for 2 h at room temperature to allow for covalent coupling of antibody to latex beads.
5. Wash the beads three times with 0.5 M MES at 16,100 × *g* for 3 min each.
6. Quantify the protein concentration of the antibody-bound latex beads using a BCA assay, and determine the efficiency of binding (*see* **Note 1**).

7. Resuspend the beads in 450 μl of bead storage buffer (*see* **Note 2**).
8. Centrifuge an aliquot of anti-IgG Fc-coated beads, appropriate for 500 ng of beads per sample, at 16,100 × *g* for 3 min and resuspend in antibody binding buffer (*see* **Note 3**).
9. Add anti-CD21/35 or isotype control antibody to aliquots of anti-IgG Fc beads, bringing the antibody to a final concentration of 0.3 mg/ml, mix, and incubate for 2 h at room temperature.
10. Wash the coated beads in wash buffer three times at 16,100 × *g* for 3 min each time and resuspend in wash buffer at a concentration of 250 ng/μl. The beads are ready at this step and cannot be stored for later use.

3.2 Preparation of B Cells

1. Obtain a single-cell suspension of mouse splenocytes in a 15 ml conical tube, and use ACK to lyse the red blood cells as described in **steps 1–4** of the Chap. 24: *Detection of Complement Receptors 1 and 2*.
2. Wash the splenocytes in 10 ml of RPMI 1640 three times at 800 × *g* for 10 min each time. Resuspend the cells in RPMI 1640, that has been pre-warmed to room temperature, at a concentration of 1×10^7 cells/ml. Aliquot a 1 ml volume of 1×10^7 cells to be sampled for analysis.
3. Add Fluor-4 AM in DMSO to the cells bringing the Fluo-4 AM to a final concentration of 3 μg/ml (*see* **Note 4**). Mix with gentle vortexing, and incubate for 30 min in the dark at 37 °C. All steps from now on should be done taking care to limit the amount of exposure of the samples to light.
4. Centrifuge the cells at 300 × g for 5 min and resuspend in 1 ml of pre-warmed RPMI 1640. Resuspend each sample in 1 ml of RPMI 1640, transfer to a 75 × 12 mm conical bottom tube, and keep at 37 °C (*see* **Note 5**).
5. Prepare the antibody mix for identifying B cells. Dilute PE-conjugated B220 (*see* **Notes 6** and **7**) antibody to 1 μg/ml and Fc receptor block to 1 μg/ml in an appropriate volume of cell staining buffer for staining each sample in 500 μl aliquots (*see* **Note 8**).
6. Centrifuge the cells at 300 × g, and resuspend the pellet in 500 μl of antibody stain mix.
7. Centrifuge cells at 300 × g for 5 min after the addition of 1 ml of cell staining buffer. Discard the supernatant, and repeat the wash and centrifugation with 1 ml of pre-warmed RPMI 1640 three times.

8. Resuspend the cells in 1 ml of the pre-warmed RPMI 1640, and strain the cells by pipetting through a 100 μm cell strainer into a round-bottom tube.
9. A volume of 3 μl of 1 mM DAPI should be added to each 1 ml sample of cells followed by gentle vortexing in order to stain dead cells for later exclusion.

3.3 Calcium Flux Measurement

1. Define the individual positive and negative fluorescent parameters for the flow cytometer, calculate compensation, adjust the sample flow rate to obtain a rate of 200–300 cells/s, and sort stained cells using the flow cytometer (*see* **Notes 9** and **10**).
2. Analyze each sample for Fluo-4 AM intensity including only the cells that are DAPI negative (live) and B220 positive (PE positive, B cells).
3. Analyze each sample for 30 s, then pause the analysis, remove the sample, and add 5 μg of F(ab)2 anti-mouse IgM along with 500 ng of anti-CD21/35-coated beads (*see* **Note 11**). Vortex the sample, and continue analysis for 5 min. [As a positive control for maximum calcium flux substitute 1 μg/ml ionomycin, a pharmacological calcium store releasing agonist, for the F(ab)2 anti-mouse IgM- and anti-CD21/35-coated beads (*see* **Note 12**).]
4. Analyze data using flow cytometry data analysis software. Assess the calcium flux of the B cells only, by gating the live $B220^{+}$ cells and plotting time versus Fluo-4 AM intensity as shown in Fig. 1.

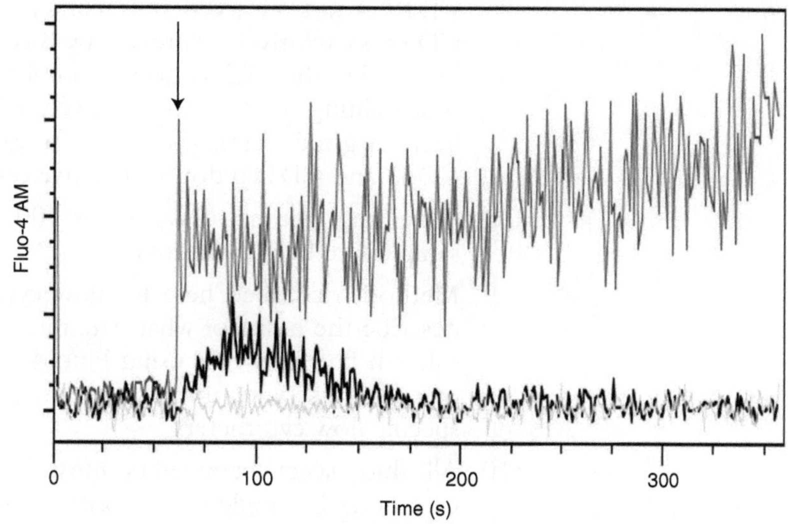

Fig. 1 B cell calcium flux measured for 300 s after B cell receptor stimulation. The *arrow* defines surface immunoglobulin cross-linking (*black line*) on Fluor-4 AM-loaded 2PK3 B cells or the addition of the positive control ionomycin (*gray line*). The *light gray line* shows unstimulated cells

4 Notes

1. A sample of beads should be assayed for protein concentration after washing, with 60–80 % retention expected [11, 12]. The protein concentration obtained here should be used as a reference to determine the quantity of coated latex beads for stimulation.
2. Protein-bound beads can reportedly be stored up to 3 months with no loss of bound antibody [11].
3. Determination of an appropriate volume of anti-IgG Fc-loaded beads for loading antibody and the final quantity of loaded beads necessary for stimulation of cells requires optimization for individual applications.
4. Reserve unstained cells for defining the non-fluorescent parameters on the flow cytometer.
5. During and after the Fluo-4 staining steps the cells should be kept at 37 °C at all times except staining. The cells must be at 37 °C before analyzing calcium flux because flux is temperature dependent.
6. B220 does not need to be a PE-conjugated antibody. Any antibody conjugated to a fluorophore that does not have an excitation/emission range of 494/506 nm (the range of common fluorophores such as GFP and FITC) can be substituted for PE-B220. Fluor-4 AM has a range of fluorescence that cannot be differentiated from GFP and FITC.
7. B220 is an accepted marker for B cells in mice; however other staining strategies may be used to suit your specific needs. CD19 is not an acceptable marker for use in this protocol. CD19 is exclusively expressed by B cells, but CD19 is directly involved in the CR2 signaling complex. Alternatively adoption of a staining method to negatively select B cells may be utilized. A good example of this is to exclude all non-B cells as CD43 and CD11b double-positive cells.
8. A staining volume of as little as 100 μl may be used if many samples are being analyzed.
9. Methods described here for flow cytometer data acquisition describe the basics of what data must be obtained to measure calcium flux in B cells using Fluo-4 AM. Consult the manual or expert users for information on proper operation of your specific flow cytometer.
10. All fluorescent parameters must be defined for the flow cytometer by single-color positive controls and an unstained negative control. All channels used must be compensated to eliminate cross-fluorescence in multiple detectors.

11. 5 μg of $F(ab)_2$ anti-IgM- and 500 ng of anti-CR2-coated latex beads are quantities that have been previously shown to activate B cells and illustrate the enhancing property of CR2 stimulation [12], but the optimal concentrations should be determined for your specific experiment.
12. Ionomycin-stimulated samples should be run last or the flow cell should be rinsed and run with 10 % bleach as well as deionized water before another sample is run on it. If residual ionomycin remains on the sample acquisition probe it will stimulate calcium flux in the subsequent samples.

References

1. Molina H, Kinoshita T, Webster CB, Holers VM (1994) Analysis of C3b/C3d binding sites and factor I cofactor regions within mouse complement receptors 1 and 2. J Immunol 153:789–795
2. Carter RH, Spycher MO, Ng YC, Hoffman R, Fearon DT (1988) Synergistic interaction between complement receptor type 2 and membrane IgM on B lymphocytes. J Immunol 141:457–463
3. Luxembourg AT, Cooper NR (1994) Modulation of signaling via the B cell antigen receptors by CD21, the receptor for C3dg and EBV. J Immunol 153:4448–4457
4. Whipple EC, Shanahan RS, Ditto AH, Taylor RP, Lindorfer MA (2004) Analyses of the in vivo trafficking of stoichiometric doses of an anti-complement receptor 1/2 monoclonal antibody infused intravenously in mice. J Immunol 173(4):2297–2306
5. Haas KM, Hasegawa M, Steeber DA, Poe JC, Zabel MD, Bock CB, Karp DR, Briles DE, Weis J, Tedder TF (2002) Complement receptors CD21/35 link innate and protective immunity during *Streptococcus pneumoniae* infection by regulating IgG3 antibody responses. Immunity 17:713–723
6. Mattsson J, Yrlid U, Stensson A, Schön K, Karlsson MCI, Ravetch JV, Lycke NY (2011) Complement activation and complement receptors on follicular dendritic cells are critical for the function of a targeted adjuvant. J Immunol 187(7):3641–3652
7. Krych-Goldberg M, Atkinson JP (2001) Structure-function relationships of complement receptor type 1. Immunol Rev 180:112–122
8. Seregin SS, Aldhamen YA, Appledorn DM, Schuldt NJ, McBride AJ, Bujold M, Godbehere SS, Amalfitano A (2009) CR1/2 is an important suppressor of Adenovirus-induced innate immune responses and is required for induction of neutralizing antibodies. Gene Ther 16:1245–1259
9. Jacobson A, Weis J, Weis J (2008) Complement receptors 1 and 2 influence the immune environment in a B cell receptor-independent manner. J Immunol 180(7):5057–5066
10. Carroll MC, Isenman DE (2012) Regulation of humoral immunity by complement. Immunity 37:199–207
11. Luxembourg AT, Cooper NR (1994) T cell-dependent, B cell-activating properties of antibody-coated small latex beads. A new model for B cell activation. J Immunol 153:604–614
12. Chakravarty L (2002) Depletion of Lyn kinase from the BCR complex and inhibition of B cell activation by excess CD21 ligation. Int Immunol 14:139–146

Chapter 26

Purification of C1q Receptors and Functional Analysis

Berhane Ghebrehiwet and Ellinor I.B. Peerschke

Abstract

The recognition subunit of C1, C1q, has emerged as an important player in various pathophysiologic conditions largely in part due to its ability to interact with pathogen-associated or cell surface expressed ligands and receptors. Identification and purification of these molecules is therefore of paramount importance if we are to procure valuable information with regards to the structure, function, and cell surface distribution. Since the interaction of C1q is better served when the receptors are purified from homologous species, we discuss here a simple guideline for the purification and characterization of the two C1q receptors, cC1qR (calreticulin) and gC1qR, from human cell lines.

Key words C1q receptor, Collagen C1q receptor, calreticulin, globular C1q receptor

Abbreviations

cC1q	The collagen domain of C1q
cC1qR	Receptor for cC1q
CRT	Calreticulin another name for cC1qR
gC1q	The globular heads of C1q
gC1qR	Receptor for gC1q

1 Introduction

Human C1q circulates in plasma as part of a multimolecular complex comprising of C1q and a Ca^{2+}-dependent tetramer, $C1r_2$–$C1s_2$. The traditional role of C1q within this complex is to serve as a unit through which C1 recognizes immune complexes or unique patterns on pathogen-associated molecular ligands. This interaction, in turn, is subsequently translated into a highly specific and orderly intramolecular rearrangement resulting in a sequential proteolytic activation—first of C1r and then of C1s—thereby triggering activation of the classical pathway [1–3]. However, information accumulated to date show that the role of C1q is not restricted to recognition of immune complexes or other molecules that activate

Mihaela Gadjeva (ed.), *The Complement System: Methods and Protocols*, Methods in Molecular Biology, vol. 1100,
DOI 10.1007/978-1-62703-724-2_26, © Springer Science+Business Media New York 2014

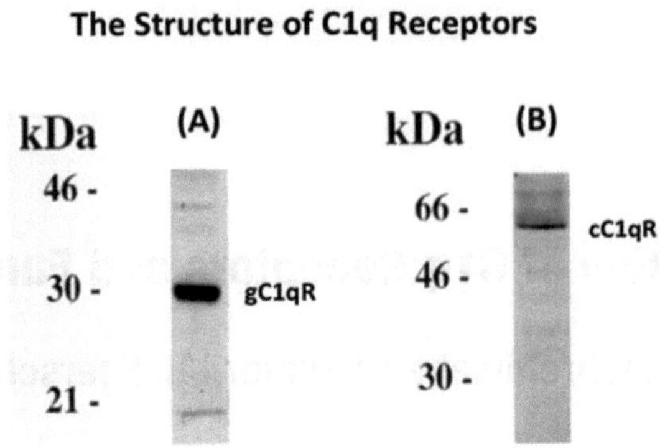

Fig. 1 Chain structure of C1qRs. Purified gC1qR (*A*) and cC1qR (*B*) were subjected to SDS-PAGE under reducing conditions

the classical pathway, but is also a key player in a rapidly expanding list of pathophysiological conditions as well as cellular functions, which contribute significantly to a plethora of inflammatory processes. These functions in turn are, by and large, mediated through the interaction of C1q with cell-associated membrane glycoproteins and surface receptors [4–7].

Because C1q is a chimeric protein comprising of a collagen-like region (cC1q) and a globular domain (gC1q), it is capable of interacting with cell surface molecules via either of its two regions. Hence, although we are witnessing an ever-increasing diversity of biologic functions mediated by C1q by virtue of its versatility to bind an increasingly long list of cell-associated molecules, there are presently two, well-characterized surface molecules that bind to either the cC1q or gC1q domains hence designated cC1qR (calreticulin) and gC1qR (p33 or p32), respectively (Fig. 1). Since receptors are involved in the control and modulation of a wide range of cellular processes, their purification from cell membranes will not only help us identify their structure and biochemical composition but also allow us to generate antibodies so that their function, cellular distribution, and structure could be assessed. In this paper, we describe a simple method for the purification of C1q receptors from cell membranes.

The two C1q receptors are ubiquitously distributed, and virtually every cell type expresses these receptors, although some cells (e.g., lymphocytes and monocytes) may express more copies per cell than quiescent endothelial cells, which need to be activated by inflammatory cytokines (e.g., LPS, INFγ, and TNFα) [9]. Therefore almost any cell type can be used as a source of C1q receptors and there appears to be no structural difference between receptors isolated from fresh circulating human cells or cultured cell lines. However since a large number of cells is required to generate a reasonable amount of membrane proteins from which quantifiable amount of protein could be recovered, it is more pragmatic to use a cultured cell line. We have successfully used both Raji cells, (a B cell line) and U937 (a monocyte-like cell line), to generate cell membrane proteins from which C1qRs were purified [4].

The purpose of purifying membrane proteins is to isolate a specific membrane receptor(s) for functional analysis and biochemical characterization. Therefore, one of the first and fundamental steps to be considered is the choice of a solubilization buffer that will keep the desired receptor in its functional state. This includes the choice of a detergent such as octyl glucoside, CHAPS, Emulphogene BC 720 (polyoxyethylene-10-tridecyl ether), and a suitable buffer medium with phosphate buffer for example being more effective than Tris buffer [10]. In addition, since the breakup of membranes releases enzymes that could potentially digest the very protein of interest, the addition of sufficient cocktail of enzyme inhibitors becomes of paramount importance although even then, one could never be sure that every enzyme released would be completely inhibited. Membrane solubilization buffers as well as cocktail mix of enzyme inhibitors are now commercially available from various sources. The example presented here uses U937 cells to isolate C1q receptors and could be adapted for the purification of other cell surface molecules as well.

2 Materials

1. Dulbecco's PBS: 0.37 M NaCl, 0.002 M KCl, 0.008 M Na_2HPO_4, 0.001 M KH_2PO_4, pH 7.4.
2. Solubilization buffer: PBS-containing enzyme inhibitors and 1 % Emulphogene BC720.
3. Coating buffer: 35 mM $NaHCO_3$, 15 mM Na_2CO_3, pH 9.6.
4. Blocking reagent: 1 % BSA in Tris-buffered saline (20 mM Tris–HCl, 100 mM NaCl, pH 7.5).
5. Alkaline-phosphatase-conjugated NeutrAvidin.
6. pNPP (ρ-nitrophenyl phosphate).
7. PMSF (phenyl-methylsulfonyl fluoride).
8. EACA, (ε-amino-*n*-caproic acid).
9. EDTA (ethylenediamine-tetraacetic acid).
10. Pepstatin.
11. Chymostatin.
12. Sulfo-NHS-LC-biotin [Sulfosuccinimidyl 6-(biotinamido) Hexanoate].
13. Surface labeling and isolation kit (Pierce).
14. Serum-free culture medium.
15. Anti-cC1qR (calreticulin).

16. Anti-gC1qR.
17. 96-Well ELISA plates.
18. ELISA reader.
19. FPLC(fast-performance liquid chromatography).
20. Mono-Q column.
21. HPLC(high-performance liquid chromatography).
22. TSK-gel DEAE-NPR column.

3 Methods

3.1 Cell Growth

1. Seed U937 cells at an initial density of 2×10^5 cells in either multiple 75 cm^2, 150 cm^2 flasks (or 1 L roller bottles) in RPMI 1640 containing 10 % heat inactivated fetal bovine serum.
2. After 3 days pour the contents onto 50 ml sterile conical test tubes and centrifuge for 10 min, at $800 \times g$, 4 °C.
3. Remove supernatants and resuspend the cell pellet from each flask in the same volume of fresh, serum-free culture medium. Transfer to 150 cm^2 flasks and incubate overnight (*see* **Note 3**).
4. After incubation, remove the flasks from the incubator and place them in BSL-2 safety hood. Remove 1 ml sample from each flask and place into corresponding sterile test tubes containing 100 μl of 0.4 % Trypan blue stain (GIBCO).
5. Mix the cells and dye, and after 1–2 min take 100 μl sample and apply it to a hemocytometer for estimation of cell density and viability. Count the cells (*see* **Note 4**).
6. Place the cells from each flask in several 50 ml sterile conical test tubes and centrifuge for 10 min at $800 \times g$, 4 °C).
7. Discard the supernatants from each tube and resuspend the cell pellets by adding 5 ml of sterile PBS pH 7.4 containing 10 mM EACA, 10 mM EDTA, 20 mM iodoacetamide, 2 mM PMSF, 1 mM pepstatin, 10 mM chymostatin, and 0.02 % NaN_3 to each tube. Pool the cells and centrifuged for an additional 10 min at $800 \times g$, 4 °C.
8. Resuspend the final cell pellet in the same buffer so that the final cell density is 1×10^8/ml. If the starting total volume was 1 L, then the final cell yield should be 1,000 ml $\times 10^6$ or 10^9 cells.
9. Remove 10^8 cells for surface labeling with sulfo-NHS-LC-biotin, a membrane impermeable reagent that labels accessible primary amino groups on surface exposed proteins (*see* **Note 5**).
10. The rest of the cells are kept frozen at −80 °C until use.

3.2 Surface Biotinylation

The surface biotinylation procedure described below can be done more efficiently using a commercially available biotinylation and purification kit (e.g., Pierce). The rationale for surface biotinylation is to ensure that the target membrane protein(s) of interest is surface expressed and binds to its target protein once purified. In addition, the surface biotinylated fraction can be mixed with the unlabeled portion and used as a tracer during large-scale receptor purification.

1. Centrifuge the cells for surface labeling for 10 min at 800 × *g*, 4 °C, discard the supernatant, and resuspend the pellet in 1 ml of PBS.
2. Biotinylation is initiated by addition of freshly prepared Sulfo-NHS-LC-biotin to a final concentration of 5 mM, and the reaction is left for 1 h at 4 °C with gentle tumble mixing.
3. After incubation, wash the labeled cells 3× in cold PBS and after the final wash lyse the cell pellet by addition of solubilization buffer, incubate on ice for 2 h to complete solubilization.
4. Centrifuge the mixture for 1 h at 45,000 × *g*, carefully collect the supernatant containing the solubilized proteins, and keep the samples frozen (−80 °C) until needed after testing the efficiency of biotinylation (see below).
5. To test the efficiency of biotinylation by ELISA, coat the wells of the microtiter plate with 100 μl of membrane protein dilutions (1:10, 1:100, and 1:1,000) in Coating buffer for 1 h, 37 °C.
6. Block for 1 h, 37 °C with Blocking reagent.
7. Visualize the bound proteins by sequential incubation with alkaline-phosphatase-conjugated NeutrAvidin for 1 h at 37 °C), followed by incubation with pNPP until color development, which is usually 10–30 min. After the final incubation, the color developed is read on a suitable ELISA reader (*see* **Note 6**).

3.3 Preparation of Cell Membranes

1. The frozen cells from Subheading 3.1, **step 4** above are quickly thawed and 1 % Emulphogene BC720 and a fresh supply of enzyme inhibitors is added. The mixture is tumbled (1–2 min), and left on ice for 2 h to complete solubilization.
2. Then, the solution is centrifuged for 1 h at 45,000 × *g*, and the supernatant containing the solubilized proteins collected. The protein concentration is then determined using the detergent compatible BCA (bicinchoninic acid) protein assay.
3. To this unlabeled solubilized protein solution is then added the biotinylated membrane proteins (Subheading 3.2, **step 4**) and the mixture dialyzed overnight at 4 °C against 20 mM

sodium phosphate buffer, pH 7.4 containing 0.1 % Emulphogene and enzyme inhibitors.

3.4 Purification of C1q Receptors on FPLC Using Mono-Q Column

1. Apply the dialyzed membrane solution from Subheading 3.3, **step 3** to FPLC fitted with a 1 ml Mono-Q column that had been equilibrated with the same buffer (10 mM sodium phosphate buffer, pH 7.4 containing 0.1 % Emulphogene BC720) as described [11].
2. Wash the column with 3× the column volume buffer (10 mM sodium phosphate buffer, pH 7.4 containing 0.1 % Emulphogene BC720), and elute the bound proteins with a linear NaCl concentration (0–1,000 mM), and collecting 1 ml fractions.
3. Under these conditions, the C1q binding activity should elute at approximately 450–500 mM NaCl (*see* **Notes** 7 and **8**).

3.5 Purification of C1q Receptors on HPLC Using DEAE Column Procedure

1. The C1q binding proteins from the Mono-Q column are pooled, dialyzed against 50 mM Tris–HCl, pH 8.0 and then subjected to HPLC purification fitted with a 1 ml TSK-gel DEAE-NPR column that has been equilibrated with the same buffer (50 mM Tris–HCl, pH 8.0).
2. Elute the bound proteins using a 0–500 mM NaCl concentration gradient in equilibrating buffer (50 mM Tris–HCl, pH 8.0) for ~10 min and then a 500–1,000 mM–1 M gradient in 50 mM Tris–HCl, pH 8.0 for an additional 5 min).
3. Test all fractions for C1q activity by the ELISA method described above.
4. Under these conditions, the 60-kDa cC1qR, which is identical to calreticulin, elutes at ~450 nM NaCl, whereas the 33-kDa gC1qR elutes at ~700 nM.
5. Concentrate each receptor fraction by ultrafiltration using a molecular weight cutoff (MWCO) of 3,000–10,000, determine the protein concentration by BCA (bicinchoninic acid) protein assay (Subheading 3.3, **step 2**), and the purity and chain structure assessed by SDS-PAGE analysis as well as by Western blot analysis using the available anti-cC1qR and anti-gC1qR antibodies.
6. Aliquot each receptor fraction and keep frozen at −80 °C.

4 Notes

1. All cell work and handling should be conducted in a sterile BSL-2 safety hood.
2. Bovine serum is more resistant to heat inactivation and therefore must be heated for at least 90 min at 56 °C.

3. This step is a precautionary measure to remove residual bovine monomeric or aggregated C1q that may interfere with receptor purification.
4. Since dead or dying cells become leaky, they will take up the dye and will appear dark blue under the microscope. Cell density is estimated as: $n \times 10^4$/ml, where n = average number of cells counted in four large quadrants. The cell density after 4 days of culture, should reach approximately 1×10^6 and viability in each flask should be ≥95 %. Flasks containing less than 90 % viability should be eliminated.
5. Surface labeling and isolation kit is available from several commercial sources (e.g., Pierce Chem Co, Rockford, IL).
6. Once the efficiency of biotinylation has been established, the biotinylated proteins can be tested by antigen-capture ELISA against C1q to detect the presence of biotinylated C1q binding protein(s) or receptor(s). Alternatively, the proteins captured by C1q can be detected using available antibodies to cC1qR/CR and/or gC1qR.
7. Fractions containing C1q binding activity are then identified by solid phase binding assay (ELISA) using C1q-coated microtiter plates and alkaline-phosphatase-conjugated streptavidin as described above.
8. The C1q-containing fractions are also tested with anti-C1q receptor antibodies to localize the position of each receptor protein.
9. Although the above described methods were those that were used to purify the known receptors, there are now alternative and much simpler approaches to these protocols. Of these affinity purification using immobilized antibodies to the desired receptor should be the most straightforward. Both monoclonal and polyclonal antibodies to cC1qR (Pierce Chem Co) and gC1qR (Abcam) are commercially available. Another approach would be to use immobilized C1q and to elute the bound receptors using NaCl concentration gradient [4].
10. Interaction of C1q with cell surface molecules induces a diversity of biological responses some of which include stimulation of leukocyte oxidative response [12], suppression of B and T cell proliferation [13], fibroblast and endothelial cell adhesion [8, 14], trophoblast cell migration [15], regulation of dendritic cells [16, 17], angiogenesis [18], and chemotaxis of eosinophils, mast cells, neutrophils, and dendritic cells [19–22]. Another interesting aspect of the C1qRs is that in addition to their cell surface expression, both are also found inside the cell including, in the case of gC1qR, in the mitochondria [23]. Since most of the surface-bound C1q can be internalized, within 30–60 min, it is believed that the receptor bound C1q

is internalized and then relayed to the intracellular receptors to induce intracellular signaling. Furthermore, both receptors are released into the pericellular milieu, by proliferating, activated, or proinflammatory cells. Because both soluble molecules are capable of activating the classical pathway, it is believed that the secreted molecules may exacerbate or even initiate the local inflammatory process. Thus, functional analysis of receptor function will depend on the availability of the F(ab'$_2$) fragment of inhibitory antibodies or receptor peptides that block the interaction between C1q and the receptor [24].

Acknowledgment

This work was supported in part by grants from the National Institutes of Health (R01 AI 060866 and R01 AI-084178).

References

1. Cooper NR (1985) The classical complement pathway: activation and regulation of the first complement component. Adv Immunol 37:151–216
2. Schumaker VN, Zavodsky P, Poon PH (1987) Activation of the first component of complement. Annu Rev Immunol 5:21–42
3. Arlaud GJ, Gaboriaud C, Thielens NM, Rossi V, Bersch B, Hernandez J-F, Fontecilla-Camps JC (2001) Structural biology of C1: dissection of a complex molecular machinery. Immunol Rev 180:136–145
4. Ghebrehiwet B, Silvestri L, McDevitt C (1984) Identification of the Raji cell membrane-derived C1q-inhibitor as a receptor for human C1q. Purification and immunochemical characterization. J Exp Med 160:1375–1389
5. Malhotra R, Reid KBM, Sim RB (1988) Studies on the isolation of C1q-receptor. Biochem Soc Trans 16:735–736
6. Malhotra R, Lu J, Thiel S, Jensenius J-C, Willis AC, Sim RB (1992) C1q receptor (collectin receptor): primary structure, homology, and interaction with ligands. Immunobiology 184:437–443
7. Ghebrehiwet B, Lim B-L, Peerschke EIB, Willis AC, Reid KBM (1994). Isolation cDNA cloning, and overexpression of a 33-kDa cell surface glycoprotein that binds to the globular 'heads' of C1q. J Exp Med 179:1809–1821
8. Ghebrehiwet B, Peerschke EIB (2004) cC1q-R (calreticulin) and gC1q-R/p33: ubiquitously expressed multi-ligand binding cellular proteins involved in inflammation and infection. Mol Immunol 41:173–183
9. Guo W-X, Ghebrehiwet B, Weksler B, Schweizer K, Peerschke EIB (1999) Upregulation of endothelial cell binding proteins/receptors for complement C1q by inflammatory cytokines. J Lab Clin Med 133:541–550
10. Hjelmeland LM, Chrambach A (1984) Solubilization of functional membrane-bound receptors. In: Venter JC, Harrison LC (eds) Receptor Biochemistry and Methodology, vol 1. Alan R Liss, New York
11. Peerschke EIB, Malhotra R, Ghebrehiwet B, Reid KBM, Willis AC, Sim RB (1993) Isolation of human endothelial cell C1q receptor (C1qR). J Leukoc Biol 53:179–184
12. Tenner AJ, Cooper NR (1982) Stimulation of a human polymorphonuclear leukocyte oxidative response by the C1q subunit of the first component of complement. J Immunol 128:2547–2552
13. Ghebrehiwet B, Habicht GS, Beck G (1990) Interaction of C1q with its receptors on cultured cell lines induces an antiproliferative response. Clin Immunol Immunopathol 54:148–160
14. Bordin S, Ghebrehiwet B, Page RC (1990) Participation of C1q and its receptor in adherence of human diploid fibroblasts. J Immunol 145:2520–2526
15. Agostinis C, Bulla R, Tripodo C, Gismondi A, Stabile H, Bossi F, Guarnotta C, Garlanda C, De Seta F, Spessotto P, Santoni A, Ghebrehiwet B, Girardi G, Tedesco F (2010) An alternative role of C1q in cell migration and tissue

remodelling: contribution to trophoblast invasion and placental development. J Immunol 185:4420–4429
16. Castellano G, Woltman AM, Schena FP, Roos A, Daha MR, van Kooten C (2004) Dendritic cells and complement: at the crossroad of innate and adaptive immunity. Mol Immunol 41:133–140
17. Hosszu KK, Santiago-Schwarz F, Peerschke EIB, Ghebrehiwet B (2010) Evidence that a C1q/C1qR system regulates monocyte-derived dendritic cell differentiation at the interface of innate and acquired immunity. Innate Immun 16:115–127
18. Bossi F, Rizzi L, Bulla R, Tripodo C, Guarnota C, Novati F, Ghebrehiwet B, Tedesco F (2011) C1q induces in vivo angiogenesis and wound healing. Molec Immunol 48:1676 (abstract)
19. Ghebrehiwet B, Gruber B, Kew RR, Marchese MJ, Peerschke EIB, Reid KBM (1995) Murine mast cells express two types of C1q receptors that are involved in the induction of chemotaxis and chemokinesis. J Immunol 155: 2614–2619
20. Kuna P, Iyer M, Peerschke EIB, Kaplan AP, Reid KBM, Ghebrehiwet B (1996) Human C1q induces eosinophil migration. Clin Immunol Immunopathol 81:48–54
21. Leigh LE, Ghebrehiwet B, Perera TP, Bird IN, Strong P, Kishore U, Reid KBM, Eggleton P (1998) C1q-mediated chemotaxis by human neutrophils: involvement of gClqR and G-protein signalling mechanisms. Biochem J 330:247–254
22. Vegh Z, Kew R, Gruber B, Ghebrehiwet B (2005) Chemotaxis of human monocyte derived dendritic cells toward C1q is mediated by gC1qR and cC1qR. Mol Immunol 43:1402–1407
23. Dedio J, Jahnen-Dechent W, Bachmann M, Müller-Esterl W (1998) The multi-ligand-binding protein gC1q-R, putative C1q receptor, is a mitochondrial protein. J Immunol 160: 3534–35542
24. Ghebrehiwet B, Hosszu KK, Valentino A, Peerschke EI (2012) The C1q family of proteins: insights into the emerging non-traditional functions. Front Immunol 3; doi:pii:52

Chapter 27

Detection of Cell Membrane-Bound CD46 Using Flow Cytometry

Martin Kolev and Claudia Kemper

Abstract

CD46 is an important regulator of the complement system by preventing unwanted deposition of the complement activation products and opsonins C3b/C4b onto self-tissue. Recently, intracellular signals mediated by CD46 activation on several distinct human cell types have demonstrated that CD46 also plays decisive roles in immuneregulation. The growing recognition of CD46 as key regulator in several vital biological processes, led to increased demand in sensitive methods for monitoring CD46 expression and changes thereof on cells and in tissues. Here we describe a method, which allows for studying CD46 expression on the surface of cells using specific antibodies in combination with fluorescence-activated cell sorting (FACS) analysis.

Key words CD46, MCP, Complement, Flow cytometry, Antibodies

1 Introduction

CD46 (also known as MCP, membrane cofactor protein) is a type I transmembrane glycoprotein expressed on all nucleated cell [1]. The CD46 gene is comprised of 13 exons and located within the so-called regulators of complement activation (RCA) gene cluster on chromosome 1q32 [2]. CD46 is commonly expressed as four different isoforms [3], of which the structures are depicted in Fig. 1. Interestingly, and the biological significance is not explained yet, some tissues only express a specific single isoform of CD46 [3]. Soluble forms of CD46 (likely generated by processing of CD46 from the cells surface via matrix metalloproteinases such as A Disintegrin And Metalloprotease family (ADAM) [4] have been observed in patients with tumors [5] or autoimmune conditions [6].

CD46 was initially discovered as a cofactor for complement factor I, which cleaves the complement proteins/opsonins C3b

Mihaela Gadjeva (ed.), *The Complement System: Methods and Protocols*, Methods in Molecular Biology, vol. 1100,
DOI 10.1007/978-1-62703-724-2_27, © Springer Science+Business Media New York 2014

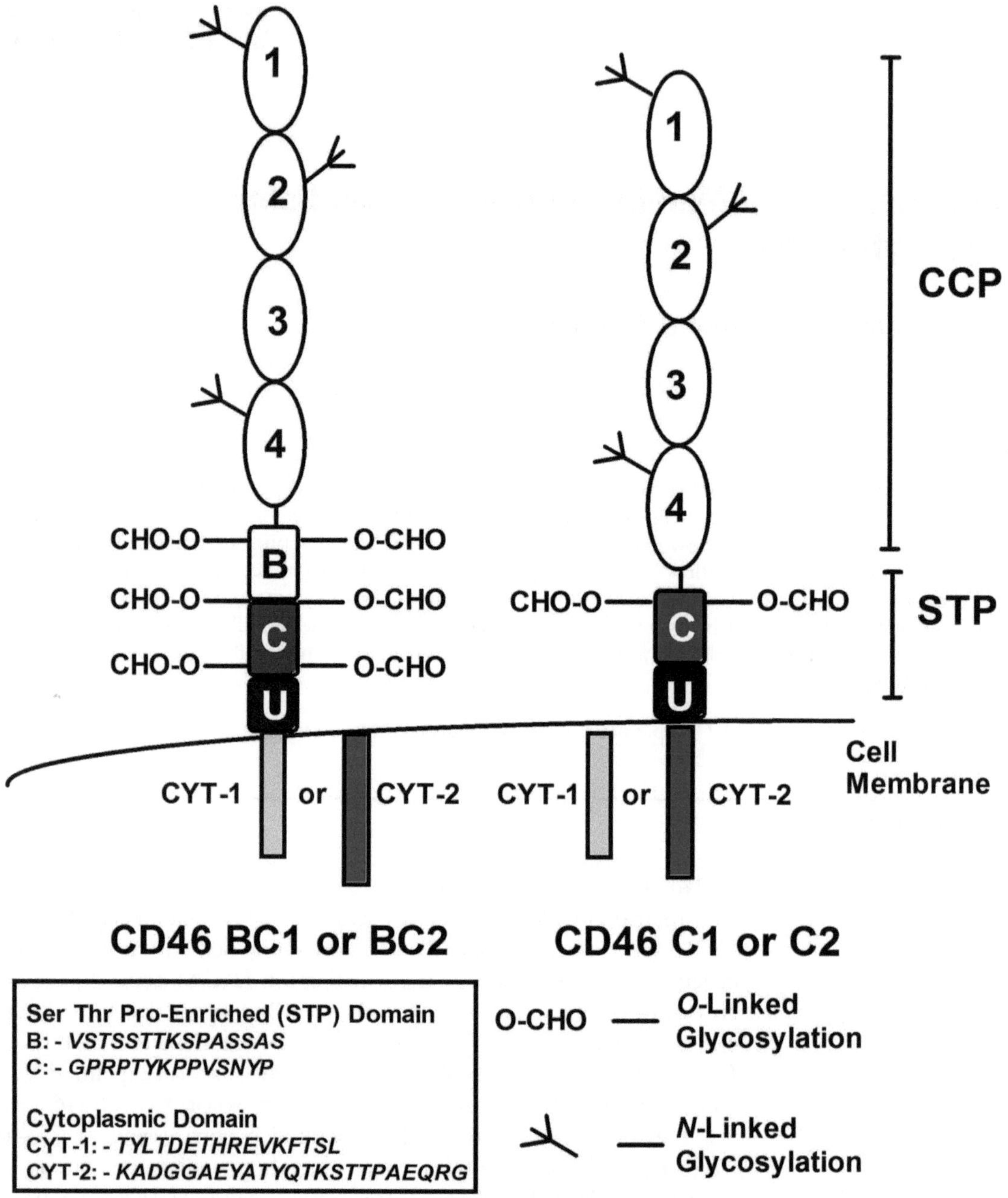

Fig. 1 Structure of CD46. CD46 consists of four extracellular complement control protein (CCP) domains termed 1–4 at the *N*-terminus, which are followed by a highly *O*-glycosylated region (O-CHO) rich in serine, threonine, and proline (termed STP). The STP region is subject to alternative splicing leading to "BC"- or "C"-containing CD46 variants. This STP region is followed by a 13 amino acid-long region of unknown function (U), a transmembrane region and then one of two possible cytoplasmic tails (CYT-1 or CYT-2). Because of the differential splicing of the STP region and the cytoplasmic tails, CD46 is expressed as at least four isoforms generally termed CD46 BC1, BC2, C1, or C2. The complement-regulatory function of CD46 resides with CCPs 2–4, while CD46-binding viruses specifically target CCPs 1–2. Figure is adapted from [3]. Full amino acid sequences of the "B" and "C" STP regions and the cytoplasmic domains, CYT-1 and CYT-2, are also shown

and C4b deposited on host tissue [1]. This complement-regulatory activity is vital as mutations in the *CD46* gene have been associated with AMD [7] and atypical hemolytic uremic syndrome (aHUS) [8, 9] and loss of protection of the epithelium or endothelium against complement deposition in an inflammatory setting.

However, in the past 20 years several biologically important "non-complement" roles of CD46 have been discovered. Some of these are briefly listed below.

CD46 is involved in the fusion of the spermatozoa with the oocyte during fertilization [10, 11], possibly explaining why mice retain CD46 expression on sperm cells, while murine somatic cells do not express CD46 [12].

Importantly, a wide range of human pathogens have chosen CD46 as cell entry receptor such as adenovirus type 11 [13], human herpesvirus 6 [14], *Streptococcus pyogenes*, *Neisseria* spp., and others described in ref. 15.

The attractiveness of CD46 to pathogens is likely based on the fact that CD46-mediated signalling events play a crucial role in T helper 1 (T_H1) effector cell regulation: CD46 also acts as a co-stimulator during $CD4^+$ T-cell activation along with CD3, which results in T_H1 like phenotype in these cells by inducing secretion of IFN-γ [16–19]. However, CD46 is also involved in the negative regulation of T_H1 responses in such that CD46 induces a switch from IFN-γ and proinflammatory cells into IL-10 coproduction and a (self)-regulatory phase. This switch is dependent on local C3a/C3b production and IL-2 [18]. The in vivo importance of this T_H1 regulative role for CD46 is attested to by the facts that defective CD46 signals have been connected with autoimmunity—as T cells from patients with rheumatoid arthritis [18] or multiple sclerosis [20] have been shown to be unable to switch to IL-10. Fully in line with an emerging novel role for CD46 in immune or tissue homeostasis is also the observation that CD46 plays a key role in epithelial cell barrier integrity and wound repair in the intestine [21].

Thus, CD46 emerges as a protein with increasing biological significance beyond mere complement regulation. Consequently, the assessment of CD46 expression on or within cells during normal homeostasis, after activation or on cells from certain patient groups, is becoming of increasing interest in immunological studies. In this chapter, we provide the protocol for a sensitive, quantitative, and simple method to measure CD46 surface expression on human cells: fluorescence-activated cell sorting (FACS) analysis. Please note that this protocol will allow detecting the surface portion of total CD46 only and does not allow for the discrimination of the isoforms expressed. Other methods for the detection of CD46 and CD46 isoforms are available, such as quantitative RT-PCR and Western blotting; however, these are not covered in this chapter.

2 Materials

Prepare all solutions using ultrapure water (prepared by deionized water to attain an electrical resistivity of 18 MΩ cm at 25 °C) and analytical or higher grade reagents. Store all reagents at 4 °C (unless indicated otherwise). Follow institutional guidelines for waste disposal.

2.1 Buffers

1. Cell detaching buffer: 4–10 mM ethylenediaminetetraacetic acid (EDTA) pH 8.0 in phosphate-buffered saline (PBS; 1×) (*see* below **items 4** and **5** for preparing stock solutions of PBS and EDTA, respectively). We do not recommend using trypsine to detach adherent cells because it may strip/cleave the molecules expressed on the cell surface.
2. FACS buffer: PBS (1×) with 1 % bovine serum albumin (BSA) and 10 mM EDTA pH 8.0 (sterile filter solution and store at 4 °C or aliquot and freeze at −20 °C) (*see* below **item 5**).
3. Cell fixing buffer: 1 % Formaldehyde in PBS (1×). Store at room temperature (*see* below **item** 7).
4. To prepare 1 l 10×PBS stock solution, weight 80.0 g NaCl, 2.0 g KCl, 2.0 g KH2PO4 and one of the following 9.2 g Na2HPO4 anhydrous OR 11.5 g Na2PO4·2H2O and resuspend into 1 l deionized water at pH 7.2.
5. To prepare 500 ml 0.5 M EDTA pH 8.0 mix 93.06 g of EDTA (MW 372.2) in ~350 ml deionized water and add NaOH pellets (approximately 10 g) until the pH reaches 8 and the EDTA dissolves. Note that EDTA is hard to dissolve at acidic pH, we therefore recommend adding the NaOH and leaving with constant stirring overnight to dissolve. Top to 500 ml with deionized water.
6. To prepare 100 ml FASC buffer dilute 10 ml of 10×PBS stock with 88 ml deionized water and then add 1 g BSA and 2 ml of 0.5 M EDTA stock solution.
7. To prepare 100 ml cell fixing buffer dilute 10 ml of 10×PBS stock with 87.3 ml deionized water and add 2.7 ml of 37 % formaldehyde. Mix well.

2.2 Antibodies and Fcγ Receptor-Blocking Reagent

1. Here, we used the anti-CD46 mouse monoclonal antibody TRA-2-10 of the IgG1κ subtype. This antibody targets CCPs1-2 of CD46. For more information on the differences between anti-CD46 antibodies please refer to **Note 1**.
2. It is sometimes desirable to use specific antibodies directly conjugated with a fluorochrome to perform a so-called "direct staining" (*see* **Note 2**). In case an antibody of choice is not available directly labelled, one can purchase kits from several

companies for the "in house" direct conjugation with a desired fluorochrome according to the manufacturer's protocol. Here, we used a fluorescein isothiocyanate (FITC) Mouse IgG1 Labeling Kit to generate a FITC-labelled TRA-2-10 antibody (*see* **Note 3**).

3. If non-labelled primary antibody is to be used, subsequent staining with an appropriate fluorochrome-conjugated secondary antibody is required. Here, we used FITC-labelled donkey anti-mouse IgG (Fab')$_2$ fragments. A protocol based on the combination of a non-labelled primary and a fluorochrome-labelled secondary antibody is usually referred to as "indirect staining".
4. In certain cases, particularly when staining dendritic cells or macrophages, the pre-incubation of cells with an Fc receptor-blocking reagent (Fc Block) is strongly suggested before adding the staining antibody. "Fc receptor blocking" is required to avoid false-positive results when staining cells that express Fc receptors as these may bind the Fc portion of the staining antibodies.

2.3 Other Materials and Equipment

1. 96-Well plates (V-bottom) with lids or adhesive film.
2. Variable volume pipettes.
3. Sterile tips.
4. Centrifuge.
5. Flow cytometer.
6. Ice.

3 Method

Grow cells as per protocol and treat or activate cells as required for your specific experiment (*see* **Note 4**). Before the experiment, assess the appearance of cells under the microscope. We do not recommend using cells that are overgrown or exhibit excessive cell death (*see* **Note 5**). This protocol allows for detection of CD46 expression on both adherent (such as epithelial) and on non-adherent cells (such as CD4$^+$ T cells). If adherent cells are used for the analysis of CD46 expression, begin with **step 1** of the protocol and if non-adherent cells are used, omit **steps 1–3** below and begin directly with **step 4**. Prepare all buffers and solutions before starting the experiment. To be able to analyze the data obtained one needs to prepare and assess controls along with the experimental staining. The controls we routinely use are listed in Table 1.

1. Wash the cells once in sterile PBS by adding 10 ml sterile PBS to T75 flask and gently tap the flask (*see* **Note 6**). Be careful to

Table 1
Routinely used negative controls

Experiment	Controls
Cells stained with directly fluorochrome-labelled anti-CD46 antibody	Non-stained cells and cells incubated with the appropriate isotype control to ensure specificity of signal
Cells stained with non-labelled primary anti-CD46 followed by staining with a fluorochrome-labelled secondary antibody	Non-stained cells and cells incubated with an isotype control and the secondary antibody and with the secondary antibody only (omit incubation with primary anti-CD46) to ensure specificity of signal

not detach the cells at this point. Aspirate the PBS by decanting or by removing with a pipet.

2. Prepare detaching solution—5 mM EDTA solution in PBS (*see* Subheading 2.1).
3. After removing the PBS used for washing, add 5–10 ml of the detaching solution to the flask of cells, swirl carefully around so that all cells are covered with the solution and incubate for 5–10 min at 37 °C in an incubator until the solution becomes cloudy (*see* **Note 6**).
4. Collect the detached cells using a pipet and transfer into a fresh tube, such as a 15 or 50 ml conical centrifuge tube. Some cells may not detached fully just by incubation in detaching solution; detachment can then often be supported by tapping the side of the culture flask against one hand or against the bench several times.
5. Pellet the cells by centrifugation at 300 × *g* for 5 min at 4 °C.
6. Resuspend the pellet in 10 ml PBS (1×).
7. Count the cells using a hemocytometer or another suitable method. Adjust cells to a minimum of 1×10^5 cells per 100 μl FACS buffer (*see* Subheading 2.1). We recommend using Trypan Blue or other live cell exclusion die to ensure that excessive cell death is not occurring prior to the experiment (*see* **Note 5**).
8. "Fc receptor block" may be required, for example when staining cells expressing Fc receptors. To block Fc receptors mix 10 μl of FcR Blocking Reagent with 90 μl FACS buffer and add up to 10^7 cells. Mix well and incubate for 10 min at 4 °C. *Note: Cell concentration can be scaled up or down depending on the particular experiment.*
9. Following incubation, wash cells by adding 1 ml of buffer per 10^7 cells and centrifuge at 300 × *g* for 5 min. Aspirate supernatant completely.

10. Dispense the cells at 1×10^5 cells/well (in 100 μl/well volume) in 96-well plate (V-bottom). Prepare as many wells as you need to perform the experiment including all non-stained and/or isotype controls and/or secondary antibody only controls (*see* Table 1).
11. Wash the cells once in 200 μl ice-cold PBS (1×) by centrifugation at 300×*g* for 5 min at 4 °C. Remove the supernatant after each wash by quickly flicking the plate upside down over a sink, then carefully tapping it on clean paper towels to remove remaining liquid.
12. While washing the cells, prepare the required amount of antibody solutions. Mix the primary FITC-labelled anti-CD46 antibody TRA-2-10 with ice-cold FACS buffer (1 μg/ml final concentration). Please refer to **Note 7** on the advantages and disadvantages of direct and indirect staining protocols. Prepare at this time also a solution with the FITC-labelled isotype control antibody (1 μg/ml final concentration). You will need 100 μl of antibody solution for each staining condition; always perform each single staining condition in duplicate. *Note: Keep all antibodies on ice at all times to avoid degradation.*
13. Add 100 μl of the diluted antibody or isotype control to each of the appropriate wells and incubate with cells for a minimum of 20 min at 4 °C in the dark. DO NOT add the primary antibody to cells that are to be used as non-stained control or as secondary antibody only control (*see* **step 16**).
14. Pellet the cells by centrifugation (300×*g* for 5 min at 4 °C).
15. Wash cells twice as in **step 11**. If you have used a directly FITC-labelled anti-CD46 antibody (FITC-TRA-2-10; direct staining), the samples are now ready for FACS analysis and you can proceed immediately to **steps 20** and **21**.
16. If you have used a non-labelled anti-CD46 TRA-2-10 antibody in **steps 12** and **13** (indirect staining), dilute the secondary FITC-labelled anti-mouse IgG antibody to 0.25 μg/ml (or 1/100 from the stock) in FACS buffer. Vortex to mix.
17. Add the secondary FITC-labelled antibody to wells containing cells stained with the anti-CD46 antibody and washed twice with PBS (1×). Also add the secondary FITC-labelled antibody to at least two wells containing isotype control-incubated and non-stained cells; these will be used as isotype control and a secondary antibody only control stainings. DO NOT forget to leave some wells without any antibody addition as non-stained cell control wells.
18. Incubate for 20 min in the dark at 4 °C.
19. Wash twice as in **step 11**.
20. If cells are to be analyzed the same day they can be resuspended in FACS buffer and kept in the dark at 4 °C for 1–2 h.

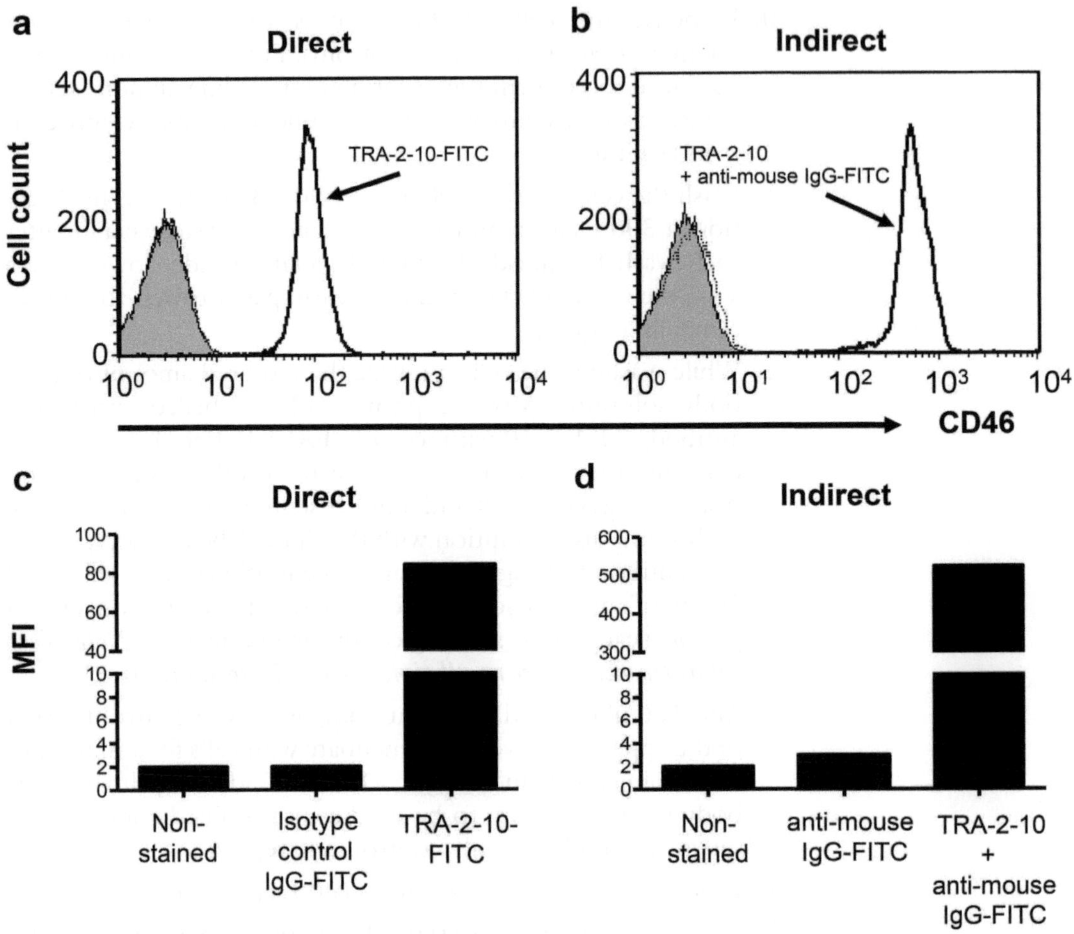

Fig. 2 Detection of CD46 on the surface of purified T cells using direct and indirect FACS staining. CD4+ T cells were purified from whole blood using the Human CD4+ T cell Isolation Kit (Miltenyi Biotec, Bergisch Gladbach, Germany). Cells were then stained following the protocol above with directly labelled TRA-2-10-FITC antibody (**a**) and indirect with TRA-2-10 antibody and secondary anti-mouse FITC-IgG (**b**) (*see arrows*). Unstained cell control are depicted in *filled grey*, while mouse IgG antibody (FITC) control and isotype IgG1κ (FITC) control are depicted in *dotted lines* in both (**a**) and (**b**). Summary of the corresponding mean fluorescence intensities (MFI) for direct and indirect stainings performed are shown in (**c**) and (**d**), respectively (*see* **Note 7**)

Alternatively, cells can be fixed with cell fixing buffer and stored at 4 °C for 2–3 days prior to analysis.

21. Analyze on a suitable flow cytometer (e.g., FACSCalibur) acquiring the non-stained cells control first, then the secondary/isotype antibody controls and the CD46-stained cells all in duplicate. Representative examples of FACS histrograms generated by staining blood-derived purified CD4+ T cells using the anti-CD46 antibody TRA-2-10 in either direct or indirect staining protocols are shown in Fig. 2.

4 Notes

1. Excellent anti-CD46 antibodies, that generate strong signals during FACS analyses, can be purchased from most major vendors such as BD Biosciences (San Jose, CA, USA), for example, clone E4.3, mouse IgG 2κ). There are two specific antibody clones that are often used by researchers addressing the functional roles of CD46 in complement regulation and in infection, GB24 [17, 22] and TRA-2-10 [17], respectively. GB24 binds to an epitope at the CCPs 3 and 4 border and blocks the complement-inhibiting function of CD46 [23]. TRA-2-10 binds to CCP1 and inhibits binding of measles virus to CD46 [24]. Some of these antibodies (GB24) though are not commercially available but can be obtained via a Material Transfer Agreement (MTA) from Dr. John Atkinson (Washington University, Saint Louis, MO, USA).
2. It is important to note that if CD46 expression analysis is to be performed on T cells that had been activated with activating antibodies to CD3 and/or CD28 of the mouse monoclonal IgG subtype, staining needs to be performed using DIRECT staining. Anti-CD3 or anti-CD3/CD28-activated T cells retain the activating antibodies on their cell surface when harvested and any mouse-specific secondary antibody used for subsequent indirect staining will interact with and detect those surface-bound antibodies.
3. For our staining here, we decided to use FITC-labelled TRA-2-10 and a FITC-labelled secondary antibody. Of course, other fluorochrome/antibody combinations can be used and the choice of those depends often on the specific experimental set up (e.g., if concurrent staining for additional surface markers is desired). Note that the appropriate controls such as fluorochrome-labelled isotype control then need to be chosen accordingly.
4. Please note that crosslinking of CD46 on cell surfaces by antibodies leads to rapid and efficient CD46 disappearance (likely via ADAM-mediated cleavage [4]) from so far any cell type tested. This CD46 downregulation serves often as a good control for successful CD46 activation as well as potential negative control for CD46 surface staining (i.e., by comparing CD46-activated vs. nonactivated cells).
5. Note that dead cells can bind antibodies nonspecifically and often give false-positive results in FACS experiments. It is therefore advisable to use cultures with a high proportion of viable cells. Cell viability can be assessed by Trypan blue staining before cell staining. Further, the forward scatter (FSC) vs. sideward scatter (SSC) pattern of the cells during FACS analysis after the

staining procedures will give a second clue about the condition of the cells (dead cells have a distinctive FSC/SSC pattern).

6. Adjust the amount of PBS used for washing and detaching buffer used for harvesting of adherent cells according to the culture vessel size used. For example, use 1 ml PBS/well for washing cells and 500 μl/well detaching solution/well when cells were cultured in 24-well plates.
7. Note that despite using the same primary antibody to CD46 (TRA-2-10), the signal strength obtained during FACS analysis differs significantly when using the direct staining (A and C) vs. the indirect staining protocol (B and D). The reason for this is that several/many fluorochrome-labelled secondary antibodies can bind to the CD46-detecting primary antibody thereby amplifying the signal obtained substantially. Though indirect staining may sometimes result in increased background (see B and D), it is often the method of choice when a rare antigen is to be detected or only a low-affinity primary antibody is available.

Acknowledgements

This work is supported by an MRC Research Grant (Grant no. G1002165 awarded to CK), the Medical Research Council Centre for Transplantation, Guy's Hospital, King's College and the Department of Health, National Institute for Health Research comprehensive Biomedical Research Centre award to Guy's & St. Thomas' NHS Foundation Trust in partnership with King's College London and King's College Hospital NHS Foundation Trust.

References

1. Purcell D, Deacon N, Andrew S, McKenzie I (1990) Human non-lineage antigen, CD46 (HuLy-m5): purification and partial sequencing demonstrates structural homology with complement-regulating glycoproteins. Immunogenetics 31:21–28
2. Liszewski M, Post T, Atkinson J (1991) Membrane cofactor protein (MCP or CD46): newest member of the regulators of complement activation gene cluster. Annu Rev Immunol 9:431–455
3. Liszewski MK, Atkinson JP (1996) Membrane cofactor protein (MCP; CD46). Isoforms differ in protection against the classical pathway of complement. J Immunol 156:4415–4421
4. Hakulinen J, Junnikkala S, Sorsa T, Meri S (2004) Complement inhibitor membrane cofactor protein (MCP; CD46) is constitutively shed from cancer cell membranes in vesicles and converted by a metalloproteinase to a functionally active soluble form. Eur J Immunol 34:2620–2629
5. Seya T, Hara T, Iwata K, Kuriyama S, Hasegawa T, Nagase Y et al (1995) Purification and functional properties of soluble forms of membrane cofactor protein (CD46) of complement: identification of forms increased in cancer patients' sera. Int Immunol 7:727–736
6. Kawano M (2000) Complement regulatory proteins and autoimmunity. Arch Immunol Ther Exp (Warsz) 48:367–372
7. Fett AL, Hermann MM, Muether PS, Kirchhof B, Fauser S (2012) Immunohistochemical localization of complement regulatory proteins

in the human retina. Histol Histopathol 27:357–364
8. Saunders R, Abarrategui-Garrido C, Frémeaux-Bacchi V, Goicoechea de Jorge E, Goodship T, López Trascasa M et al (2007) The interactive Factor H-atypical hemolytic uremic syndrome mutation database and website: update and integration of membrane cofactor protein and Factor I mutations with structural models. Hum Mutat 28(3):222–234
9. Westra D, Volokhina E, van der Heijden E, Vos A, Huigen M, Jansen J et al (2010) Genetic disorders in complement (regulating) genes in patients with atypical haemolytic uraemic syndrome (aHUS). Nephrol Dial Transplant 25:2195–2202
10. Riley RC, Kemper C, Leung M, Atkinson JP (2002) Characterization of human membrane cofactor protein (MCP; CD46) on spermatozoa. Mol Reprod Dev 62:534–546
11. Kawamoto A, Ohashi K, Kishikawa H, Zhu LQ, Azuma C, Murata Y (1999) Two-color fluorescence staining of lectin and anti-CD46 antibody to assess acrosomal status. Fertil Steril 71:497–501
12. Ruseva MM, Hughes TR, Donev RM, Sivasankar B, Pickering MC, Wu X et al (2009) Crry deficiency in complement sufficient mice: C3 consumption occurs without associated renal injury. Mol Immunol 46:803–811
13. Segerman A, Atkinson J, Marttila M, Dennerquist V, Wadell G, Arnberg N (2003) Adenovirus type 11 uses CD46 as a cellular receptor. J Virol 77:9183–9191
14. Santoro F, Greenstone H, Insinga A, Liszewski M, Atkinson J, Lusso P et al (2003) Interaction of glycoprotein H of human herpesvirus 6 with the cellular receptor CD46. J Biol Chem 278:25964–25969
15. Cattaneo R (2004) Four viruses, two bacteria, and one receptor: membrane cofactor protein (CD46) as pathogens' magnet. J Virol 78:4385–4388
16. Astier A, Trescol-Biémont M, Azocar O, Lamouille B, Rabourdin-Combe C (2000) Cutting edge: CD46, a new costimulatory molecule for T cells, that induces p120CBL and LAT phosphorylation. J Immunol 164:6091–6095
17. Kemper C, Chan A, Green J, Brett K, Murphy K, Atkinson J (2003) Activation of human CD4+ cells with CD3 and CD46 induces a T-regulatory cell 1 phenotype. Nature 421:388–392
18. Cardone J, Le Friec G, Vantourout P, Roberts A, Fuchs A, Jackson I et al (2010) Complement regulator CD46 temporally regulates cytokine production by conventional and unconventional T cells. Nat Immunol 11:862–871
19. Le Friec G, Sheppard D, Whiteman P, Karsten CM, Al-Tilib Shamoun S et al (2012) The novel Jagged1 and CD46 interaction on T lymphocytes mediates a critical defence mechanism of human adaptive Th1 immunity. Nat Immunol 13:1213–1221
20. Astier AL, Meiffren G, Freeman S, Hafler DA (2006) Alterations in CD46-mediated Tr1 regulatory T cells in patients with multiple sclerosis. J Clin Invest 116:3252–3257
21. Cardone J, Al-Shouli S, Kemper C (2011) A novel role for CD46 in wound repair. Front Immunol 2:28
22. Hofman P, Hsi B, Manie S, Fenichel P, Thyss A, Rossi B (1994) High expression of the antigen recognized by the monoclonal antibody GB24 on human breast carcinomas: a preventive mechanism of malignant tumor cells against complement attack? Breast Cancer Res Treat 32:213–219
23. Cho SW, Oglesby TJ, Hsi BL, Adams EM, Atkinson JP (1991) Characterization of three monoclonal antibodies to membrane co-factor protein (MCP) of the complement system and quantification of MCP by radioassay. Clin Exp Immunol 83:257–261
24. Manchester M, Valsamakis A, Kaufman R, Liszewski MK, Alvarez J, Atkinson JP et al (1995) Measles virus and C3 binding sites are distinct on membrane cofactor protein (CD46). Proc Natl Acad Sci U S A 92:2303–2307

Chapter 28

Detection of CD59 Using Flow Cytometry

Martin Kolev

Abstract

CD59 is the single regulator of the terminal complement pathway. It has been implicated in disease such as Paroxysmal nocturnal hemoglobinuria (PMH) and cancer. Expression of CD59 protects normal and malignant cells from the cytotoxic potential of the complement system. Here we describe a method, which allows for studying its expression on the surface of cells.

Key words CD59, Complement protection, Flow cytometry, Antibodies

1 Introduction

Human CD59 is a small (~19 kDa), heavily glycosylated, globular GPI-anchored protein [1]. CD59 has also been found as a secreted soluble form shed from apoptotic cells [2]. The soluble form isolated from urine retains its specific complement binding activity, but exhibits greatly reduced ability to inhibit the complement membrane attack complex (MAC) assembly on cell membranes [3]. CD59, the only membrane-bound inhibitor of the complement MAC, acts by binding to the C8 and/or C9 components of the assembling MAC thereby preventing incorporation of the multiple copies of C9 required for complete formation of the osmolytic pore [4, 5]. CD59 has also other roles than simply complement regulation—it has been shown to down-modulate $CD4^+$ T cells in response to polyclonal and Ag-specific stimulation in both mouse [6] and human [7]. The roles of the CD59 not directly involved in regulation of complement system have been extensively reviewed [8–10].

In this chapter a flow cytometry-based technique that can be used to detect CD59 on the cell surface of normal or malignant cells will be discussed. It has to be noted that other methods for detection of CD59 expression exist, such as western blot and quantitative PCR. However, flow cytometry is the most sensitive

Mihaela Gadjeva (ed.), *The Complement System: Methods and Protocols*, Methods in Molecular Biology, vol. 1100,
DOI 10.1007/978-1-62703-724-2_28, © Springer Science+Business Media New York 2014

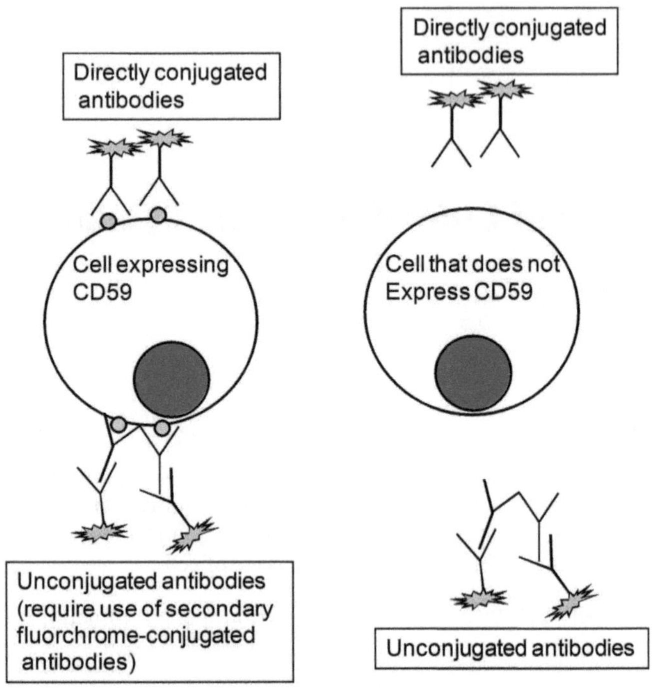

Fig. 1 Schematic representation of the staining of cells for flow cytometry. The cells could either express the antigen of interest or not. Staining could be done using directly conjugated antibodies or non-conjugated antibodies in which case a secondary antibody labeled with fluorochrome is required

protein-based and quantitative method for determining expression of CD59.

Flow cytometry (or *F*luorescence *A*ctivated *C*ell *S*orting, shortly FACS) is routinely used to study surface expression of antigens [11]. For a review of the recent advances in flow cytometry *see* ref. 12. When cells are analyzed by flow cytometry, only the cells expressing the marker of interest will manifest fluorescence (*see* Fig. 1). The amount of fluorescence on the cell surface is directly correlated with the expression of the antigen that is being studied. Unbound antibodies are then washed away from the cell surface and either fluorescently labeled secondary antibody is added (if the primary one is not conjugated to a fluorochrome) or cells are fixed and analyzed using a flow cytometer such as FACS Calibur or FACS Canto.

2 Materials

Prepare all solutions using ultrapure water (prepared by deionized water to attain an electrical resistivity of 18 MΩ cm at 25 °C) and analytical or higher grade reagents. Store all reagents at 4 °C (unless indicated otherwise).

2.1 Buffers

1. Cell detaching buffer: (10 mM EDTA pH8.0 in 1 × PBS).
2. FACS buffer: (1 × PBS, 1 % BSA, 10 mM EDTA). Sterile filter and freeze at –20 °C.
3. Cell fixing buffer: (1 × PBS, 4 % formaldehyde). Store at room temperature.

2.2 Antibodies

1. We use monoclonal mouse anti-human CD59 (clone HelC1, raised in house) but good anti-CD59 antibodies (detecting both human and mouse CD59a) can be purchased from most major vendors (*see* **Notes 1** and **2**).
2. Secondary antibody directly conjugated to FITC was donkey anti-mouse IgG (Fab')$_2$ fragments (*see* **Note 3**).

2.3 Other Materials

1. 96-Well plates (U- or V-bottom) with lids.
2. Variable volume pipettes.
3. Sterile tips.

3 Methods

To be able to analyze the data obtained one need to prepare and run controls along with the test staining. The controls we routinely use are listed in Table 1. Before starting the experiment refer to **Note 4**.

1. Wash the cells once in sterile 1× PBS.
2. Add 5 ml of the detaching solution (*see* Subheading 2.1, **item 1**) to T75 flask of cells and incubate for 5–10 min at 37 °C in incubator until the solution becomes cloudy.
3. Count the cells using hemocytometer or other suitable method. Adjust cells to have a minimum of 1×10^5 cells per 100 μl. We recommend using not more than 5×10^5 cells per well.
4. Dispense 1×10^5 cell per well (or 100 μl/well) in 96-well plate (U- or V-bottom).

Table 1
Suggested negative controls for the detection of CD59 by flow cytometry

Type of control	Notes
Unstained cells	To check for dead cells using FCS/SSC plots
Cells stained with secondary antibody or isotype control antibody	Control for nonspecific binding of secondary or isotype controls to cells of interest
Cells that does not express CD59 (if desired)	Control for nonspecific binding of anti-CD59 antibody

5. Wash the cells twice in 200 μl ice-cold 1 × PBS by centrifugation at 250–300 × *g* for 5 min at 4 °C. Remove the supernatant after each wash by gently turning over the plate and tapping it on clean paper to remove remaining liquid. Be careful not to loose the cells.
6. While washing, prepare the antibody solution by mixing ice-cold FACS buffer (*see* Subheading 2.1, **item 2**) with the required primary antibody (10 μg/ml final concentration). The final volume of the mix we typically use is 100 μl per well, but this could be scaled to from 50 to 250 μl if desired. If the antibody is directly labeled dilute also the isotype control at this step. *Note that the final concentration of the staining antibody and the isotype control should be the same.*
7. Add 100 μl of the diluted antibody to each well and incubate with cells for a minimum of 30 min at 4 °C. DO NOT add the antibody to cells that are to be used as secondary and unstained cells control.
8. Pellet the cells by centrifugation (spin at 250 × *g*, 4 °C for 5 min).
9. Wash twice as in **step 5**.
10. If using the unlabelled primary, dilute the secondary anti-mouse IgG-APC 0.3 μg/ml (or 1/100 from stock) in FACS buffer. Gently vortex to mix.
11. Add secondary anti-mouse IgG-APC to cells stained for CD59 and to cells, which will be used as a secondary antibody control. DO NOT add to unstained cells control.
12. Incubate for at least 30 min in the dark at 4 °C.
13. Wash twice as in **step 5**.
14. If cells are to be analyzed the same day they can be resuspended in FACS buffer and kept at 4 °C in dark. Alternatively cells can be fixed with cell fixing buffer (*see* Subheading 2.1, **item 3**) and stored in the fridge for 2–3 days prior to analysis.
15. Analyze on a suitable flow cytometer (e.g., FACS Calubur, FACS Canto II) acquiring the non-stained cells control first, then the secondary/isotype antibody controls and the CD59-stained cells. Example FACS plots are shown in Fig. 2.

4 Notes

1. Anti-CD59 antibodies can be purchased from most major such as Abcam (clone MEM-43), BD Biosciences, BioLengend (directly conjugated to FITC), etc. Anti-CD59 antibodies such as the mouse monoclonal antibody clone BRIC 229 can block the complement-inhibiting function of CD59 and thus

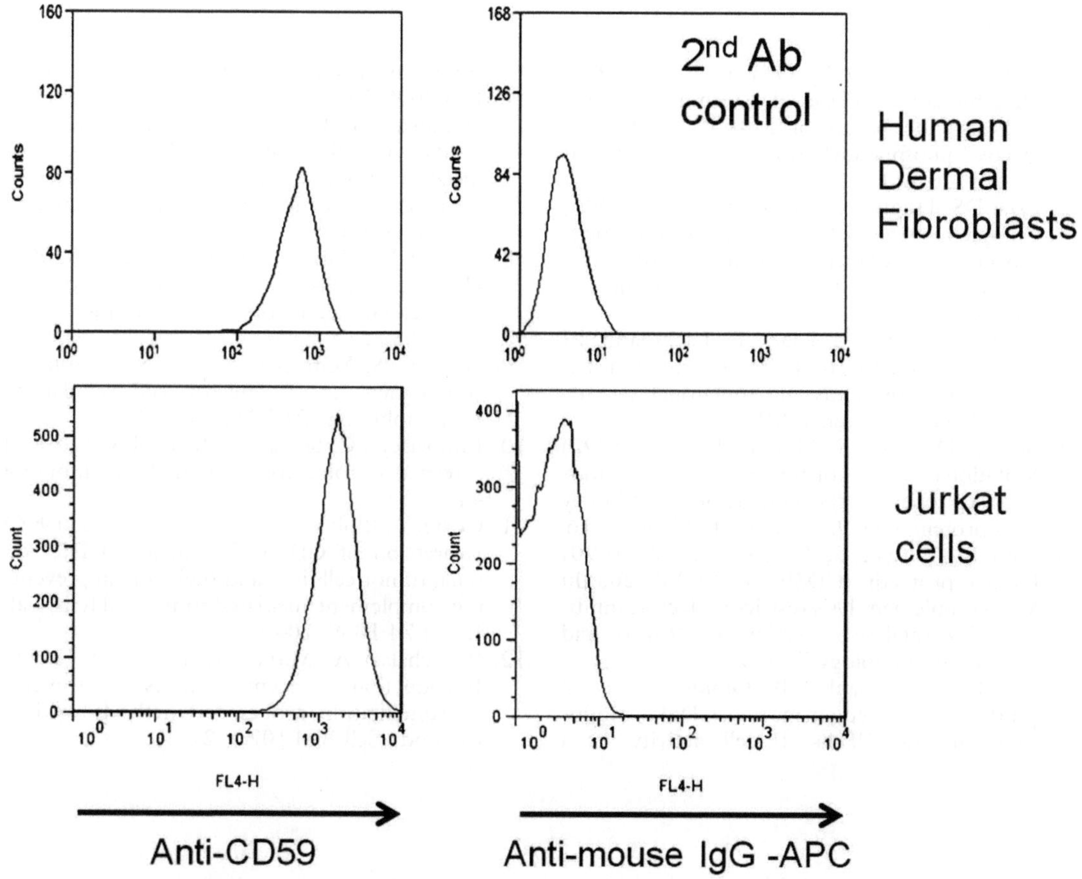

Fig. 2 Detection of CD59 on the surface of Jurkat and human dermal fibroblast cells. Indirect staining with anti-CD59 (clone HelC1) antibody (shown on the *left*) and secondary anti-mouse IgG-FITC. Cells stained with the secondary antibody are shown on the *right*

can be used in functional assays evaluating the role of CD59 in complement protection.

2. For detection of mouse CD59a, a mouse anti-mouse CD59a monoclonal antibody is supplied by HyCult Biotechnology (clone 7A6).
3. The secondary goat-anti-mouse antibody (Jackson laboratory) we typically used has minimal reactivity to Human, Bovine, Rat, Rabbit, and other immunoglobulins. This antibody can be used to detect both antihuman and anti-mouse antibodies because they are raised in mouse.
4. Grow cells as per protocol. Replace the media on the day before experiment. If cells growing in suspension are used skip **steps 1** and **2**. If adherent cells are to be analyzed start from **step 1**.

References

1. Sugita Y, Nakano Y, Oda E et al (1993) Determination of carboxyl-terminal residue and disulfide bonds of MACIF (CD59), a glycosyl-phosphatidylinositol-anchored membrane protein. J Biochem 114:473–477
2. Cole DS, Hughes TR, Gasque P et al (2006) Complement regulator loss on apoptotic neuronal cells causes increased complement activation and promotes both phagocytosis and cell lysis. Mol Immunol 43:1953–1964
3. Meri S, Vakeva A, Laari T, Lachmann PJ (1991) Soluble forms of CD59-antigen: distribution in body fluids and functional activity. Complement Inflammat 8:193
4. Bodian D, Davis S, Morgan B et al (1997) Mutational analysis of the active site and antibody epitopes of the complement-inhibitory glycoprotein, CD59. J Exp Med 185:507–516
5. Meri S, Morgan B, Davies A et al (1990) Human protectin (CD59), an 18,000–20,000 MW complement lysis restricting factor, inhibits C5b-8 catalysed insertion of C9 into lipid bilayers. Immunology 71:1–9
6. Longhi M, Sivasankar B, Omidvar N et al (2005) Cutting edge: murine CD59a modulates antiviral CD4+ T cell activity in a complement-independent manner. J Immunol 175:7098–7102
7. Sivasankar B, Longhi M, Gallagher K et al (2009) CD59 blockade enhances antigen-specific CD4+ T cell responses in humans: a new target for cancer immunotherapy? J Immunol 182:5203–5207
8. Longhi M, Harris C, Morgan B et al (2006) Holding T cells in check – a new role for complement regulators? Trends Immunol 27: 102–108
9. Heeger PS, Kemper C (2011) Novel roles of complement in T effector cell regulation. Immunobiology 217(2):216–224
10. Kimberley FC, Sivasankar B, Paul MB (2007) Alternative roles for CD59. Mol Immunol 44:73–81
11. Gorter A, Blok VT, Haasnoot WH et al (1996) Expression of CD46, CD55, and CD59 on renal tumor cell lines and their role in preventing complement-mediated tumor cell lysis. Lab Invest 74:1039–1049
12. Pierzchalski A, Mittag A, Tárnok A (2011) Introduction A: recent advances in cytometry instrumentation, probes, and methods – review. Methods Cell Biol 102:1–21

Chapter 29

Functional Analysis of CD59 Using Complement-Dependent Cytotoxicity Assay

Martin Kolev

Abstract

CD59 overexpression has been shown to confer the resistance of tumors to complement lysis. Complement lysis is one of the two major killing mechanisms of therapeutic anticancer antibodies. This chapter provides a method that allows studying the extent of complement protection of tumors by CD59.

Key words Complement-dependent cytotoxicity, Fab fragments, Normal human serum, Anti-disialoganglioside GD2 antibody, Cancer, Cell lines

1 Introduction

Complement-dependent cytotoxicity (CDC) is a mechanism of complement activation in the presence of complement-activating antibodies. It is one of the main mechanisms of action of anticancer monoclonal antibodies [1, 2]. Rituximab (humanized anti-CD20 antibody used in the treatment of non-Hodgkin lymphoma) has been shown to have CDC as one of the main mechanisms of action [3].

CDC is routinely employed to investigate the resistance of cancer cells to complement lysis. Limiting factor for CDC is the expression of membrane-bound complement regulators (mCReg), namely, CD46, CD55 and CD59 [2, 4].

A schematic representation of steps involved in CDC is shown in Fig. 1. Briefly, the target cells were first incubated with the fluorescent viability dye calcein AM for 30 min at 37 °C in complete RPMI 1640 media. Following two washes in plain RPMI 1640 (without serum), cells were incubated for 30 min at 4 °C with complement-activating antibody anti-disialoganglioside GD2 (short GD2), and in some cases Fab fragments of polyclonal anti-CD59 antibody were also added. GD2 antigen is expressed on the

Mihaela Gadjeva (ed.), *The Complement System: Methods and Protocols*, Methods in Molecular Biology, vol. 1100,
DOI 10.1007/978-1-62703-724-2_29, © Springer Science+Business Media New York 2014

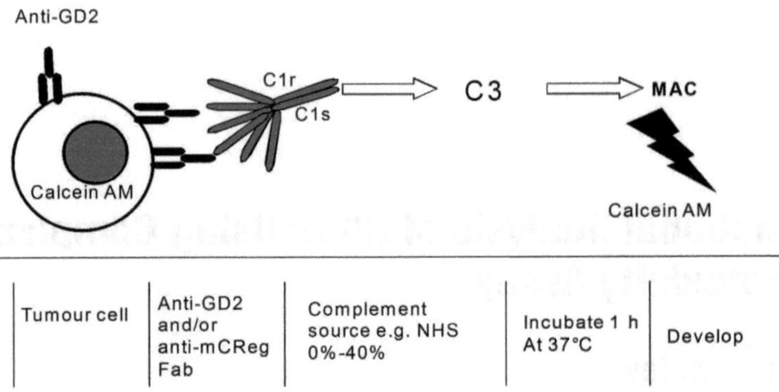

Fig. 1 Schematic representation of the steps involved in complement-dependent cytotoxicity assay. The assay is based on loading the cells with viability dye such as calcein AM prior to the binding of antibody. Serum is then added as a complement source. At the end of the assay free calcein AM in the cell supernatant is detected

surface of many tumor cells such as melanoma, neuroblastoma, and small cell lung carcinoma. Unbound antibody is then removed by washing with plain RPMI 1640 media, and a source of complement is added for 1 h at 37 °C. Normal human serum (NHS) was used as a source of complement. Cells are then pelleted and supernatants analyzed for fluorescence using plate reader. For alternative target cells refer to **Note 1**.

2 Materials

Please carry out all steps in sterile conditions under laminar flow cabinet unless otherwise stated to avoid contamination. Follow all waste disposal regulations when disposing waste materials. Typically no sodium azide was added to the reagents to ensure that cells are not harmed by its toxic effect.

1. RPMI 1640. Supplement the media with 10 % fetal calf serum, sodium pyruvate (5 mM), streptomycin (50 U/ml), penicillin (50 U/ml), and L-glutamine (2 mM). Store at 4 °C.
2. DMEM. Supplement the media as in **item 1** for RPMI 1640. Store at 4 °C.
3. Tumor cell lines or primary cells to be used as target cells for complement-dependent lysis. We have used melanoma cell line G361 and neuroblastoma cell line IMR32.
4. Calcein AM. *See* **Note 1** for dilution and storage recommendations.
5. NHS (*see* **Note 2** for instructions on how to prepare NHS). Store at −80 °C.
6. Cell detaching buffer. 10 mM EDTA in PBS. Store at 4 °C.

7. Cell lysis buffer. 10× solution, 2 % Tritone X100 in PBS (*see* **Note 2** for preparation instructions). Store at 4 °C.
8. Anti-disialoganglioside GD2 antibody (Millipore). Store at 4 °C.
9. Fab fragments of anti-CD59 antibody in-house made. Alternatively use any polyclonal anti-human CD59 to make sure that all epitopes of CD59 are blocked. *See* **Note 3** for the protocol used for preparation of Fab fragments. Store at 4 °C.
10. 96-Well U- or V-bottom plates.
11. Plate reader capable of recoding fluorescence (we used FLUOstar Optima).
12. Incubator capable of maintaining 37 °C and 5 % CO_2 humidified atmosphere.

3 Methods

Before starting the method follow instructions in **Note 4** to prepare working calcein AM solution. Follow **Notes 3** and **5** to prepare NHS and Fab fragments, respectively.

Prepare a scheme of the experimental setup. Use Fig. 2 for guidance.

1. Grow the cells in appropriate media until 70 % confluent. IMR32 was maintained in RPMI 1640, while DMEM was used for G361 cells (for more information on cell lines *see* **Note 6**). DO NOT allow the cells to overgrow.
2. On the day before experiment replace the media with a fresh one.

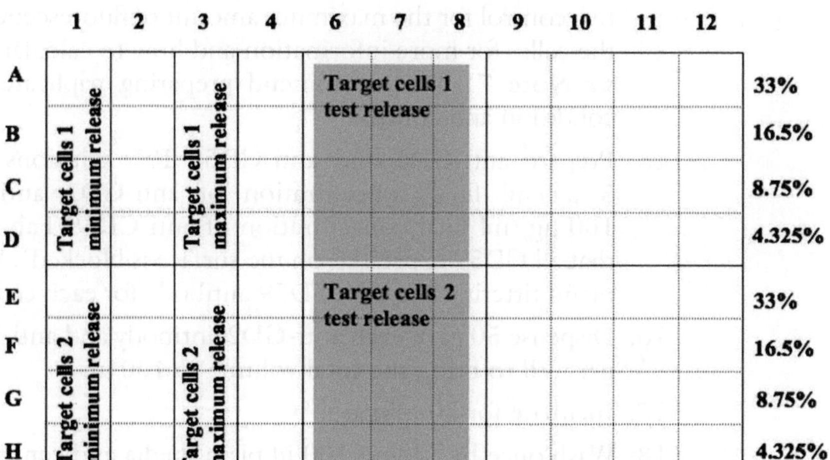

Fig. 2 Example plate setup. The drawing represents a 96-well plate containing the experimental and control wells necessary for the CDC assay. Perform each experimental and control reaction in at least triplicate

3. Next day add to the cells 5 ml cell detaching solution. Incubate for 5–10 min at 37 °C.
4. Wash the cells once by adding 10 ml 1× PBS to the cells from one T75 mm^3 flask containing detaching solution.
5. Spin down the cells at 250×*g* for 5 min at room temperature.
6. Remove the supernatant and resuspend in 10 ml 1× PBS.
7. Count the cells using hemocytometer or other suitable method.
8. Adjust the cell counts to 1×10^6 cells/ml in plain RPMI 1640.
9. Add 15.2 μl of stock calcein AM solution to 1 ml of the cellular suspension. For preparation of stock calcein AM *see* **Note 4**.
10. Incubate for 30 min at 37 °C. Resuspend the cells by gently tapping the vial every 10 min to ensure that the dye is loaded evenly.
11. Add plain RPMI 1640 up to 20 ml and spin down at 250×*g* for 5 min at room temperature. Remove the supernatant.
12. Repeat **step 11** once more.
13. Add 5 ml of plain RPMI 1640 to cell pellet and mix by pipetting up and down gently.
14. Dispense 50 μl of cells per well in 96-well U-bottom plate. When preparing for the assay, make sure to have spare wells for the controls as suggested in Fig. 2. Required controls are cells only in media and cells treated with cell lysis buffer (*see* **Note 2**, for preparation of stock solution, dilute ten times to working concentration (0.2 % Trition X100)). Cells with media are the background control for spontaneous release of the fluorescent dye in the media, while cells with 1× lysis buffer are the positive control for the maximum amount of fluorescence taken by the cells (for more information and how to calculate % of lysis *see* **Note 7**). We recommend preparing triplicates for each condition and control.
15. Prepare anti-GD2 and anti-CD59 Fab solutions. We used 5 μg/ml final concentration of anti-GD2 antibody and 100 μg/ml final concentration of anti-CD59 Fab (to ensure that all CD59 expressed on the surface is blocked). We recommend tittering the anti-CD59 antibody for each cell line used.
16. Dispense 50 μl of each anti-GD2 antibody and anti-CD59 Fab per well to bring the total volume to 100 μl.
17. Incubate for 30 min at 4 °C.
18. Wash once by adding 100 μl plain media and centrifuging for 5 min at 250×*g*. Add 100 μl plain media to the wells.

19. 5 min before the end of incubation time thaw the NHS in water bath and dilute it as required. Start from neat NHS (100 %), and make several twofold dilutions with RPMI 1640 to obtain dilution curve (*see* also Fig. 2 for recommended final dilutions of the serum). Alternatively the serum can be kept in the same concentration, and the GD2 antibody or the CD59 Fab fragments can be tittered.
20. Add 50 μl of undiluted or diluted NHS to the wells. Total volume then should be 150 μl. Also at this step add 35 μl of media and 15 μl of cell lysis buffer (to make 1×) to maximum release wells. For the background control wells add 50 μl plain media.
21. Spin down the plate for 5 min at 250×*g* at room temperature.
22. Incubate for 1 h at 37 °C.
23. Spin down the plate at 250×*g* for 5 min.
24. Using multichannel pipette remove very carefully 75 μl of the supernatant, and dispense it into fresh microtiter flat-bottom plate. DO NOT disturb the pellet.
25. Record fluorescence at 480/520 nm.

Some typical cytotoxicity curves are given in Fig. 3. Refer to **Note** 7 for how to calculate the percent of lysis.

4 Notes

1. Mouse or rat cells can be used in this assay. In these cases we recommend using mouse or rat serum as the source of complement. The other two complement regulators can also be blocked in order to dissect the mechanism of protection against complement in the same way as shown below.
2. Dilute 2 ml of 100 % stock Triton X100 in 98 ml PBS to obtain 2 % (10× concentrated) stock. Store at 4 °C.
3. Before starting the digestion, check the integrity of the antibody on SDS-PAGE. One mg of anti-CD59 (rabbit anti-human polyclonal antibody), made in-house against whole soluble CD59 molecule, is dialyzed against Fab digestion buffer (17 mM cysteine-HCl, 0.1 M Na_2HPO_4, 10 mM EDTA; pH 7.0) overnight at 4 °C and then incubated with 250 μl of a papain slurry (Pierce) for 2–3 h at 37 °C with shaking. Following incubation, the samples are centrifuged to remove the slurry. Digestion can then be verified on nonreducing and reducing 10 % SDS-PAGE gels, with Fab fragments appearing as 50 kDa band (nonreducing) or around 30 kDa (reducing conditions).

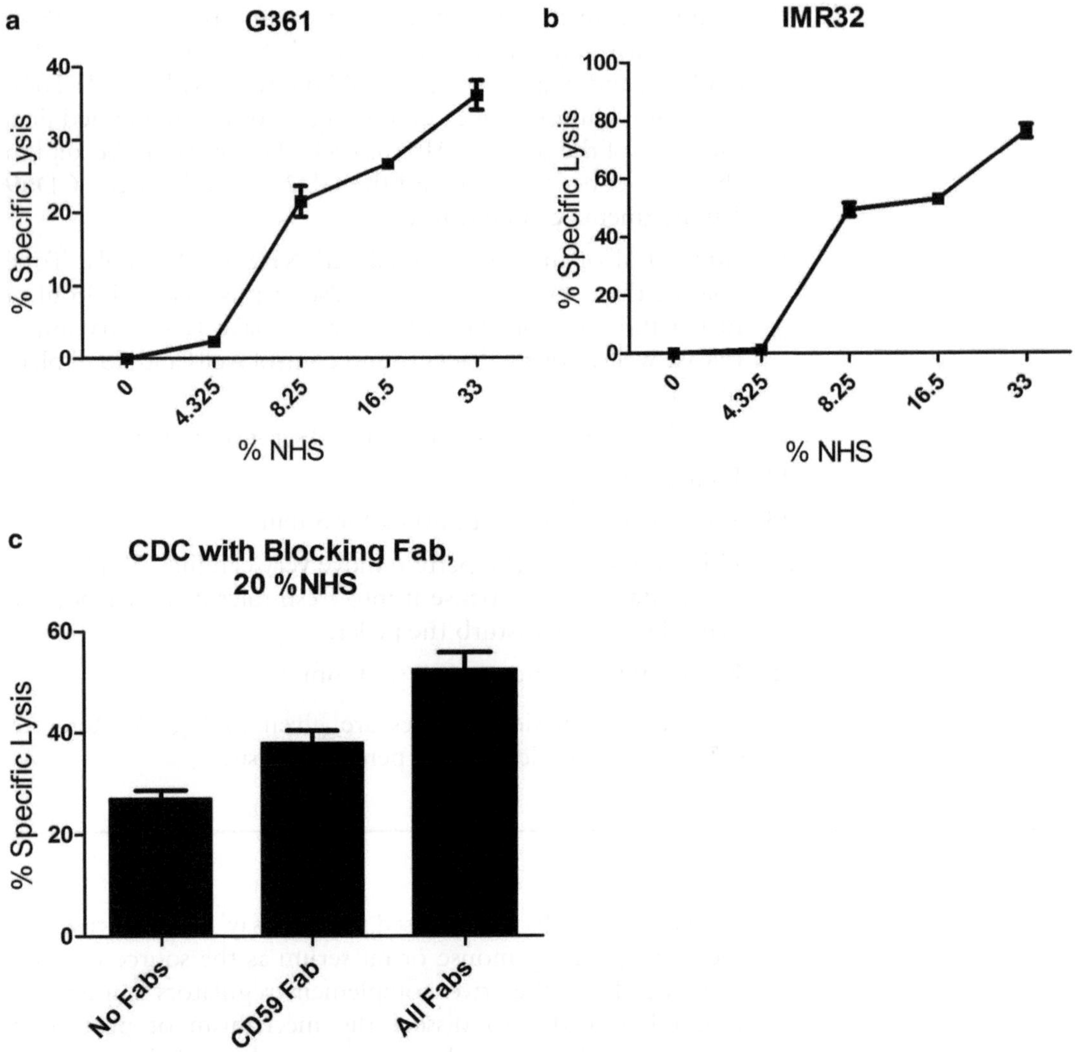

Fig. 3 Typical killing curves. (**a**) G361 cells were incubated with GD2 antibody as per protocol. Serum was titrated from neat to 4.325 % using twofold dilutions. Percent of specific lysis was calculated as mean ± SD from each triplicate condition as explained in **Note 6**. (**b**) Same as for (**a**) but using a different target cell line—IMR32. (**c**) CDC assay with blocking Fabs. The assay was repeated in the same serum concentration (20 %), and cells were preincubated with either no Fabs or blocking Fab fragments against either CD59 or all mCregs (CD46, CD55, and CD59). Results indicate that the addition of either CD59 or all Fabs increased % of lysis significantly compared to non-treated cells indicating that these regulators protect the cells from complement killing

4. Dilute one 50 mg vial of calcein AM (Special packaging, Molecular Probes) with 50 μl sterile DMSO (1 mg/ml concentration) in sterile conditions. Use 15.6 μl of stock for 1 ml or 7.4 μl for 500 μl media.
5. NHS is prepared from fresh blood. Serum is blood plasma without fibrinogen or the other clotting factors. Collect blood

in glass flasks, and allow clotting at room temperature for 1 h with occasional stirring using a glass stick. After clotting incubate the blood on ice for a further 30 min–1 h to promote clot contraction. After a 5-min spin at $650 \times g$ in a bench-top centrifuge collect the serum supernatant and transfer into new vial for another $650 \times g$ spin but this time for 10 min. Serum appearance should be yellow with little evidence of hemolysis. Aliquot the serum and store at −80 °C until required. Thaw only once to ensure maximal activity.

6. The cell lines listed are used due to their variable mCRegs and availability of complement fixing antibody—GD2 (supplied by Millipore). IMR32 only expresses very little CD46 and CD59, and while G361 expresses all mCReg, CD59 seems to be conferring its resistance to CDC. Other cell lines or primary cells can be adapted to be used with this protocol.

7. To calculate the percent of specific lysis use the following formula:

   $\%\text{ lysis} = 100 \times (\text{Test}_{F480/520} - 0\,\%_{F480/520}) / (100\,\%_{F480/520} - 0\,\%_{F480/520})$

   where

   Test—Fluorescence of the experimental wells

   0 %—Fluorescence background in wells where only cells and media were present (background control)

   100 %—Fluorescence of cells incubated with detergent to determine maximum killing (maximum release)

References

1. Gelderman K, Tomlinson S, Ross G et al (2004) Complement function in mAb-mediated cancer immunotherapy. Trends Immunol 25:158–164
2. Kolev M, Towner L, Donev R (2011) Complement in cancer and cancer immunotherapy. Arch Immunol Ther Exp (Warsz) 59:407–419
3. Di Gaetano N, Cittera E, Nota R et al (2003) Complement activation determines the therapeutic activity of rituximab in vivo. J Immunol 171:1581–1587
4. Gelderman KA, Blok VT, Fleuren GJ et al (2002) The inhibitory effect of CD46, CD55, and CD59 on complement activation after immunotherapeutic treatment of cervical carcinoma cells with monoclonal antibodies or bispecific monoclonal antibodies. Lab Invest 82:483–493

Chapter 30

Detection of Soluble CR3 (CD11b/CD18) by Time-Resolved Immunofluorometry

Gitte Krogh Nielsen and Thomas Vorup-Jensen

Abstract

In the cell membrane complement receptor 3 (CR3) consists of one alpha chain (CD11b) and one beta chain (CD18). CR3 participates in many immunological processes, especially those involving cell migration, adhesion, and phagocytosis of complement-opsonized microbes. Recent findings of soluble CR3 in body fluids and in culture supernatant from experiments in vitro point to the involvement of ecto domain shedding as a part of the CR3 biology. To monitor such shedding on a quantitative basis, we have developed time-resolved immunofluorometric assays (TRIFMA) to detect soluble CD11b and CD18 in plasma or serum of either human or murine origin. Compared with most enzyme-linked immunosorbent assays methodologies, TRIFMA possesses prominent advantages, including better dynamic range and reproducibility. These assays may contribute to the understanding of the role of shedding of CR3 and other cell adhesion molecules in human disease and animal models involving inflammation.

Key words Complement, Integrin, CR3, CD11b, CD18, TRIFMA

1 Introduction

The complement receptor 3 (CR3) is a member of the β_2 subfamily of integrins consisting of heterodimeric cell membrane-anchored receptors. The β_2 subfamily comprises four known members that share a common β_2 subunit associated non-covalently with either of the four distinct, but structurally similar, α-subunits to form the receptors CR3 (also named $\alpha_M\beta_2$, CD11b/CD18, or Mac-1), $\alpha_L\beta_2$ (also known as LFA-1 or CD11a/CD18), $\alpha_X\beta_2$ (CD11c/CD18, CR4, p150,95), and $\alpha_D\beta_2$ (CD11d/CD18) [1]. The β_2 integrins play a crucial role in the immune system as demonstrated in patients with leukocyte adhesion deficiency (LAD). Such individuals have a global deficiency in phagocyte-mediated acute inflammatory responses due to deficiency of CD18 [1–3]. Consequently, they suffer from recurrent infections due to the malfunction of their macrophages and neutrophil granulocytes [4, 5].

Mihaela Gadjeva (ed.), *The Complement System: Methods and Protocols*, Methods in Molecular Biology, vol. 1100, DOI 10.1007/978-1-62703-724-2_30,

The CR3 is an abundant β_2 integrin receptor in the cell membrane of neutrophiles, macrophages, and monocytes and participates in many immunological processes, especially those involving cell migration, adherence, and phagocytosis [1, 6–8]. Via the I-domain located in the N-terminal ectodomain of the α-subunit, CR3 binds a wide variety of ligands in a divalent cation-dependent manner [9–11]. Notably, CR3 binds the fragment of complement component C3 generated by complement factor I cleavage, namely, iC3b [12, 13], providing one of the links between the complement system and cellular immunity. By recognizing iC3b-opsonized particles the CR3 triggers phagocytosis resulting in clearance of pathogens and apoptotic cells [14, 15]. Other ligands include the intercellular adhesion molecule (ICAM) family of intercellular adhesion molecules [11]. The binding of CR3 to ICAMs plays a key role in the molecular mechanisms supporting leukocyte migration and diapedesis through the endothelial barrier and accumulation at sites of tissue injury [16, 17]. The list of CR3 ligands has gradually been expanding, however, and now includes more than 50 molecules of considerable structural and chemical diversity [18, 19]. The ability of the receptor to interact with proteins, polymers of nucleic acids, and lipopolysaccharides was suggested to originate from a relatively high affinity for at least certain acidic moieties such as the γ-COOH of the glutamate side chains as well as the carboxyl groups found in the uronic acid residues in heparin [20, 21].

In the past, the main focus has been on the cell surface expression of CR3 and ligand binding properties in connection to its role in leukocyte adhesion and migration. However, recently the finding of soluble (s)CR3 in various body fluids suggested the functional importance of shedding. Results from our laboratory demonstrated that the concentration of sCD11/CD18 is elevated in synovial fluid as consequence inflammatory arthritis while such fluid under conditions with less or no inflammation has a significantly lower concentration sCD11/CD18 [22]. Systemic alterations, i.e., in the plasma concentration, were also found in inflamed patients compared with healthy volunteers. Although the distribution of the four alpha chains in these complexes is unclear, CD11a was easily detectable in complexes found in human plasma while, by contrast, CD11b was barely detectable and CD11c was not detected. However, in addition to the relative concentration of these species, this finding may at least in part reflect properties of the monoclonal antibodies utilized for detection as well. Other investigations presented evidence that proteolytic cleavage of the extracellular domain serves as an important mechanism for leukocyte detachment after initial cell adhesion and transmigration in both humans and mice [23]. Kinetic studies showed that the cleavage of CD11b is positively correlated with polymorphonuclear leukocyte detachment and subsequent transmigration [24–27].

Cross-immunoprecipitation using CD11b and CD18 antibodies further suggested that the cleaved CD11b and CD18 fragments were at least partially associated with one another, suggesting a potential biological function for the soluble integrin fragments [23]. Specific cleavage of the CD18 ectodomain by MMP-9 further supports a functional importance of soluble β_2 integrins [28]. Likewise, specific anti-CD11b antibodies that recognize the I-domain are applicable for detecting the soluble ectodomain suggesting that these possess a ligand binding activity [23]. Indeed, in humans sCD11/CD18 was found to be able to bind ICAM-1 immobilized on plastic surfaces, although in this case the binding was most likely contributed by sCD11a/CD18 [22].

In light of the above-described findings and the possible functional importance of CR3 ectodomain shedding in different conditions, we have developed a time-resolved immunofluorometric assay (TRIFMA) to detect sCD11b and sCD18 in serum of both human and murine origin (Fig. 1). The TRIFMA assay is a method for detection of specific analytes very similar to ELISA but with prominent advantages. The long-lasting fluorescence of the europium ions is measured by photon counting with better sensitivity, dynamic range, and reproducibility as compared to the enzymatic based reaction of ELISAs. In addition, the fluorescence emitted from the europium ions upon reading can be measured following storage of the microtiter plates at 4 °C for several days. We believe that these assays may add new tools for understanding the role of cell adhesion molecules in human disease and animal models involving inflammation, notably those involving CR3.

2 Materials

All buffers and solutions are made with analytic grade reagents and ultrapure water prepared by purifying deionized water to attain a resistivity of 18 MΩ cm at 25 °C. Buffers are typically supplemented with 10 mM NaN_3 to preserve sterility and are stored at 4 °C until use.

1. 96-Well microtiter plates, e.g., FluoroNunc Maxisorp™ microtiter plates (*see* **Note 1**).
2. Plastic container.
3. Paper towels.
4. Coating antibody: Monoclonal (m) antibody (Ab) anti-CD11b (e.g., mAb anti-mouse CD11b, clone 5c6) or anti-CD18 antibodies of choice (mAbs, anti-human CD18 antibody, clone KIM185, and anti-mouse CD18 antibody, clone 313903) (*see* Table 1).
5. Detection antibody: Biotin-labeled mAb anti-CD11b-antibody (e.g., mAb anti-mouse CD11b antibody, clone M1/70.15) or

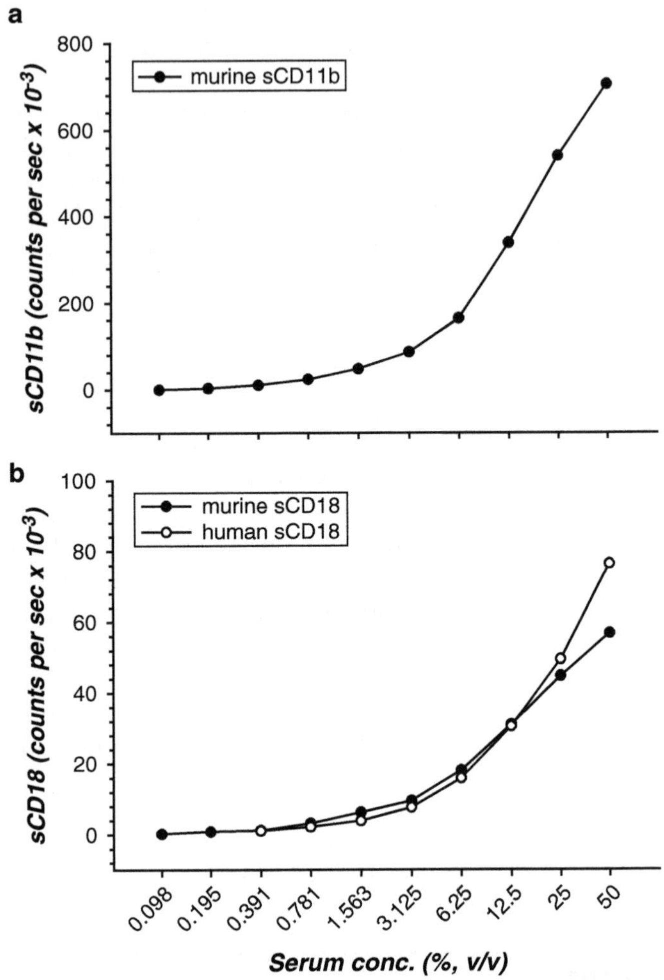

Fig. 1 Detection of sCD11b and sCD18 by TRIFMA. Serum samples from either male C57BL/6 mice or human volunteers were titrated as indicated in the lower abscissa axis (in serum volume percentage). (**a**) Serum samples from male C57BL7/6 mice were applied to wells coated with rat mAb anti-mouse CD11b antibody (clone 5c6) followed by development with biotinylated mAb anti-mouse CD11b antibody (clone M1/70.15). (**b**) Serum samples from human volunteers were applied to wells coated with KIM185 and developed with biotinylated antibody KIM127. Rat mAb anti-mouse CD18 antibody (clone 313903) was used to coat wells to detect CD18 in serum from male C57BL/6 mice, whereas the biotinylated rat mAb anti-mouse CD18 antibody (clone C71/16) was used for development

biotin-labeled monoclonal anti-CD18-antibody of choice (e.g., mAb anti-human CD18 antibody, clone KIM127, and anti-mouse CD18 antibody, clone C71/16) (*see* Table 1).

6. Phosphate-buffered saline (PBS): 137 mM NaCl, 2.5 mM KH_2PO_4, 6.9 mM $K_2HPO_4 \cdot 3H_2O$, pH 7.4.
7. Tris-buffered saline (TBS): 10 mM Tris–HCl, pH 7.4, 145 mM NaCl, 15 mM NaN_3.

Table 1
List of recommended anti-CD11band anti-CD18 monoclonal Abs and their characteristics

Antibody (clone)	Immunogen	Isotype (Ig class)	Specificity	Reactivity	References	Provider (cat. no.)
Anti-human CD18						
Monoclonal mouse anti-human CD18 (KIM185)	Human CR3 immunopurified from human white cell lysate. Human CR3 immunized BALB/c mouse spleen cells fused with Sp2/0 cells	IgG_1, κ	Integrin β_2/CD18	Human	[22]	
Monoclonal mouse anti-human CD18 (KIM127)	Human CR3 immunopurified from human white cell lysate. Human CR3 immunized BALB/c mouse spleen cells fused with Sp2/0 cells	IgG_1, κ	Integrin β_2/CD18	Human	[22]	
Anti-mouse CD18						
Monoclonal rat anti-mouse CD18 (313903)	CHO-derived rmIntegrin β_2 (Gln24-Asn702) accession # P11835	IgG_{2a}	Integrin beta 2/CD18	Mouse	[29]	R&D Systems (MAB2618)
Monoclonal rat anti-mouse CD18 (C71/16)	Cell membrane glycoproteins from mouse T-cell lymphoma BW5147	IgG_{2a}, κ	CD18	Mouse	[30, 31]	BD Pharmingen (557439)
Anti-mouse CD11b						
Monoclonal rat anti-mouse CD11b (5C6)	Thioglycollate-elicited peritoneal macrophages (TPM)	IgG_{2b}	Recognizes mouse complement type 3 receptor (CR3) and precipitates a heterodimer of 165 and 95 kD	Human, mouse	[32]	AbD Serotec (Cat# MCA711)
Monoclonal rat anti-mouse CD11b (M1/70.15)	T cell-enriched splenocytes from B10 mice	IgG_{2b}	Recognizes the murine CD11b cell surface antigen	Human, mouse, rabbit	[32, 33]	AbD Serotec (Cat# MCA74)

8. TBS/Tw: TBS with 0.05 % (v/v) Tween-20.
9. Human serum albumin (HSA) (*see* **Note 2**).
10. Serum or plasma samples for analysis (store in aliquots at −80 °C until use).
11. Heat-aggregated human IgG (*see* **Note 3**).
12. Bovine IgG, rat IgG, and mouse IgG.
13. Assay binding buffer: TBS/tw, 1 mM $CaCl_2$, 1 mM $MgCl_2$, 100 μg/ml heat-aggregated human IgG, 100 μg/ml bovine IgG, 100 μg/ml rat IgG, 100 μg/ml mouse IgG (*see* **Note 4**).
14. Biotinylated Ab binding buffer: TBS/Tw, 1 mM $CaCl_2$, 1 mM $MgCl_2$.
15. Streptavidin-Eu^{3+}.
16. TBS/Tw/EDTA: TBS with 0.05 % (v/v) Tween 20 and 25 μM EDTA.
17. Enhancement solution: Mix 5.7 ml of glacial acetic acid with a sufficient amount of 0.1 M potassium hydrogen phthalate to reach pH 3.2. Add 1 ml Triton X-100, and adjust the volume to 1 l with distilled water. Just before use, add 2 μl of a solution containing 15 μM 2-naphthoyltrifluoracetate (2-NTA) and 50 μM tri-*o*-octylphosphine oxide (TOPO) per ml of the acetic acid/potassium hydrogen phthalate mixture (*see* **Note 5**).

3 Methods

Carry out all procedures at room temperature unless otherwise specified.

3.1 Detection of Soluble CR3 by TRIFMA

Detection of sCD11b and sCD18 in serum samples is carried out by TRIFMA using a "sandwich" technique with pairs of polystyrene-coated and biotinylated mAbs applied for the detection of either the CD11b chain or the CD18 chain of CR3.

1. Coat the wells of a 96-well microtiter plate by adding the captured mAb diluted in PBS buffer to each well using a total volume of 100 μl per well. The mAb anti-mouse CD11b (clone 5c6) is used in a concentration of 0.5 μg per ml PBS, whereas the optimal concentration of mAb anti-mouse CD18 (clone 313903) is 1 μg per ml PBS. In assay for human samples the mAb anti-human CD18 antibody (clone KIM185) is used at a concentration of 1 μg per ml PBS (*see* Table 1 for information about the antibodies).
2. Incubate at 4 °C overnight in a moist chamber (*see* **Note 6**).
3. Empty the wells by tapping the plate on a layer of paper towels, and block nonspecific binding by adding 200 μl of TBS containing 0.05 % (v/v) Tween 20 to each well. Incubate for 1 h at

20 °C. After incubation, empty wells and wash three times with 200 μl of TBS containing 0.05 % (v/v) Tween 20 (*see* **Note 7**).

4. Dilute samples of serum (or plasma) 1:10 or 1:20 in binding buffer for antigen assay. Add 100 μl to each well of the coated plate. Incubate in moist chamber overnight at 4 °C. At the end of incubation, empty wells by repeated tapping of the plate on a layer of paper towels, and then wash wells three times with TBS containing 0.05 % (v/v) Tween 20.
5. Dilute the biotinylated mAb in TBS containing 0.05 % (v/v) Tween 20. Rat anti-CD11b antibody (clone M1/70.15) is diluted to 0.25 μg/ml, whereas rat anti-CD18 antibody (clone C71/16) is used at a concentration of 1 μg/ml. The biotinylated mAb anti-human antibody (KIM127) should be used in a concentration of 1 μg/ml. Add 100 μl of the diluted antibody to each well and incubate for 1–2 h at 20 °C in the moist chamber. At the end of incubation, empty wells by tapping the plate repeatedly on a layer of paper towels, and then wash wells three times with TBS containing 0.05 % (v/v) Tween 20.
6. Dilute streptavidin-Eu^{3+} appropriately (e.g., 1:1,000) in TBS containing 0.05 % (v/v) Tween 20 and 25 μM EDTA. Add 100 μl to each well and incubate for 1–2 h at 20 °C in the moist chamber. At the end of incubation, empty wells by repeated tapping of the plate on a layer of paper towels, and then wash wells three times with TBS containing 0.05 % (v/v) Tween 20.
7. Add 200 μl enhancement solution per well, and incubate plate for 5 min with shaking at room temperature. Read the signals developed in a machine equipped for TRIFMA measurements (*see* **Note 8**).

4 Notes

1. For example, FluoroNunc Maxisorp™ microtiter plates with a low background fluorescence. The maxisorp surface is a modified, highly charged polystyrene surface with high affinity to molecules with polar or hydrophilic groups, which implies that when coating with antibodies the hydrophilic Fc region of the antibody is more likely to be bound, thereby leaving the fab region intact for detection of a specific analyte.
2. HSA can be added to the TBS/TW buffer used as blocking buffer to reduce background fluorescence signal. When necessary, we use HSA at a concentration of 1 mg/ml to reduce background fluorescence noise signal.
3. The IgG is heat-aggregated prior to use in the assay by incubation of TBS with 10 mg/ml IgG at 63 °C for 30 min followed

by centrifugation for 10 min at 3,000 × *g* to remove insoluble complexes (grossly aggregated IgG). The supernatant is then used. Addition of heat-aggregated IgG reduces interference by rheumatoid factor (RF) in the assay.

4. Since immunoglobulin-reactive antibodies are found in sera from humans as well as other species, the inclusion of aggregated human IgG and IgGs from mouse, rat, and cow is a mean of avoiding an influence of the immunoglobulins binding to antibodies applied for antigen detection. The presence of these immunoglobulin-reactive antibodies may cause a false-positive signal through the binding and capture of the antibodies applied for antigen detection. We find that it is best to prepare the assay binding buffer fresh each time.
5. Store both the acetic acid/potassium hydrogen phthalate solution and the NTA/TOPO solutions up to 3 months at 4 °C. Once the solutions are mixed, the complete enhancement solution should be used within a month. Furthermore, it is advisable to check the background fluorescence signal of the enhancement buffer just after preparation. Counts per second should not exceed 1,000.
6. The humid chamber consists of a closed plastic container with a moist paper towel at the bottom.
7. If the plates are to be stored for later use, add 200 μl TBS per well and store at 4 °C in a moist chamber.
8. Measurements of TRIFMA signals can be done using a Victor® plate reader available from PerkinElmer.

Acknowledgements

We would like to thank Drs. Jens C. Jensenius and Steffen Thiel, Dept. of Biomedicine, Aarhus University, for their support and excellent advice on applications of TRIFMA. This work was financially supported by grants from the Lundbeck Foundation (LUNA), the Danish Multiple Sclerosis Association, and the Danish Council for Independent Research | Medical Sciences.

References

1. Arnaout MA (1990) Structure and function of the leukocyte adhesion molecules CD11/CD18. Blood 75(5):1037–1050
2. Hibbs ML, Wardlaw AJ, Stacker SA, Anderson DC, Lee A, Roberts TM, Springer TA (1990) Transfection of cells from patients with leukocyte adhesion deficiency with an integrin beta subunit (CD18) restores lymphocyte function-associated antigen-1 expression and function. J Clin Invest 85(3):674–681
3. Wardlaw AJ, Hibbs ML, Stacker SA, Springer TA (1990) Distinct mutations in two patients with leukocyte adhesion deficiency and their functional correlates. J Exp Med 172(1):335–345
4. Kishimoto TK, Hollander N, Roberts TM, Anderson DC, Springer TA (1987) Heterogeneous mutations in the beta subunit common to the LFA-1, Mac-1, and p150,95 glycoproteins cause leukocyte adhesion deficiency. Cell 50(2):193–202

5. Anderson DC, Springer TA (1987) Leukocyte adhesion deficiency: an inherited defect in the Mac-1, LFA-1, and p150,95 glycoproteins. Annu Rev Med 38:175–194
6. Dana N, Styrt B, Griffin JD, Todd RF 3rd, Klempner MS, Arnaout MA (1986) Two functional domains in the phagocyte membrane glycoprotein Mo1 identified with monoclonal antibodies. J Immunol 137(10):3259–3263
7. Ross GD, Yount WJ, Walport MJ, Winfield JB, Parker CJ, Fuller CR, Taylor RP, Myones BL, Lachmann PJ (1985) Disease-associated loss of erythrocyte complement receptors (CR1, C3b receptors) in patients with systemic lupus erythematosus and other diseases involving autoantibodies and/or complement activation. J Immunol 135(3):2005–2014
8. Park JY, Arnaout MA, Gupta V (2007) A simple, no-wash cell adhesion-based high-throughput assay for the discovery of small-molecule regulators of the integrin CD11b/CD18. J Biomol Screen 12(3):406–417
9. Lee JO, Rieu P, Arnaout MA, Liddington R (1995) Crystal structure of the A domain from the alpha subunit of integrin CR3 (CD11b/CD18). Cell 80(4):631–638
10. Beller DI, Springer TA, Schreiber RD (1982) Anti-Mac-1 selectively inhibits the mouse and human type three complement receptor. J Exp Med 156(4):1000–1009
11. Diamond MS, Staunton DE, de Fougerolles AR, Stacker SA, Garcia-Aguilar J, Hibbs ML, Springer TA (1990) ICAM-1 (CD54): a counter-receptor for Mac-1 (CD11b/CD18). J Cell Biol 111(6 Pt 2):3129–3139
12. Rosen H, Law SK (1990) The leukocyte cell surface receptor(s) for the iC3b product of complement. Curr Top Microbiol Immunol 153:99–122
13. Ross GD, Vetvicka V (1993) CR3 (CD11b, CD18): a phagocyte and NK cell membrane receptor with multiple ligand specificities and functions. Clin Exp Immunol 92(2):181–184
14. Tsuji S, Kaji K, Nagasawa S (1994) Activation of the alternative pathway of human complement by apoptotic human umbilical vein endothelial cells. J Biochem 116(4):794–800
15. Ezekowitz RA (2002) Local opsonization for apoptosis? Nat Immunol 3(6):510–512
16. Ross GD (2000) Regulation of the adhesion versus cytotoxic functions of the Mac-1/CR3/alphaMbeta2-integrin glycoprotein. Crit Rev Immunol 20(3):197–222
17. Dunne JL, Collins RG, Beaud et al, Ballantyne CM, Ley K (2003) Mac-1, but not LFA-1, uses intercellular adhesion molecule-1 to mediate slow leukocyte rolling in TNF-alpha-induced inflammation. J Immunol 171(11):6105–6111
18. Vorup-Jensen T (2012) On the roles of polyvalent binding in immune recognition: perspectives in the nanoscience of immunology and the immune response to nanomedicines. Adv Drug Deliv Rev 64(15):1759–1781
19. Tan SM (2012) The leucocyte beta2 (CD18) integrins: the structure, functional regulation and signalling properties. Biosci Rep 32(3): 241–269
20. Vorup-Jensen T, Carman CV, Shimaoka M, Schuck P, Svitel J, Springer TA (2005) Exposure of acidic residues as a danger signal for recognition of fibrinogen and other macromolecules by integrin alphaXbeta2. Proc Natl Acad Sci U S A 102(5):1614–1619
21. Vorup-Jensen T, Chi L, Gjelstrup LC, Jensen UB, Jewett CA, Xie C, Shimaoka M, Linhardt RJ, Springer TA (2007) Binding between the integrin alphaXbeta2 (CD11c/CD18) and heparin. J Biol Chem 282(42):30869–30877
22. Gjelstrup LC, Boesen T, Kragstrup TW, Jorgensen A, Klein NJ, Thiel S, Deleuran BW, Vorup-Jensen T (2010) Shedding of large functionally active CD11/CD18 Integrin complexes from leukocyte membranes during synovial inflammation distinguishes three types of arthritis through differential epitope exposure. J Immunol 185(7):4154–4168
23. Zen K, Guo YL, Li LM, Bian Z, Zhang CY, Liu Y (2011) Cleavage of the CD11b extracellular domain by the leukocyte serprocidins is critical for neutrophil detachment during chemotaxis. Blood 117(18):4885–4894
24. Evans BJ, McDowall A, Taylor PC, Hogg N, Haskard DO, Landis RC (2006) Shedding of lymphocyte function-associated antigen-1 (LFA-1) in a human inflammatory response. Blood 107(9):3593–3599
25. Mechtersheimer S, Gutwein P, Agmon-Levin N, Stoeck A, Oleszewski M, Riedle S, Postina R, Fahrenholz F, Fogel M, Lemmon V, Altevogt P (2001) Ectodomain shedding of L1 adhesion molecule promotes cell migration by autocrine binding to integrins. J Cell Biol 155(4):661–673
26. Phillipson M, Heit B, Colarusso P, Liu L, Ballantyne CM, Kubes P (2006) Intraluminal crawling of neutrophils to emigration sites: a molecularly distinct process from adhesion in the recruitment cascade. J Exp Med 203(12): 2569–2575
27. Phillipson M, Heit B, Parsons SA, Petri B, Mullaly SC, Colarusso P, Gower RM, Neely G, Simon SI, Kubes P (2009) Vav1 is essential for mechanotactic crawling and migration of neutrophils out of the inflamed microvasculature. J Immunol 182(11):6870–6878
28. Vaisar T, Kassim SY, Gomez IG, Green PS, Hargarten S, Gough PJ, Parks WC, Wilson CL, Raines EW, Heinecke JW (2009) MMP-9 sheds the beta2 integrin subunit (CD18) from macrophages. Mol Cell Proteomics 8(5):1044–1060
29. Gomez IG, Tang J, Wilson CL, Yan W, Heinecke JW, Harlan JM, Raines EW (2012)

Metalloproteinase-mediated shedding of integrin beta2 promotes macrophage efflux from inflammatory sites. J Biol Chem 287(7):4581–4589
30. Springer TA (1990) Adhesion receptors of the immune system. Nature 346(6283):425–434
31. Springer TA (1994) Traffic signals for lymphocyte recirculation and leukocyte emigration: the multistep paradigm. Cell 76(2):301–314
32. Rosen H, Gordon S (1987) Monoclonal antibody to the murine type 3 complement receptor inhibits adhesion of myelomonocytic cells in vitro and inflammatory cell recruitment in vivo. J Exp Med 166(6):1685–1701
33. Halle A, Hornung V, Petzold GC, Stewart CR, Monks BG, Reinheckel T, Fitzgerald KA, Latz E, Moore KJ, Golenbock DT (2008) The NALP3 inflammasome is involved in the innate immune response to amyloid-beta. Nat Immunol 9(8):857–865

Chapter 31

Analysis of the Complement Activation in Mice

Nirmal K. Banda and Kazue Takahashi

Abstract

Complement activation is an important immune mechanism in mice like in humans. Murine complement is also activated via three pathways, the classical, lectin, and alternative. Complement proteins are serine proteases; thus activation of complement is proteolytic cleavage of complement proteins, which are both soluble and deposited forms. Therefore, complement pathway activation can be assayed by measuring deposited cleaved complement proteins on materials that are known to activate each pathway. In this chapter, we describe how we assay activation of these three pathways in murine system.

Key words Complement, Mouse, ELISA, Assay, Activation, Pathway

1 Introduction

Mice, like humans, have three complement pathways, the alternative, classical, and lectin. Complement proteins are serine proteases; thus activation is essentially proteolytic cleavage of complement protein, resulting in generation of complement protein fragments. The classical and lectin pathways activate C4, in resulting proteolytic cleavage of C4 to generate C4b, which is deposited on the targets. Although these two pathways activate C4 they are initiated by distinctive two upstream pathways. The classical pathway is via the activation of C1q on immunoglobulins, such as IgG and IgM. The lectin pathway is via the activation of mannose-binding lectin (MBL)-associated serine proteases (MASP), which form complexes with complement-activating lectins, including MBL. MASP activation occurs upon binding of MBL and ficolins, which are similar to MBL, to its ligand, including mannan and *N*-acetyl-D-glucosamine. Therefore, activation of these two complement pathways can be assayed by measuring amounts of deposited C4b on pathway-specific ligands. The alternative pathway is spontaneously activated on its targets, including bacteria and bacterial components like zymosan, resulting in deposition of mainly C3b in mouse. Thus the alternative pathway can be assayed by measuring amounts of deposited C3b. Serum is commonly used to assess complement

Mihaela Gadjeva (ed.), *The Complement System: Methods and Protocols*, Methods in Molecular Biology, vol. 1100,
DOI 10.1007/978-1-62703-724-2_31, © Springer Science+Business Media New York 2014

activation; however, body fluids (for example, synovial fluid) and cell culture supernatants also can be used. In this chapter, we describe complement activation assay using murine serum in ELISA. For chromogenic substrate, we describe *p*-nitrophenyl phosphate (pNPP, sodium salt) and 3,3′,5,5′-tetramethylbenzidine (TMB) for alkaline phosphatase (AP)- and horseradish peroxidase (HRP)- conjugated detecting antibodies, respectively. These soluble chromogenic products are widely used and are measured by OD 405 and 450 nm, respectively. The methods described here have been previously published [1–3].

2 Materials

2.1 Serum

Collect blood by cardiac puncture from euthanized mice using a 1 ml syringe attached to a G25 needle and transfer to a microcentrifuge tube. Blood also can be collected by retro-orbital bleeding or tail-bleeding; however these methods are generally performed on anesthetized mice. Incubate blood at room temperature for 2 h (*see* **Note 1**) and then spin at 12,000 rpm (11,750 × *g*) for 10 min at room temperature. Transfer the supernatant, which is serum, to a new microcentrifuge tube and store in the −80 °C freezer. Discard serum if it appears reddish due to hemolysis. Make aliquots in order to avoid repeated freeze–thaw cycles.

2.2 Stock Buffers (See Note 2)

Prepare all reagents using pure water (resin purified, distilled, double distilled, or bottled). Many stock and working solutions are available from commercial vendors. Similarly many reagents (ready to use) are also commercially available.

1. 1 M Tris, pH 7.4: Weigh 121 g of Trizma base (MW 121.14) and add 900 ml water. Adjust pH to 7.4 with HCl (*see* **Note 3**) and make up to 1 L with water.
2. 1 M Tris, pH 9.5: Prepare Tris as above and adjust pH to 9.5.
3. 5 M NaCl: Weigh 290 g of NaCl (MW 58.44), add 900 ml water, and leave the solution on a magnetic stir till NaCl is dissolved. Make up to 1 L with water.
4. 1 M $CaCl_2$: Weigh 111 g of $CaCl_2$ (MW 110.98), add 900 ml water, and leave the solution on a magnetic stir till $CaCl_2$ is dissolved. Make up to 1 L with water.
5. 1 M $MgCl_2$: Weigh 95 g of $MgCl_2$ (MW 95.21), add 900 ml water, and leave the solution on a magnetic stir till $MgCl_2$ is dissolved. Make up to 1 L with water.
6. 0.4 M Barbital, pH 7.4: Weigh 8. 3 g of barbital sodium salt (MW 206.2) and dissolve in 100 ml of water.
7. 0.5 M Ethylene glycol tetraacetic acid (EGTA): Weigh 190 g of (MW 380.4) and add 900 ml of water. Adjust pH to 8.0 with NaOH (*see* **Note 4**) and make up to 1 L with water.

8. Tween20, 50 %: Mix 20 ml of 100 % Tween and 20 ml of water.
9. 5× Barbital-buffered saline (BBS): Mix 50 ml of 0.4 M Barbital, 140 ml of 5 M NaCl, and 810 ml of water.
10. 10 % Bovine serum albumin (BSA): Dissolve 50 g of BSA into 500 ml of water. Dissolving takes a while. It can be left at 4 °C (such as the cold room) with gentle agitation overnight. Aliquot 10 or 40 ml per 15 or 50 ml tubes, respectively, and store them at −20 °C.

2.3 Working Solutions

1. Coating buffer (0.1 M carbonate/bicarbonate buffer, pH 9.5): Weigh 1.6 g of Na_2CO_3 and 2.9 g of $NaHCO_3$ and dissolve in 1 L of water. Adjust pH as needed.
2. Wash buffer: For the classical and lectin pathway assay: TBS/Ca^{2+}/tw buffer (10 mM Tris, pH 7.4, 140 mM NaCl, 10 mM $CaCl_2$, 0.05 % Tween20): Mix 10 ml of 1 M Tris, pH 7.4, 10 ml of 1 M CaCl2, 28 ml of 5 M NaCl, and 1 ml of 50 % Tween20 (*see* **Note 5**). Make up to 1 L with water. For the alternative pathway assay: Use PBS (without Ca2+ and Mg2+) instead of TBS/Ca2+.
3. TBS/Ca2+ buffer (100 mM Tris, pH 7.4, 140 mM NaCl, 10 mM CaCl2): Mix 100 ml of 1 M Tris, pH 7.4, 10 ml of 1 M CaCl2, and 28 ml of 5 M NaCl. Make up to 1 L with water.
4. TBS/NaCl/Ca2+ buffer (100 mM Tris, pH 7.4, 1 M NaCl, 10 mM CaCl2): Mix 100 μl of 1 M Tris, pH 7.4, 10 ml of 1 M CaCl2, and 200 ml of 5 M NaCl. Make up to 1 L with water.
5. Blocking buffer (0.1 % BSA in TBS/Ca2+): Mix 1 ml of 10 % BSA into 100 ml of TBS/Ca2+. Prepare fresh from stock or store diluted at −20 °C.
6. BBS2+ (1× BBS, 5 mM CaCl2, 5 mM MgCl2): Mix 200 ml of 5× BBS, 5 ml of 1 M CaCl2, and 5 ml of 1 M MgCl2. Make up to 1 L with water.
7. PBS/EGTA/Mg2+ (PBS/5 mM MgCl2/10 mM EGTA): Mix 5 ml of 1 M MgCl2 and 10 ml of 0.5 M EGTA into 1 L of PBS (Mg2+ and Cl2+ free).
8. AP buffer (0.1 M Tris, pH 9.5, 0.1 M NaCl): Mix 100 ml of 1 M NaCl, pH 9.5 and 20 ml of 5 M NaCl. Make up to 1 L with water.

2.4 Reagents Required for the Lectin Complement Pathway Assay

1. Mannan, 100 μg/ml in coating buffer: Dilute from 10 mg/ml stock solution in water.
2. Mouse serum samples: Dilute mouse serum in TBS/NaCl/Ca^{2+} buffer between 10- and 400-folds.
3. Complement standard: Prepare serial dilutions (40, 20, 10, 5, 2.5, 1.25, 0.625, 0 U/ml) of complement standard (human

MBL standard, State Serum Institute, Denmark) in TBS/NaCl/Ca^{2+} buffer. Human MBL standard is arbitrarily assigned as 1,000 U/ml.

4. Human C4, 1 μg/ml in BBS2+: Dilute 1:1,000 from 1 mg/ml stock solution in BBS2+.
5. Rabbit anti-human C4c antibody, 1 μg/ml (*see* **Note 6**): Dilute 1:5,000 of a stock solution (5 mg/ml) with TBS/Ca2+. The antibody is sold as anti-human C4c but reacts on C4b.
6. Biotinylated goat anti-rabbit antibody: Dilute 1:7,500 with TBS/Ca2+.
7. ABC-AP (alkaline phosphatase-conjugated avidin): Mix two drops each of reagent A and reagent B in 10 ml of TBS/Ca2+ (*see* **Note 7**). Prepare the reagent about 30 min prior to use.
8. pNPP substrate: Dissolve 5 mg tablet to 0.5 mg/ml with 10 ml of AP buffer (*see* **Note 8**).

2.5 Reagents Required for the Classical Pathway Assay

1. IgG, 10 μg/ml in coating buffer: Dilute 1:100 from 1 mg/ml stock solution of human IgG.
2. Mouse serum samples: Dilute mouse serum 1:10- and 1:400-folds in TBS/Ca2+ buffer.
3. Prepare the following reagents as in Subheading 3.1: Complement standard, human C4, rabbit anti-human C4c antibody, biotinylated goat anti-rabbit antibody, and pNPP substrate.

2.6 Reagents Required for the Alternative Pathway Assay

1. Zymosan 2×10^8 particles/ml in coating buffer: Dilute 1:10 from 10^9 particles/ml stock solution with the coating buffer. Stock is made at 50 mg/ml in water, which is approximately 10^9 particles/ml because 1 mg solid contains approximately 2×10^7 particles (*see* **Note 9**).
2. Mouse serum samples: Dilute mouse serum 1:10 in PBS/EGTA/Mg2+ buffer.
3. HRP-conjugated goat anti-mouse C3 antibody: Dilute 1:2,000 of stock solution with PBS, 0.05 % Tween20.
4. 2 N H2SO4 solution: Dilute 1:18 from sulfuric acid (36 N) with water.
5. TMB substrate: Mix 1:1 volume of TMB with 1 % H_2O_2.

3 Methods (*See* Note 10)

3.1 The Lectin Complement Assay

1. Coat a 96-well assay plate by incubating wells with 100 μl of mannan (100 μg/ml) in coating buffer overnight at 4 °C.
2. Rinse wells. Shake off mannan coating buffer. Add 300 μl/well wash buffer and shake off, and repeat this step four times.

After the last wash shake off excess wash buffer by tapping plates upside down against a pad of paper towels.

3. Block wells by incubating wells with 300 μl/well of blocking buffer at room temperature for 10 min with agitation.
4. Shake off excess blocking buffer as in **step 2**.
5. Add standard and samples in 100 μl/well and incubate at room temperature for 1 h with agitation.
6. Rinse wells as in **step 2**.
7. Add 100 μl/well of human C4 (1 μg/ml) and incubate at 37 °C for 1.5 h.
8. Rinse wells as in **step 2**.
9. Add 100 μl/well of rabbit anti-human C4c antibody, 1 μg/ml, and incubate at room temperature for 1 h.
10. Rinse wells as in **step 2**.
11. Add 100 μl/well of biotinylated goat anti-rabbit antibody (1:7,500) and incubate at room temperature for 1 h.
12. Rinse wells as in **step 2**.
13. Add 100 μl/well of ABC-AP reagent and incubate at room temperature for 1 h.
14. Rinse wells as in **step 2**.
15. Add 100 μl/well of pNPP substrate and incubate at room temperature for 15 min or till pale yellow color is seen.
16. Read OD at 405 nm using a ELISA plate reader. Results are expressed as units/ml.

3.2 The Classical Complement Assay

1. Coat 96-well assay plates by incubating wells with 100 μl of IgG (10 μg/ml) in coating buffer overnight at 4 °C.
2. Rinse wells. Shake off mannan coating buffer. Add 300 μl/well wash buffer and shake off, and repeat this step four times. After the last wash shake off excess wash buffer by tapping plates upside down against a pad of paper towels.
3. Block wells by incubating wells with 300 μl/well of blocking buffer at room temperature for 10 min with agitation.
4. Shake off excess blocking buffer as in **step 2**.
5. Add standard and samples in 100 μl/well and incubate at room temperature for 1 h with agitation.
6. Rinse wells as in **step 2**.
7. Perform **steps 7** through **16** as in Subheading 3.1 above.

3.3 The Alternative Pathway Complement Activity

1. Coat 96-well assay plates by incubating wells with 100 μl of zymosan 2×10^8 particles/ml in coating buffer overnight at 4 °C.
2. Rinse wells. Shake off zymosan coating buffer. Add 300 μl/well wash buffer and shake off, and repeat this step four times.

After the last wash shake off excess wash buffer by tapping plates upside down against a pad of paper towels.

3. Block wells by incubating wells with 300 μl/well of blocking buffer at room temperature for 10 min with agitation.
4. Shake off excess blocking buffer as in **step 2**.
5. Add serum samples in 100 μl/well and incubate at 37 °C for 45 min with agitation.
6. Rinse wells as in **step 2**.
7. Add HRP-conjugated goat anti-mouse C3 antibody and incubate at room temperature for 1 h.
8. Rinse wells as in **step 2**.
9. Add 100 μl/well of TMB solution and incubate for 15–25 min or till yellowish orange color is seen.
10. Add 50 μl/well of 2 N H_2SO_4.
11. Read plates were read at 450 nm subtracting the values at 550 nm.

4 Notes

1. This process is to complete gentle coagulation, which also aggregates cellular component in contrast to plasma preparation, in which anticoagulants are used.
2. NaN_3 (1–2 mM) can be added for storage to prevent contamination, except for buffers to dilute enzyme-conjugated antibodies.
3. Add 12 N HCl while mixing (use a magnetic stir) to lower pH at the beginning, and then use 1 N HCl to adjust pH to 7.4.
4. Add 10 N NaOH while mixing (use a magnetic stir) to bring up pH at the beginning, and then use 1 N NaOH to adjust pH to 8.0.
5. Add Tween20 after the solution is mixed to avoid excess bubbling.
6. This polyclonal antibody cross-reacts on cat, cow, dog, goat, guinea pig, horse, mink, mouse, rat, sheep, and swine, according to the vendor data sheet.
7. Two drops equal roughly 100 μl. For example, if you need only 2 ml mix 20 μl each of A and B into 2 ml of TBS/Ca^{2+}.
8. We have been using pNPP as this is simple and easy. However, there are many other AP substrates for ELISA. This is the same for TMB substrate.
9. Zymosan needs to be boiled in order to inactivate properdin, which activates C3. Follow the instructions. Briefly suspend

zymosan at 1 % in saline in a polypropylene tube, place it in the boiling water bath for 1 h, and then spin at 10,000 × *g* for 1 min. Resuspend the pellet in water, aliquot, and store in the freezer.

10. These assays can be performed in 384-well plates by reducing volume to 15 or 20 μl/well. 96-Well plate assay can also be performed with 50 μl/well volume; however extra caution may be required in order to make sure that all well surface is covered by buffers and reagents.

References

1. Petersen SV, Thiel S, Jensen L, Steffensen R, Jensenius JC (2001) An assay for the mannan-binding lectin pathway of complement activation. J Immunol Methods 257:107–116
2. Banda NK, Takahashi K, Wood AK, Holers VM, Arend WP (2007) Pathogenic complement activation in collagen antibody-induced arthritis in mice requires amplification by the alternative pathway. J Immunol 179:4101–4109
3. Shi L, Takahashi K, Dundee J, Shahroor-Karni S, Thiel S, Jensenius JC et al (2004) Mannose-binding lectin-deficient mice are susceptible to infection with *Staphylococcus aureus*. J Exp Med 199:1379–1390

Chapter 32

Opsonophagocytic Assay

Markryan Dwyer and Mihaela Gadjeva

Abstract

The opsonophagocytic killing (OPK) assay is used as a correlate for protection to measure the functional capacities of vaccine-candidate-raised antibodies. This in vitro assay aids selecting promising vaccines by demonstrating whether the vaccine-induced antibodies drive efficient complement deposition and subsequent opsonophagocytic killing. Here, we describe two protocols for an OPK assay using either human-derived PMNs or cultured HL-60 cells.

Key words Complement, Phagocytosis

1 Introduction

Since its initial publication by Romero-Steiner et al. [1], the opsonophagocytic killing (OPK) technology has been widely used to evaluate the efficacy of vaccine candidates. OPK data allows establishing an OPK titer. This is the reciprocal value for a serum dilution derived from immunized patients at which the OPK assay documents efficient bacterial killing. These values correlate well with the potency of vaccine candidates to generate protection. Due to these characteristics, the OPK assay was adopted both by Wyeth, to evaluate the *Streptoccocal pneumonia* vaccine [2], and by Glaxo Smith Kline, as they evaluated their pneumococcal conjugate vaccine [3].

Pathogen-specific monoclonal antibodies drive activation of the Classical Complement activation pathway, stimulating opsonization of the target with C4b and C3b fragments. The deposition of these Complement components onto the target greatly enhances phagocytosis (opsonophagocytosis) and killing by immune cells. In addition to evaluating vaccine candidates, the OPK assay can be used to test the efficacy of newly generated, pathogen-specific monoclonal antibodies as described by Cerca et al. [4].

Mihaela Gadjeva (ed.), *The Complement System: Methods and Protocols*, Methods in Molecular Biology, vol. 1100, DOI 10.1007/978-1-62703-724-2_32, © Springer Science+Business Media New York 2014

Here, we outline two methods to perform an OPK assay with comparable outcomes using either purified PMNs or cultured HL-60 cells [5].

2 Materials

2.1 Material for PMN Isolation

1. Blood collection set: sterile kit, including 21 gauge needle for venipuncture. 0.75″ length, attached to 12″ of tubing with luer adapter (*see* **Note 1**).
2. Sodium heparin 10 ml blood collection tubes 15 and 50 ml polypropylene conical tubes.
3. Polymorph density gradient.
4. 0.45 % and 0.9 % NaCl solutions.
5. Red blood cell depletion buffer: 0.83 % w/v ammonium chloride in 10 mM HEPES buffer, pH 7.2.
6. Hanks Balanced Salt solution supplemented with calcium chloride and magnesium chloride (HBSS++).
7. 10× PBS: 100 mM sodium phosphate, 20 mM potassium phosphate, 27 mM potassium chloride, 1.37 M sodium chloride, pH 7.4.
8. Hemacytometer.
9. Trypan Blue and Turks cell counting stains.
10. 1.5 or 2 ml Eppendorf or similar tubes.
11. 50 and 15 ml polypropylene Falcon tubes.

2.2 Materials for HL-60 Cell Culture

1. RPMI 1640 Media.
2. Heat-Inactivated Fetal Bovine Serum (HI-FBS).
3. Penicillin–Streptomycin (P/S) (100× stock).
4. Dimethylformamide (DMF).
5. HL-60 cells.
6. T-150 tissue culture-treated, filter-cap stationary flasks.
7. Trypan Blue cell viability stain.
8. Growth Media: RPMI supplemented with 15 % HI-FBS and 100 U/ml of penicillin–streptomycin.

2.3 Materials for OPK Assay

1. Hank's balanced balt solution, supplemented with calcium chloride and magnesium chloride (HBSS++).
2. Hank's balanced salt solution, without calcium chloride, magnesium chloride, and magnesium sulfate (HBSS−−).
3. Macconkey agar plates or other types of agar plates, appropriate for bacterial culturing.

4. MEM Media.
5. Fetal Bovine Serum.
6. Triton X-100.
7. 1.5 or 2 ml Eppendorf or similar tubes.
8. Round-bottom polypropylene tubes.
9. Trypan Blue cell viability stain.
10. OPK buffer: HBSS++, 0.1 % gelatin.
11. Complement source: human or rabbit serum.
12. Heat-Inactivated Complement: heat-inactivate the Complement source by incubating at 56 °C for 30 min.
13. Bacteria-specific purified monoclonal antibodies or antisera.
14. Tryptic Soy Broth (TSB).
15. Dilution buffer: MEM, 5 % FBS, 0.01 % Triton X-100; filtered sterilize on the day of use.
16. Differentiation media: RPMI supplemented with 15 % HI-FBS and 70 mM DMF (final concentration in media).
17. 10 ml glass culture tubes.

3 Method

3.1 PMN Isolation (See Note 2)

1. Draw 15 ml of human blood and collect in Heparin blood collection tubes. Invert the blood-filled tubes slowly for a few times.
2. Slowly layer 5 ml of blood on the top of 5 ml of Polymorthprep reagent in a 15 ml conical tube. Do not disturb the Polymorph/blood interface.
3. Transfer the tubes into a swing-bucket centrifuge and spin samples at $500 \times g$ for 30 min at room temperature, with the brake turned off.
4. Transfer the PMN layer into a fresh 15 ml conical tube. The PMN layer is the second white, puffy layer from the top of the separated blood.
5. Immediately add equal volume of water to the PMN suspension to restore normal osmolarity. Invert tubes to mix.
6. Bring volume of PMN suspension to 15 ml with 9 % NaCl.
7. Centrifuge tubes at $400 \times g$ for 10 min at RT using centrifuge with a swing-out bucket rotor.
8. Discard supernatant and resuspend PMN pellet with 5 ml red blood cell depletion buffer. Incubate at room temperature for 10 min.

9. Centrifuge tubes at 400×*g* for 10 minutes at room temperature.
10. Wash PMN pellet twice, using 0.9 % NaCl solution, before resuspending in 5 ml of HBSS Count cells immediately.
11. Perform two counts: in Trypan Blue to determine viability and in Turks buffer to determine the PMNs-specific count. A dilution of 1:50 of cells in counting dye is recommended and in Turks buffer to determine the PMNs-specific count.

3.2 HL-60 Growth and Differentiation

1. Seed the HL-60 cells at a density 5×10^5 cells/ml in growth medium.
2. Grow the cells in suspension without agitation at 37 °C with 5 % CO_2 in T-150 flasks, standing-up. Culture the cells until they reach density of 2×10^6 cells/ml. The typical growth culture schedule asks for a feeding and seeding pattern every 48–72 h (*see* **Note 3**).
3. To terminally differentiate the HL-60s into neutrophil-like cells, spin the cells down for 5 min at 450×*g* to remove the conditioned growth media (*see* **Note 4**).
4. Seed the cells at 1×10^6 cells/ml in a total volume of 120 ml in differentiation media. Culture the cells for 4–5 days before using in OPK experiments.

3.3 OPK Assay

1. Pre-warm plates for bacterial growth to room temp or 37 °C.
2. Prepare bacterial dilutions in OPK buffer; inoculate bacteria directly from the agar culture plate into the pre-autoclaved glass culture tubes containing 5 ml of HBSS++ buffer so that OD650 reaches 0.45 (*see* **Note 5**). Use 100 μl of bacterial suspension containing 2×10^6 cfu per reaction tube for multiplicity of infection (MOI) of 1 (*see* **Note 6**).
3. Spin the PMNs or the HL-60 cells at 450×*g* for 5 min and resuspend in OPK buffer at 2×10^7 cells/ml (*see* **Note 7**).
4. Pipet 100 μl of PMNs or HL-60 cells into 1.5 or 2 ml Eppendorf tubes (*see* **Note 8**).
5. Add 100 μl of diluted Complement or HI Complement (*see* **Notes 9** and **10**).
6. Add 100 μl of bacteria-specific purified antibody or antisera (*see* **Note 11**).
7. At Time zero (T0) remove 25 μl from each reaction tube and dilute with 225 μl dilution buffer. This is your 1:10 (10–1) dilution. Make tenfold serial dilutions. Be sure to change pipette tips between dilutions!! Plate 10 μl drops (in duplicate) on Macconkey agar plates. Do not allow the drop to run to the

edge of the plate; if running fast invert the plate 180° and let the liquid run back along the same path.

8. Rotate the remaining OPK reactions at 37 °C for 90 min end-over-end at 20 cycles per minute.
9. Make tenfold serial dilutions in dilution buffer and plate 10 μl drops (in duplicates) on Macconkey agar plates after the completion of the incubation period (i.e., the 10–1, 10–2, or 10–3 dilutions are most often used, but this may vary depending on the MOI at which the OPK is assembled, the pathogenic strain, and its growth characteristics).
10. Incubate the Macconkey agar plates agar plates 10–11 h at 37 °C, next day count the dilutions having between 20 and 100 bacteria per 10 μl drop, if feasible.
11. To evaluate the OPK efficiency, control samples with HI-serum or lacking pathogen-specific antibodies should be included. The percent OPK may be calculated using the following equation:

$$\%OPK = \left(1 - \frac{\textit{Average cfu in samples with serum, PMNs, and Ab}}{\textit{Average cfu in samples with serum and Ab}}\right) \times 100$$

Significant killing is usually defined as reduction of bacterial cfu more than 40 %.

4 Notes

1. We use Becton Dickinson Vacutainer Safety-Lok blood collection set.
2. This protocol provides activated PMNs.
3. We do not recommend extending the HL-60 passaging beyond passage 35, although, it was reported that the use of 20 % HI-FBS in the media relieves this requirement.
4. To determine whether the HL-60s are properly differentiated, flow cytometry analysis is strongly recommended. Typically, the differentiated cultures should show 80 % viability estimated using Trypan blue staining or 65 % viability using PI staining. The cell surface markers that confirm the acquisition of the differentiated phenotype is maturation markers (e.g., CD35 and CD11b) and proliferation markers (e.g., CD71) (Fig. 1). More than ≥55 % of the cells in the cultures should express CD35 and CD11b and less than 20 % of the cells should maintain CD71 expression. The cultures should not have abundance of apoptotic cells which can be determined using Annexin V and PI staining. Less than 25 % of the cells in culture should appear Annexin V^+ and PI^- [6].

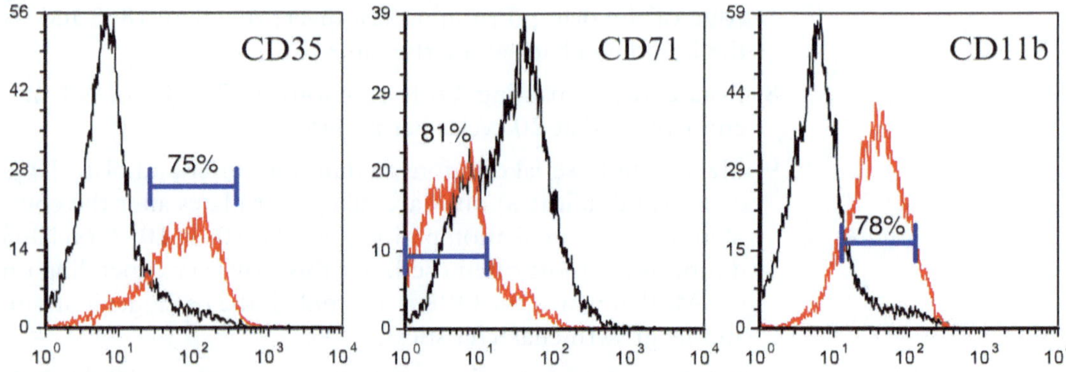

Fig. 1 Differentiated phenotype is maturation markers and proliferation markers

5. The bacterial culture density can be estimated using OD_{650} measurements. Typically, when $OD_{650} = 0.45$, then the culture density is 1×10^9 bacteria/ml.
6. MOI is defined as a ratio of bacterial cfu versus number of neutrophils.
7. Avoid placing the HL-60s or PMNs on ice.
8. The bacteria:neutrophil ratio may vary and testing the OPK assay at a wide MOI range is advisable (e.g., MOI of 1–0.004).
9. Dilution of the Complement source may vary with the target strain and type of growth. Usually the dilution will range between 1:2 and 1:10 in Complement dilution buffer. Include samples with HI Complement to quantify the Complement-specific opsonophagocytosis.
10. Avoid repeated freeze–thaw cycles of the Complement source; the Complement thioester containing proteins C3 and C4 are sensitive to temperature changes. Make sure that you keep the Complement source on ice as you prepare for the experiment. Store Complement at −80 °C.
11. The concentration of pathogen-specific antibody or antisera at which an effective OPK occurs depends on the class/subclass of the antibody, and its affinity for the antigen. Therefore, we suggest testing a range of antibody concentrations for example starting from 0.1 to 20 μg/ml. Make sure that the antibody source matches the serum source to avoid antibody anti-isotypic interactions and Complement activation which may interfere with the OPK.

References

1. Romero-Steiner S, Libutti D, Pais LB, Dykes J, Anderson P, Whitin JC, Keyserling HL, Carlone GM (1997) Standardization of an opsonophagocytic assay for the measurement of functional antibody activity against *Streptococcus pneumoniae* using differentiated HL-60 cells. Clin Diagn Lab Immunol 4:415–422
2. Fleck RA, Romero-Steiner S, Nahm MH (2005) Use of HL-60 cell line to measure opsonic capacity of pneumococcal antibodies. Clin Diagn Lab Immunol 12:19–27
3. Guttormsen HK, Liu Y, Paoletti LC (2008) Functional activity of antisera to group B streptococcal conjugate vaccines measured with an opsonophagocytosis assay and HL-60 effector cells. Hum Vaccin 4:370–374
4. Cerca N, Maira-Litran T, Jefferson KK, Grout M, Goldmann DA, Pier GB (2007) Protection against *Escherichia coli* infection by antibody to the *Staphylococcus aureus* poly-N-acetylglucosamine surface polysaccharide. Proc Natl Acad Sci U S A 104: 7528–7533
5. Nahm MH, Burton RL (2011) Protocol for multiplexed opsonophagocytic killing assay (UAB-MOPA) for antibodies against *Streptococcus pneumoniae*. Online manual
6. Hu BT, Yu X, Jones TR, Kirch C, Harris S, Hildreth SW, Madore DV, Quataert SA (2005) Approach to validating an opsonophagocytic assay for *Streptococcus pneumoniae*. Clin Diagn Lab Immunol 12:287–295

INDEX

Mihaela Gadjeva (ed.), *The Complement System: Methods and Protocols*, Methods in Molecular Biology, vol. 1100, DOI 10.1007/978-1-62703-724-2, © Springer Science+Business Media New York 2014

N

P

Q

R

S

T

MIX
Papier aus verantwortungsvollen Quellen
Paper from responsible sources
FSC® C105338

If you have any concerns about our products,
you can contact us on
ProductSafety@springernature.com

In case Publisher is established outside the EU,
the EU authorized representative is:
Springer Nature Customer Service Center GmbH
Europaplatz 3, 69115 Heidelberg, Germany

Printed by Libri Plureos GmbH
in Hamburg, Germany